Donna Summer, "Queen of the Disco"

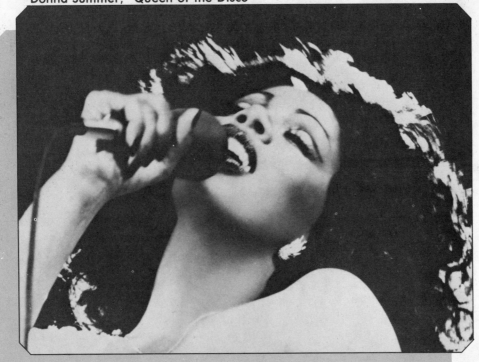

The Complete Book on
DISCO
and Ballroom Dancing

by
Ann T. Kilbride
and
A. Algoso

Hwong Publishing Company
10353 Los Alamitos Blvd.
Los Alamitos, CA. 90720
U.S.A.

International Standard Book Number: 0-89260-149-3 (PB)
0-89260-150-7 (HB)
Library of Congress Catalog Card Number: 78-73545

ACKNOWLEDGMENTS

ANN KILBRIDE:

Ann Kilbride, a dance aficionado, received her M.A. in English from the University of Virginia. Ann's passionate interest in dance has led her to explore such diverse forms as ballet, modern interpretive, and disco. As an editor and free-lance writer, Ann has worked on more than 35 trade and educational books. She also writes poetry and fiction.

ANGELO ALGOSO:

Angelo Algoso, an expert dancer and choreographer in tap, jazz, ballroom, and disco dancing, is currently organizing and syndicating dance studios in the Philippines and the United States. A well known disco champion from L.A., Angelo has performed in numerous competitions and exhibitions. In addition to preparing for a series of television performances, Angelo is currently choreographing a disco special.

Contributors

We would like to thank the following dancers and dance studios for their invaluable advice and guidance:

DANCE EXPERTS

DORIS ARNDT:

Doris Arndt taught dance for more than 20 years at Arthur Murray Dance Studios. She now owns and operates two of her own dance studios in Laguna Beach and Newport Beach.

THE LOCKERS:

Creators of wild free-form dances such as the *Robot, Slow Motion, Skeeter Rabbit, Stop and Go, Samba Splits,* and the *Scoobie Doo,* the Lockers sport an all-star cast of seven: Don Campbellock Campbell, Tony "Go-Go" Lewis, Alfa Scobot Anderson, Stan "The Man" Rodarto, Doreen Rivera, Lewis Deputy Green, and Slim "The Robot" Williams. The group's name, by the way, was culled from their unique free-style technique in which they would "lock joints into position," while experimenting with every conceivable type of rhythm. This dynamic group has made guest appearances on innumerable television shows such as: *Johnny Carson, Dinah, Carol Burnett, What's Happening, Saturday Night Live, Merv Griffin, American Bandstand, Soul Train, In Concert,* and, *The Midnight Special.*

BUDDY SCHWIMMER:

Buddy Schwimmer, proponent of the *Unit System,* has been both State Rock Champion and California State Disco Champion. Owner of Buddy's Dance Clinic in Costa Mesa, Buddy conducts dance workshops and exhibitions throughout the entire country.

SKIPPY BLAIR:

Skippy Blair devised the *Unit System* (copyright 1963) to ameliorate the teaching and learning of dance. After modifying and refining the system for ten years, Skippy simplified the *Unit System* into three basic units, which apply to all patterns used in ballroom, jazz, and rock dances. A member of the Golden State Dance Teachers' Association, Skippy owns her own dance studio and has written a book on dance, entitled *Disco to Tango and Back.*

CATHY SHEPHERD:

Cathy Shepherd received her M.F.A. from Western Michigan University in Detroit, Michigan. Cathy has specialized in classical, ballet, jazz, tap, and flamenco dancing. A professional dance champion in both Latin and Ballroom divisions, Cathy has also performed in disco exhibitions on national television and in feature films. At the present time, Cathy is a studio manager for Fred Astaire Dance Studios in Los Angeles.

DANCE STUDIOS

Fred Astaire Dance Studio
Arthur Murray Dance Studio
Backstage Dance Studio
Earl Manning Dance Studio
Fantasia Dance Studio

STAFF

publisher
Jack Hwong

editorial director
Ann T. Kilbride

art director
Larry Safady

senior editor
Barbara Van Hoven

associate editor
Sarah Keating

assistant editor
Sharon Mekaru

illustrator
Lindy Reilley

photographers
Dave Gooley
D. Hsiao

video specialists
Steve Hitter & Associates

design associate
Judy Chow

production assistants
Dave Garcia
Joe Zeni
Victoria Fuller

administrative assistants
Margorie Kustra
Tina Vasquez

CONTENTS

PART III: FREE-STYLE DISCO

CHAPTER 8
DISCO BODY DANCES

CHAPTER 9
FREE-STYLE COMBINATION DANCES

CHAPTER 10
LINE DANCES

PART IV: BALLROOM DANCES

CHAPTER 11
WALTZ

PART I

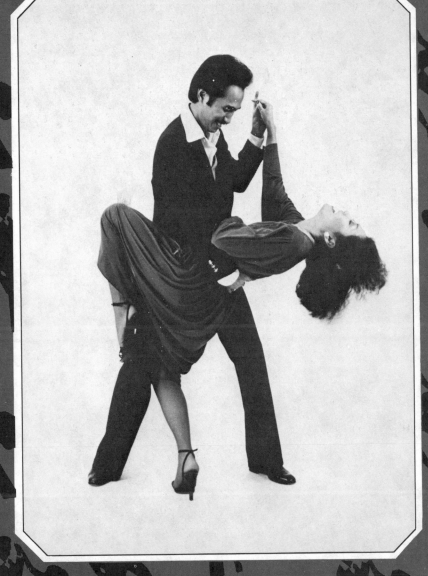

INTRODUCTION

CHAPTER 1
INTRO TO DISCO

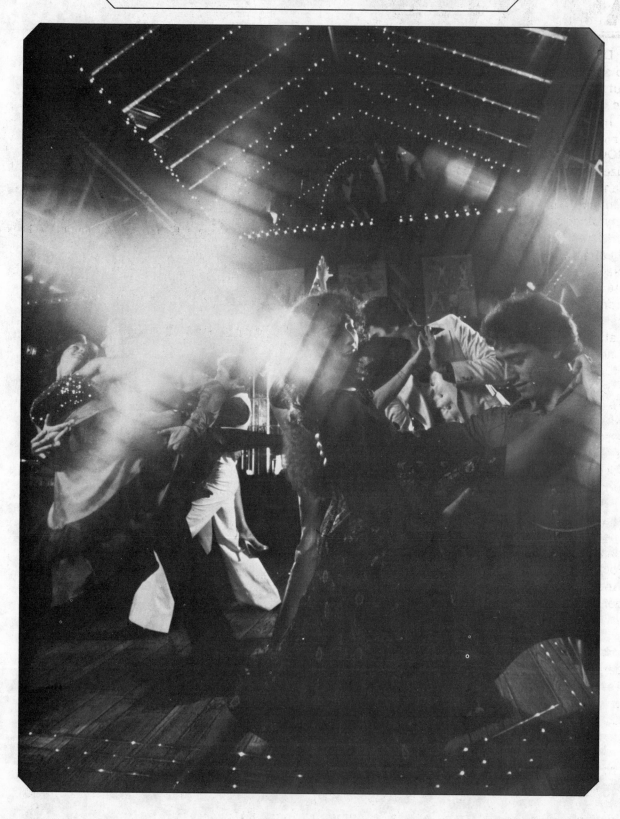

SECTION A:
GET DOWN AND BOOGIE!

Do you want to be a disco champ? Do you want to spit fire as a free-form winner? Do you want to cut ice as the world's best touch dancer? In short, do you want to become king or queen of the disco?

Impossible? Not anymore, because you own THE COMPLETE BOOK ON DISCO AND BALL-ROOM DANCING. This book examines the shape, size, and form of every conceivable type of disco dance. In terms of content alone, this book contains more information than can be found in any other dance book on the market.

More than 100 popular touch dances are illustrated with hundreds of photographs, step diagrams, and illustrations. This book takes you step-by-step through partner dances that range from disco fast to disco slow. Just a few of the partner dances explored include the New York — Latin Hustle, Tango Hustle, Cha-Cha Hustle, Continental Hustle, Latin Street Hustle, Two-Step Hustle, Newporter Salsa, and Cuban Salsa.

But step patterns alone do not a dancer make. To add style and class, you also need to know where, how, and when to turn. Thus, this book describes at least 45 different turn variations, including the Cradle, Scarecrow, Pretzel, Flair, Airplane, Chase, Corkscrew, Boomerang, Death Drop, Dip, Whip, and Pinwheel.

If single is your thing, this book covers more than 25 free-style or free-form disco dances. For the sensualist there's a chapter on disco body dances that show you how to snap, freak, freeze, rock, roll, bounce, bump, shimmy and shake. Another chapter describes popular line dances that get you hoofing to the Disco Duck, the Bus Stop, and the Midnight Fever, among other wild and crazy line patterns. For the fancy steppers a third chapter contains a slew of free-style combination dances such as the Pivot Pendulum, Funky Glide, Taxi Driver, Split Pivots, Disco Swivel, and a stack of other variations which teach you how to strut, tap, kick, pivot, swivel and spin like there's no tomorrow.

But no dance book would be complete without a thorough examination of the major ballroom dances. Most, if not all, disco touch dances have their roots firmly planted in the social dance tradition. The Two-Step Hustle is an up-dated version of the Samba; the New York-Latin Hustle takes bits and pieces from Swing; the saucy

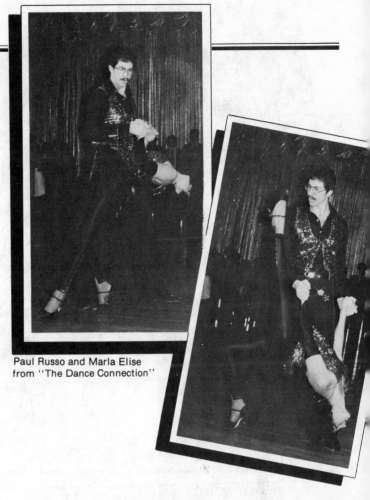

Paul Russo and Marla Elise from ''The Dance Connection''

Salsa contains a smidgen of the Merengue. To add the finishing touch, therefore, this book contains more than 40 ballroom variations that explore the elegant Waltz, the foxy Fox Trot, the slinky and sensuous Tango, the jive talking Swing, the hip flipping Rumba, the red hot Samba, the mellow yellow Merengue, and the far out Cha-Cha.

This explosive book — researched, written, and designed with the aid of 12 dance experts, 4 major dance studios, 3 professional writers, and 7 artists — is the most comprehensive guide to dance ever published. Read this book, and you'll know how to get down and boogie! If nothing else, heed the advice given to the readers of *Memphis,* a local city magazine: ''At least know the names of current dances. Memphis dancers are about a year behind New York and Los Angeles. To be behind Memphis is to be hopeless.''

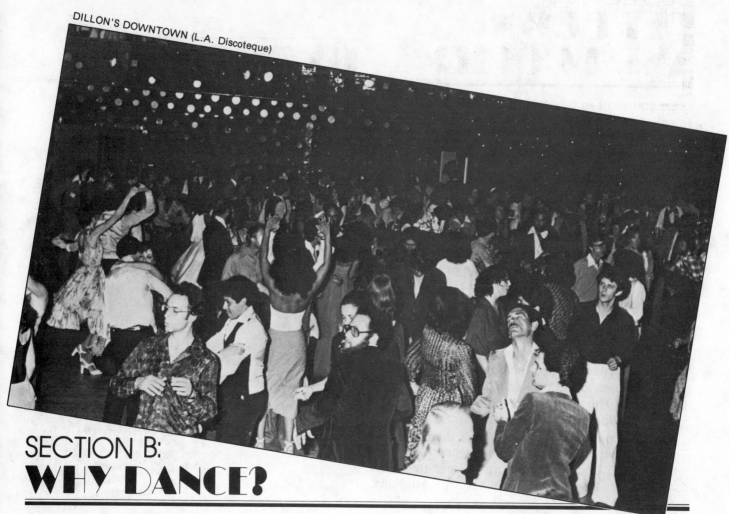

DILLON'S DOWNTOWN (L.A. Discoteque)

SECTION B:
WHY DANCE?

Many people, at least during the early 1970s, could not see much point in stylized dancing. Perhaps the height of the anarchistic approach to dance found expression in the Woodstock "Happening" in the summer of '69. True, the free-form expression of dance was, to some extent, more communal, more personal, and less restrictive. Nevertheless, this free-floating form of dance fell by the wayside with other, less desirable habits, such as free-floating anxiety. In short, we were bored with doing nothing, but trying to make it look like something.

The disco revolution brought couple dancing back into style. Now we want to know how to dance, and how to dance well! We want to pick up a partner, any partner that strikes our fancy, and boogie like never before. We want to reach out, touch somebody, and communicate through our bodies. And nothing, but nothing, has the power of communication like gliding, sliding, and hustling through a series of perfectly attuned, perfectly synchronized steps.

Needless to say, dancing is a fantastic form of exercise. Dr. Maxim Asa, a noted physiologist and

director of the New York Stress and Research Center, claims that "continuous disco dancing is the equivalent to running an eight or ten-minute mile. For every ten minutes that you are continuously disco-ing, you are running a mile." Moreover, disco dancing forces the heart muscles to pump harder, keeps the body well oxygenated, and strengthens flabby leg and stomach muscles.

The disco experience intermingles myth with magic. Dressing up for a night of dancing is no longer the ignominy it was just a few years back. Instead, the ritualistic event transforms the dancer, whether one dons snazzy jeans studded with rhinestones, or a ritzy black tuxedo topped with a ruffled silk shirt. Costumes, masks, and disguises are all part of the mystical, mythical world of dance.

Most important, dancing is fun. It's common knowledge among club owners that most disco dancers are light imbibers. Dancers become so completely immersed in the total dancing experience that they tend to be "naturally high." Yes, disco dancing is ecstasy! 🕺

SECTION C:
HISTORICAL ROOTS OF DANCE

EARLIEST DANCE FORMS

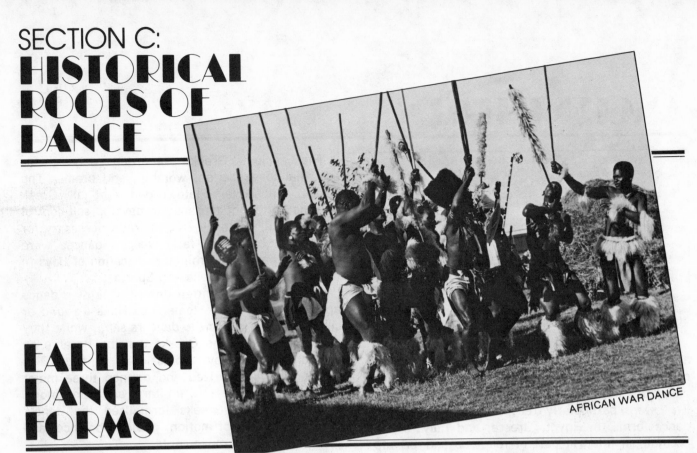

AFRICAN WAR DANCE

Dancing is one of the oldest forms of human expression. Prehistoric paintings of dancers found on cave walls in Africa and Southern Europe may be more than 20,000 years old. Historians and anthropologists theorize that religious ceremonies which combined dance, music, and drama, probably played an instrumental part in the lives of prehistoric people. These ceremonies may have been held to propitiate the gods. Ceremonial dances may have also functioned as a means to heal the ill, mourn the dead, or celebrate a victory in battle.

Rudolph Laban, a pioneer in dance education, identifies five universal types of body movements: (1) *gesture* (any movement not connected with supporting the body's weight); (2) *stepping* (the transfer of weight from one support to another); (3) *locomotion* (movement of the body from one place to another); (4) *jumping* (movement without a point of support); and (5) *turning* (changing position in a circular direction). These five movements have been incorporated into an endless variety of dances.

Although no one knows when or how dancing started, most historians agree that the earliest form of dance was performed in a *circle*. Primitive people would dance around symbolic objects placed in the center of a circle. These circle dances were used to ward off illness, as well as to pray for rain, bountiful harvests, and fertility.

Another ancient form of dance involved *pantomime*. Most primitive courtship dances, for example, started with the pantomime of wooing. Another type of mimetic dance was the weapon dance in which performers staged mock battles. Masks, of course, were a necessary part of these mimetic or representational dances. In the courtship dances of Northern Melanesia, for instance, both the men and the women wore masks, as they moved towards, then away from each other. Disguises freed the dancer from inhibitions. Masks also added a touch of magic and mystery.

The *line* dance, which evolved from the circle dance, was considered appropriate for celebrating the themes of love or war. Participants in these dances would stand and face each other, as they pretended to woo or to fight. Moreover, in the Renaissance the couple dance evolved from mimetic wooing dances performed in a line. Line dances became particularly functional in hierarchical societies, because they enabled all dancers in a line to turn and face the chief or the king of the society. Peter Buckman, author of *Let's Dance*, explains that the "Chinese, in the days of feudalism, allotted an exact number of lines of dancers where the homage was to be performed: eight rows for the emperor, six for the top princes, and four for mandarins. As an advanced civilization, they codified the dance and reduced it (or raised it) from a spontaneous activity to an art based on precisely regulated movements and gestures."

INTRO TO DISCO

ANCIENT TIMES

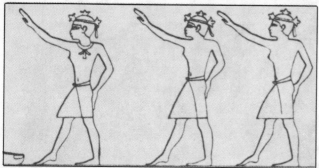

EGYPTIAN DANCERS

Most dance historians concur that both sacred and nonreligious dancing existed in ancient civilizations. Societies which evolved in regions along the Mediterranean Sea and in the Middle East were particularly receptive to a variety of dance forms. In Egypt, Greece, and Italy dance became an integral part of religious and private celebrations.

Information concerning early Egyptian dancing is evident in numerous paintings, sculptures, and writings. Decorative carvings in Egyptian tombs, for example, indicate that dances were performed during funerals, parades, and religious ceremonies. Moreover, major Egyptian religious festivals involved dances honoring Osiris, the god of vegetation. Dancing was also used as a form of private entertainment in which Egyptian slaves danced to entertain wealthy members of the society.

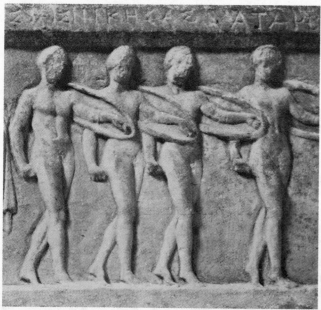

GREEK PYRRHIC DANCE

The ancient Greeks regarded dancing as essential to education, worship, and drama. The Greek philosopher Plato urged that all Greek citizens be taught to dance to develop self-control and physical dexterity — two traits necessary for success in battle. In fact, weapon dances were taught as part of the military education of boys in the city-states of Athens and Sparta.

One of the first written descriptions of a dance appears in the *Iliad*. Homer describes a round or circle dance in which the dancers sang, while they danced. Through the Greeks dancing became an art form taught by professional dancers. The Greeks also categorized and defined three major types of dances: sacred, military, and celebratory. And finally, the Greeks formalized the dance, requiring fluidity of motion, graceful balance, and well-proportioned movements.

There were several types of dances popular in ancient Greece. The *emmeleia* were dignified round or circle dances, performed primarily by women. The *hyporchemata* were mimetic choral dances dedicated to Apollo as the patron god of poetry and music. The Greeks also performed dances called *paians,* which were used to ward off illness. Another type of dance, *gymnopaidiai*, was a wrestling dance performed by naked boys.

In addition to staging serious dramas or tragedies, the Greeks also produced comedies and short, humorous plays called *satyrs*, which included some boisterous dances. The frenzied Bacchic dances, for example, were dedicated to the god of wine, known as Dionysus to the Greeks, but later called Bacchus by the Romans. In the Great Dionysia, a festival of music and drama, men masquerading as satyrs wore beards and tails and danced around the women.

By the time the Romans conquered Greece in 197 B.C., they had already adopted much of the Greek culture, including Greek dancing. The Romans, however, transformed the dances of the Greeks into mere entertainment performed by paid professionals and slaves. Many entertainers combined dancing with juggling and acrobatics.

Dancing also became a desirable social accomplishment for upper class Romans, and most well-to-do families kept a dancing teacher on their

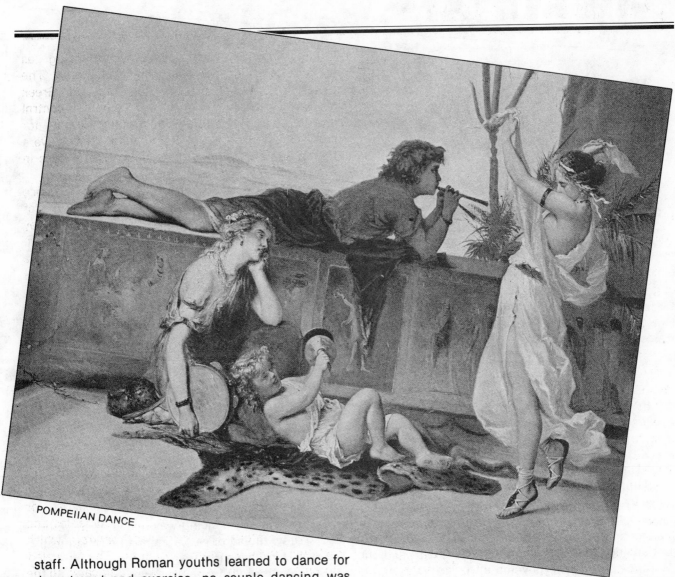

POMPEIIAN DANCE

staff. Although Roman youths learned to dance for deportment and exercise, no couple dancing was done, and usually men and women had their own separate dances.

During the same period, professional dancing developed a loyal public following. Rival dancers were as fanatically supported by their admirers as rival professional football teams are now. Once professional dancers appeared, critics of dancing were not far behind. Dance was condemned for showing disrespect for sacred things and for exciting lustful desires. In the words of the famous orator Cicero, "No man dances unless he is drunk or insane."

MIDDLE AGES

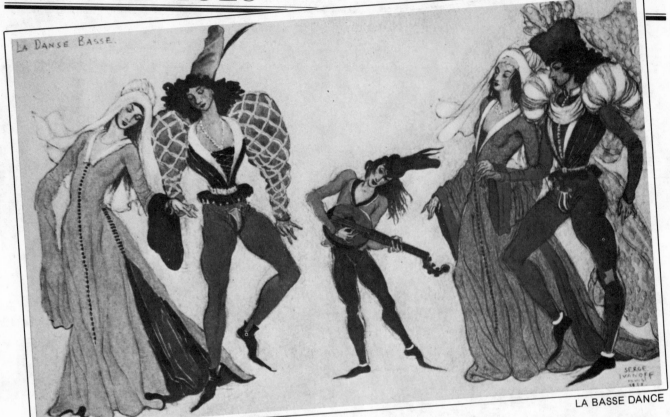

LA DANSE BASSE.

LA BASSE DANCE

During the Middle or "Dark" Ages, a period in history which lasted approximately a thousand years, dancing was viewed as decadent. Since the paid professional dancers of the Romans concentrated on the sensuous, erotic aspects of their dancing to attract and keep their audiences, dancing began to develop an unsavory reputation. Through its association with public entertainments, dancing became increasingly shocking and disgusting to the well-bred Roman. As the empire declined and the fathers of the Christian Church came to power, dancing was further condemned. In 300 A.D. the Church announced that anyone connected with the circus, with mimicking (make-believe acting), or dance would not be baptized.

Although information about dance during the period 200 A.D. to 1200 A.D. is meager, dancing did survive. Many pagan ways were kept alive in Medieval Europe by traveling entertainers, poets, musicians, and dancers. Dance itself was frequently denounced by church authorities who tried very hard to stamp out what they called: "This evil, this lascivious madness in man called dance which is the devil's business."

On the other hand, the Church did encourage composers to create music to accompany the liturgy. The participants in group social dancing often sang, while they danced in a circle or a line. This type of dancing was known then as the carol. Later, the carol was accompanied by music played on wind instruments.

By the 11th century, dancing was once again accepted at the feudal courts and in the houses of the rich lords. During the 12th century, feudalism took deeper root, emphasizing piety, bravery, loyalty and honor. Knightly codes of romantic love and chivalry arose, reinforced by the sons of the troubadours. Rules of proper etiquette began to dominate living. A knight, admired for his strength and skill during the day's tournaments, was now expected to show equal ability on the dance floor in the evening.

Until this point in history, dance forms provided few opportunities for dancing courtiers or knights to show off their skill in courting the opposite sex—a necessary part of courtly love. Thus, a new type of couple or partner dance was needed. Of course, the couple dance would soon become an integral part of the courtship ritual.

The first recorded couple dance is the estampie of the 12th century. This dance consisted of a leading couple stepping sedately around the room in a rhythm so slow that the dancers could have balanced a glass of wine on their heads while they were dancing. One reason for the slowness of the movement was, no doubt, the heavy velvet and brocade skirts worn by the women. Such gowns did not lend themselves to quick, lively movement.

The earliest existing dance book which contained written dance steps is *Le Livre des Basse-Danses.* This instructional book, a Burgundian work, may have been written in the 14th century. In *basse danse* ("low dance") the dancer kept his feet on or close to the ground, whereas in *haut danse* ("high dance") the dancer performed a series of leaps, kicks, and other exuberant movements.

Directly derived from the estampie, the *basse danse* contained five distinct parts. One part of the *basse danse* alternated quick with slow rhythms. Another part, the *branle double*, introduced an 8-bar musical phrase for the first time.

An Italian version of the *basse danse* was the saltarello. The saltarello (Latin for leaping or jumping) had a pattern in which the man performed a solo of hopping movements in front of his lady. Afterwards, the woman performed a similar, but more restrained solo for the man.

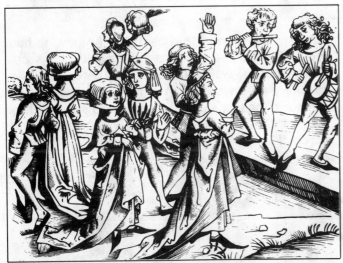

15th CENTURY DANCERS

The couple dance developed slowly and did not become widely popular before the early 16th century. Nevertheless, the emerging couple dance marked a distinction between theater dance (couple dance) and folk dance (ritualistic, entertainment dance). The folk dances performed by the peasants were jubilant, active, ring-shaped group dances, in which the peasants sang and danced at the same time. Theater dances were sedate, used set dance patterns, expressed refined pleasure, were performed solo or by couples, and were usually accompanied by instrumental music. Although the spontaneity marking the dances of the peasants was not entirely missing from the dances of the nobility, the court dances were subjected to innumerable rules. Moreover, these two kinds of dancing did not merge again for nearly 300 years.

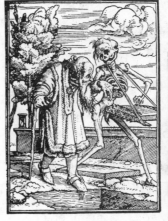

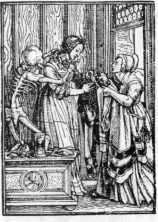

"The Old Man" and "The Countess" from Han Holbein's DANCE OF DEATH.

During the 14th century, a plague known as the *Black Death* swept across Europe and wiped out at least a fourth of the population. A bizarre dancing epidemic concurrently broke out in many European countries, including Germany and Italy. Many have attempted to explain the function of this dancing madness in the Middle Ages, but no one answer appears complete. Some dance historians claim that the people sang and danced frantically in graveyards, because they superstitiously believed such acts would drive away the demons of death. Other historians claim that the plague itself brought on high fevers, convulsions, and uncontrollable twitchings that resembled a strange dance. For many victims, the *danse macabre* became a portent of death.

THE RENAISSANCE

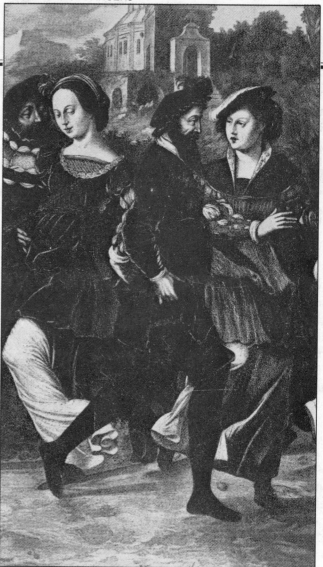

The Renaissance was a fervid period of economic growth and cultural expansion. The Renaissance began in Italy in the late 1300s, then spread throughout most of Europe by the 1600s. During the Renaissance, many people believed that harmony of skilled dance movement reflected harmony in government, nature, and the universe.

In Italy throughout the late 15th and early 16th centuries Italian nobles hired professional dancing masters to create original court spectacles that included dances called *balletti*. These spectacles combined poetry, dancing, music, scenic effects, fireworks, and parades. Leading composers wrote the music, and renowned artists such as Leonardo da Vinci (1452-1519) designed the costumes and stunning special effects.

The Italians also accentuated the division between stage dancing, court dancing and folk dancing. A further distinction was made between ordinary couple dances (*danzi*) and couple panto-mimic dances (*balli*). Anyone could participate in the *danzi*, but *balli* was reserved for the nobility. In *balli*, the nobility acted out the court ritual of advance, retreat, and encirclement. In time, the *balli* was taken over by professionals who transformed this dance into the elegant and sophisticated ballet.

In 1547 Catherine de Medici, a member of the ruling family of Florence, Italy, became Queen of France. Not surprisingly, Catherine was the one who introduced Italian dance and spectacle to the French Court. For a royal wedding in Paris in 1581, Catherine commissioned a group of Italian artists to produce the spectacular *Ballet Comique de la Reine,* one of the first ballets ever produced.

In addition to producing magnificent spectacles, dancing masters taught social dancing to the nobility. By the mid-16th century, the pavane had replaced the *basse danse* as the major court dance. A slow dance, well-suited to court ceremony, the pavane was performed in a forward progression. Although the steps to this dance were simple, they allowed the men to perform a strut that would show off their legs and feet.

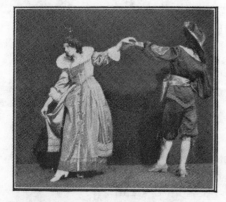

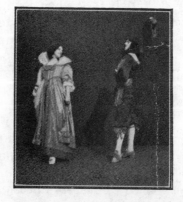

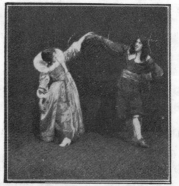

PAVANE

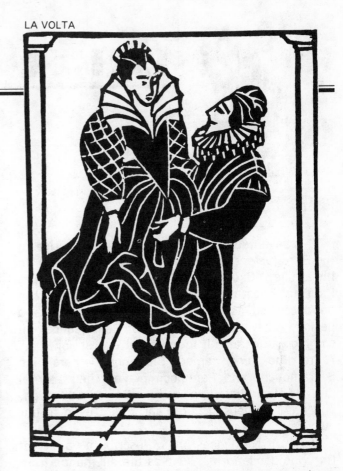

Another dance which underwent a transformation at court was the saraband. The saraband, which originated sometime in the 12th century in Seville, Spain, was once a sexual pantomime in which partners twisted their bodies to the rhythm of castanets. By the time the dance arrived in Italy, the dancers were allowed to collide, until their lips met in a kiss. But by 1588, after the dance was introduced to the French Court, the saraband had turned into a gliding, processional dance, devoid of all erotic elements.

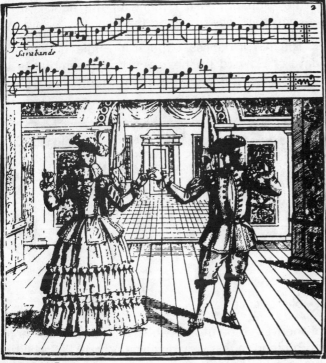

SARABAND

La Volta ("turning dance") was also being performed by the 16th century. This dance, believed by some to be the forerunner of the waltz, was considered highly indecent because of the close body contact required on the leaping step. In La Volta partners held each other closely, while they performed two hopping and turning steps together, before the woman lept high into the air. To keep the woman balanced during the lift, the man wrapped his left arm around her right hip, jammed his left thigh against her right thigh, and placed his right hand below the front part of her corset. After the leap, the man was rewarded with a kiss.

Outside the court, folk dances remained popular.

In England during the late 16th century, there were many vigorous kinds of round and line dances. Some of these folk dances contained complicated figures performed by several sets of couples, who exchanged positions as they danced. These dances often had fanciful names: "Pepper is Black," "Greensleeves," "Basilino," "Turkey Loney."

Kissing was an important part of English dance. The Puritan, Philip Stubbes, wrote in his *Anatomie of Abuses* (1583): "For what clipping, what culling, what kissing and bussing, what smooching and slavering one of another, what filthie groping and uncleane handling is not practised in those dancings?"

The country dances that have survived to the present day were designed for group, rather than partner, dancing. The only known exception to the group folk dance was the jig. The jig provided an opportunity for the country dancer to whirl about at high speeds and to do so either alone or with a partner.

11   *INTRO TO DISCO*

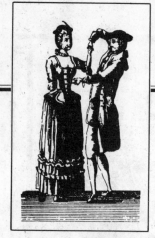

ALLEMANDE

17TH CENTURY

The seventeenth century witnessed the rise of the Baroque period in art, literature, and dance. In his article, "Exoticism in the Baroque Dance," Dr. Paul Nettl postulates that the "Baroque, which can be described as a state of mind, as well as a period, was the decay of the Renaissance. In commedia dell'arte it found great expression. . . . A terrible turk named Cucurucu, others like Scaramouche and Pantaloon played their eternal dramas of conflict on the commedia dell'arte stage, and have influenced mime and dance even to our own day."

Dr. Paul Nettl goes on to describe a variety of Baroque dance forms, such as the allemande from Germany, the courant from France, the hornpipe from England, and the sarabande from Spain. Most exotic dances of the Baroque period, such as the furlana, the tarantella, the chaconne, the passacaglia, and the folia, were influenced by African and South American rhythms. Moreover, most of these dances were characterized by the repetition of a brief motif with a definite beat.

The tarantella, an "endless, continuous dance like the furlana, or the dances of the Orient," came from Naples. Since the 17th century, this dance has often been mentioned in connection with Tarantism, a type of frenzied dance similar to that of St. Vitus during the Plague. Some people believed that the cause of Tarantism was the bite of the Apulian spider, although the names for both the dance and the spider were derived from the town of Taranto in Sicily.

One of the most unusual dances of the Baroque period was the moresche. The moresche, a fertility dance originally performed by either Africans or Moors, involved a pantomime of one or more persons wearing masks. At most festivities, including coronations and weddings in the 17th century, the moresche was danced. Moreover, many masquerades popular during this century were labelled "moresche" or "morescha."

The main characteristics of the moresche were bells, castanets, and masks. In his *Orchesographie* (1588), Arbeau, the French theoretician, describes his impressions of the moresche:

"In my youth I had an opportunity to see how often in good society, after supper was over, a youth with blackened face and a white or yellow taffeta ribbon over his forehead, bells on his ankles, perform the Morescha. . . . Formerly, one stamped one's foot in addition. Since this was rather difficult for the dancers, they substituted a tapping of the heels but kept their toes firmly on the floor."

The morris dances, popular in England since the days of Edward III, bear a strong resemblance to the moresche. According to Dr. Nettl, the "music

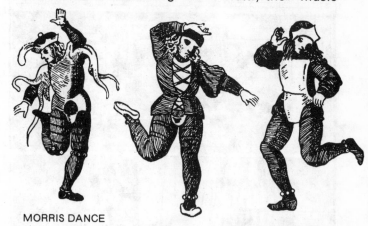

MORRIS DANCE

of the Morescha of Arbeau is played note for note in England to this very day as a Morris." Sachs, in his *World History of the Dance,* points out that, like the moresche dancers, the English morris dancers appeared in groups of six and wore bells. Moreover, in the morris dances, the hobby-horse, an age-old symbol of fertility, plays an important part.

Another exotic dance popular in Spain during the 17th century was the canario, a dance imported from the Canary Islands in the 16th century. This dance, mentioned in Caroso's *Ballarino* (1601), contained lively but bizarre movements, accompanied by hops and heel clicks. To perform the canario, according to Arbeau, "a young man chooses a lady and dances with her to the end of the hall. Then he leaves her and dances backward and forward. The lady performs similarly."

18TH CENTURY

BARN DANCE

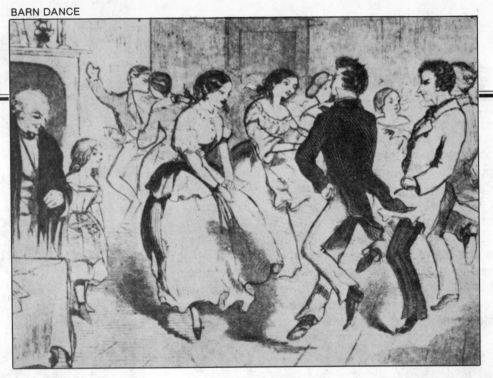

While folk dancing was being enjoyed by the country people, Louis the XIV (The "Sun King") ascended the French throne in 1643. During his reign of 72 years, Louis transformed France into the cultural center of Europe. He gave extravagant balls which were avidly copied in other countries. By 1700, people of the upper classes in Europe and America had adopted the practice of throwing magnificent balls.

During Louis' reign ballet changed significantly. A formalized system of movements was performed by professional dancers. Moreover, ballet performances were gradually moved from the royal ballroom to the theater. The theater contained a *proscenium arch* which framed the stage and separated the dancers from the audience, thus effecting a separation between performer and spectator.

The most popular social dances of the 1700s included the gavotte, the allemande, and the minuet. In the original version of the gavotte, dancers stood in a line or circle. After taking a few jumps, one couple would perform alone, saluting each other with a kiss. After the couple finished their performance, the man would kiss all of the women in the line, while the other men would take turns kissing their own partners. Gradually, however, all kissing was eliminated, until the gavotte became quite sedate.

The minuet, written in 3/4 time, originated from a *franle* portion of the *basse danse.* The pattern for the minuet contained 4 steps with a timing of slow, quick, quick, slow. In many ways, this elegant court dance resembled a highly stylized ritual. Nevertheless, the dignified minuet survived for more than 150 years.

During the 18th century dance became more diffuse and affected all segments of society. Lively English folk dances called *country dances* became favorites of the middle and upper classes throughout Europe. Furthermore, the invention of written systems of *dance notation* enabled people to learn dances by following diagrams printed in books. In addition, wealthy merchants and plantation owners in America imported dance masters from Europe to teach dancing and other social graces to their families.

Moreover, dancing went public. In 1750 two places of public amusements opened in London: the Pleasure Gardens of Vauxhall, and the Ranelagh in Chelsea. These two establishments might be considered the forerunners of our modern night clubs. Anyone who could afford the admission fee was permitted to enter, allowed to listen to the music, have dinner in one of the boxes around the amphitheater, or participate in the dancing. A more exclusive London gathering place, called Almack's, opened in 1765, and the aristocracy went there to dance and gossip. These gathering places, called assembly rooms, soon became popular in Europe and America. While the gentry visited assembly rooms, however, the American country folk enjoyed themselves at lively barn dances, where they often danced to the music of the fiddle. ♣

INTRO TO DISCO

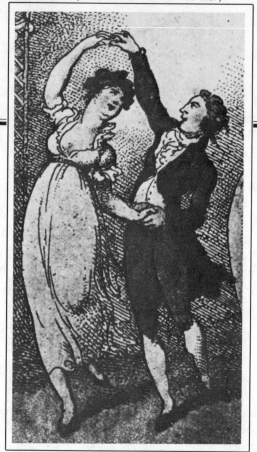

19TH CENTURY

The French Revolution may have proclaimed the end of an era. With the Revolution, many changes occurred in clothing, ideas, and manners. The old ponderous ways sank from sight. Knee breeches gave way to less restrictive trousers. The hooped, heavy skirts were replaced by softer, more sensual dresses of the French Empire. Wigs were abandoned for natural hair. Footwear became lighter and easier to dance in. Lastly, music underwent a radical change as the classic music fell before a growing flood of romantic music. New melodies, harmonies, and rhythms shattered the old ways forever.

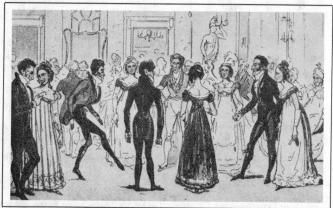

THE POLKA (From *Godey's Lady's Book*)

New York took an early lead in creating fabulous social entertainments in which dancing was featured. The assemblies of the 18th century were replaced by glamorous balls, held by all kinds of groups. Moreover, dancing was finally considered a respectable form of entertainment, as well as an excellent form of indoor exercise. Acceptance of dance disappeared, however, after the waltz and the polka burst onto the scene.

While everyone else was performing slow courtly dances, the Germans continued to perform their traditional wooing dances which contained wild turns and a close embrace. The name, *Waltzer*, which crops up in the middle of the 18th century, is derived from the Latin word *volvere*, which means "revolving." But for a long time most turning dances were lumped under the name *Deutsche* (German).

Some dance historians speculate that the waltz evolved from these German wooing dances. With its 3/4 time and fantastic first beat, the waltz contained a giddy turn which necessitated a close

body hold for maintaining the dancers' balance. Many partners discovered the thrill of embracing closely, while they whirled madly around the dance floor. After Napoleon brought the waltz to France as part of his booty from Germany, this dance spread throughout Europe and reached the U.S. by 1815.

The polka, written in 2/4 time, originated in Bohemia and was popularized by the French. The name polka probably comes from the Czech word,

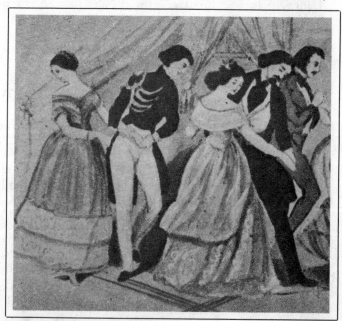

BALL AT ALMACK'S (By Cruikshank)

"pulka," which means half, because the half-step was an integral part of this dance. The polka, which contained a lively rhythm (the fast da-da-dum, da-da-dum), required a close body hold that excited dancers, but incited hostility from critics.

By 1860, people were amusing themselves more in private and less in public. Society balls were held in the houses of rich hostesses, rather than in exclusive assembly rooms. Dances began to trickle upward into high society, instead of dribbling down into the masses. Dance halls that catered to the public in general seemed to spring up overnight. One dance that reflected the new trend was the Barn Dance, which contained three sliding steps and a hop, performed while partners advanced hand-in-hand and side-by-side.

Another dance popular in the late 19th century was the lively two-step. The most famous two-step was created for the Washington Post March, composed by John Philip Sousa in 1891. This march, dripping with patriotism, caught on even in Europe. Of course, not all two-step dances required such unrelenting energy. But the extreme simplicity of the two-step (a quick marching step, followed with skips) made this dance a perennial favorite.

New forms of theatrical dancing developed or first became popular among the working class and the poor in America during the late 19th century. Black dancers developed tap-dancing by combining traditional African dances with the Irish jig and the English folk dance called the *clog*. Black performers tap-danced in taverns and on street corners. By the 1870s they appeared in traveling variety shows. At the same time, chorus girls danced the high-kicking cancan in dance halls along the American frontier. ♣

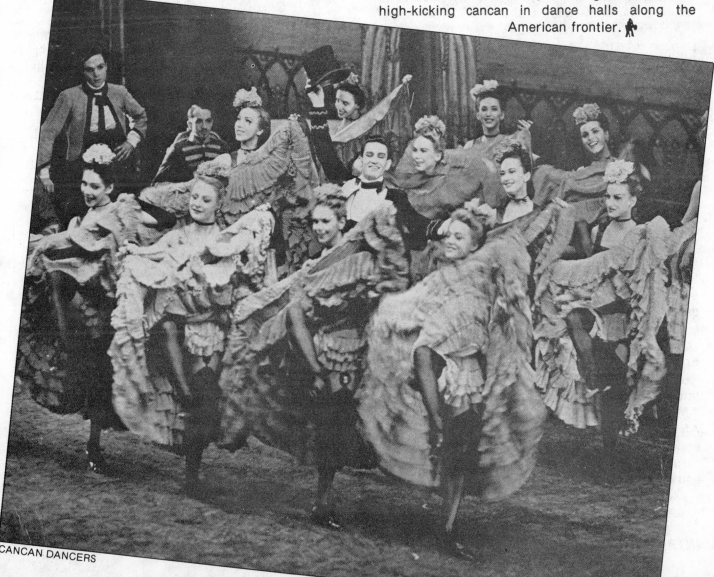

CANCAN DANCERS

20TH CENTURY

Two trends were apparent in the 20th century before World War I: tradition and innovation. Some people tried to revive older traditions by whirling through faster waltzes and galops. Other, more daring dancers, searched frantically for revolutionary and self-expressive dance forms.

Indeed, the early part of this century was a veritable hotbed of new theories and new forms of dance. The ballet was infused with new life under the leadership of Russian impresario, Sergey Diaghilev. Diaghilev produced powerful, even shocking ballets during the early 1900s. One of his most famous productions, *The Rite of Spring* (1913), contained primitive-style dances by the great Russian choreographer and dancer, Vaslav Nijinsky, as well as radical music by the Russian composer Igor Stravinsky. At the opening performance of this ballet in Paris, the innovative elements set off a riot in the audience.

Another group of dancers, led by Isadora Duncan, created a different form of dance dubbed "modern dance." Modern dancers revolted against the cramped artificiality of Romantic ballet. Isadora Duncan initiated changes that expanded the types of movement that could be used effectively in dance. Although the beginnings of modern dance were happening before Isadora Duncan, she was the first person, according to James Penrod and Janice Gudde Plastine, "to bring the new dance to general audiences. . . Her search for a natural movement form sent her to nature. She believed movement should be as natural as the swaying of the trees and the rolling waves of the sea, and should be in harmony with the movements of the earth." Isadora Duncan's unique dancing style and revolutionary theories on dance as a natural art form influenced other pioneers in the modern dance movement, including Loie Fuller, Ruth St. Denis, Martha Graham, Emile Jacques-Dalcroze, and Rudolf van Laban.

Popular music in the 20th century began to be infused with Caribbean, Latin American, and African rhythms. The overwhelming popularity of Afro-American rhythms radically changed the entire spirit and style of social dancing. As a result, social dancing became freer, more relaxed, and intimately sensual.

Moreover, the black influence on American music and dance from soul to disco has been

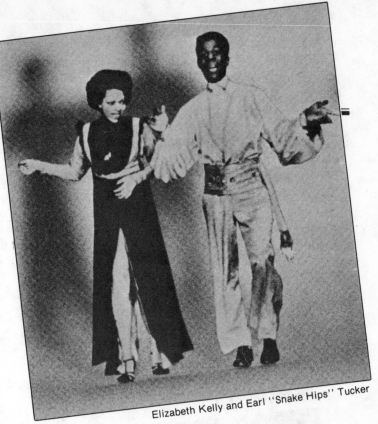
Elizabeth Kelly and Earl "Snake Hips" Tucker

phenomenal. Just two of the most outstanding black dancers, popular in the early part of this century, were Earl "Snake Hips" Tucker and Perry Bradford. Before Elvis Presley was out of diapers, Earl Tucker had stormed the nightclubs of Harlem in the 1920s with his hip slithering, tassle hassling gyrations, which earned him the name of "freak dancer."

Perry Bradford, on the other hand, was a self-made dancer, born in Atlanta in 1890. "Touring the south in them days," Bradford once said,

"I saw a million steps in a million tonks. The dancers had all kinds of names and no names for them, and I just took over the steps I liked and put them in my act. Once in awhile, if the step went over big, I'd work up a tune and lyrics that explained how to do it, have it printed, and sell it to the audience after my act."

In the field of music, black musicians were the innovators and trend-setters. In the U.S. during the early 1900s, there existed a subculture of the black musical establishment. These "underground" musicians blended African rhythms with traditional country music to create a unique form of syncopation. This syncopation resulted in two types of music — *ragtime* and *jazz.*

1900-1910

The advent of ragtime radically changed the structure and sound of American music. In ragtime music, the right hand played the tune, while the left hand kept up a regular beat, with syncopation included in the melody. The origin of the word ''ragtime'' has puzzled many dance historians. Peter Gammond, Scott Joplin's biographer, suggests that the music is called ''ragged'' because of the syncopation. The music was originally called ''jig time,'' but the word ''rag'' eventually replaced the word ''jig.'' Although ragtime music had been around for many years, the first tune to contain the word ''rag'' in its title was William H. Krell's ''Mississippi Rag'' which appeared in 1897.

Of course the greatest ragtime musician of all time was Scott Joplin who was born in November 1868. Scott's father was a railroad worker who had been born and raised a slave, becoming legally free only five years before Scott was born. By the time Scott Joplin was eleven, he had already earned a reputation as a proficient musician who could play the guitar, the bugle, and the piano. Joplin himself said: ''It is never right to play Ragtime fast.''

Ragtime music created a demand for new dance forms. One of the earliest ''rag'' dances was the cakewalk. Before ragtime, the cakewalk had been a strutting walk or promenade which concluded a minstrel show. A prize — candy, ice cream or a cake — was given to the couple who devised the most ingenious steps. After the introduction of ''ragged'' music, however, the cakewalk changed significantly. Performed to syncopated music, the revised cakewalk alternated wild jumps with sedate processional steps.

Ragtime music was also responsible for the rise in the popularity of animal dances, in which the dancers imitated the gait and mannerisms of various animals. Many of these animal dances were free-style dances which contained a series of jerky steps, suggestive body movements, and a lewd grinding of the hips. The names for these animal dances ranged from the bizarre to the ridiculous: for instance, there was the crab, the kangaroo dip, the horse trot, the bunny hug, the fish trail, the eagle rock, and the buzzard lope, to name just a few.

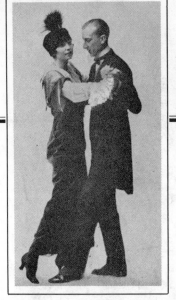

Irene and Vernon Castle

1910-1920

In 1911, ''Alexander's Ragtime Band,'' a song composed by Irving Berlin, became the first worldwide best-selling record. In that same year, two unforgettable dance teachers, Vernon and Irene Castle, changed the face of ballroom dance. Irene Castle shocked American society by wearing no corset, styling her hair in a short, simple cut, and dressing in long, flowing clothes. In addition to standardizing dance steps, the Castles also invented their own dance called the Castle walk. The Castle walk contained a strutting step performed on the balls of the feet, with the knees kept straight.

In the Ziegfeld Follies of 1914 music hall performer Harry Fox performed a trotting dance to ragtime music. The fox trot, a more sophisticated type of ''animal dance'' contained a series of four slow walk steps, followed with eight fast running steps. Gradually, however, the jerky steps were smoothed out and replaced with less frenetic variations, such as the butterfly, the twinkle, and the chassé.

Another dance that rose in popularity during the early 1900s was the tango. Sociologist Frances Rust maintains that the tango was probably an odd mixture of the tangano (a dance brought by African slaves to Haiti and Cuba in the 18th century) and the habanera (a 19th century Cuban dance).

In 1910, the tango was introduced to Paris and popularized by French dancer Camille de Rhynal. But the tango, with its exotic mixture of African and South American rhythms, plus erotic body movements had to be toned down, before it could be accepted into English society in 1912. Although the infamous Castles standardized the tango steps for American dancers in 1914, it was Valentino's flashy style in the 1920s that finally ignited public enthusiasm for this particular dance.

INTRO TO DISCO

1920-1930

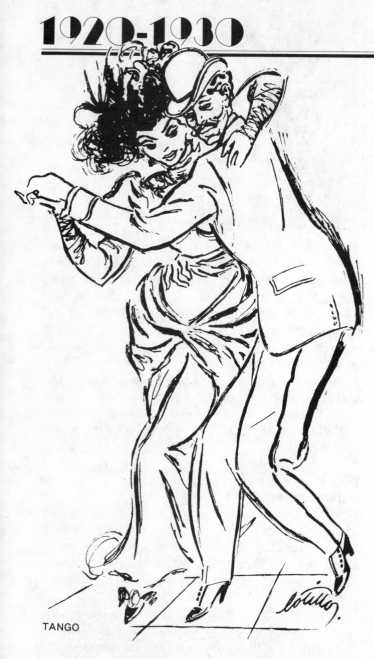

TANGO

range of instruments: for instance, a typical jazz band would include a banjo, clarinet, cornet, tuba, trombone, saxophone, and drums. But most important, jazz was improvisational music which, unlike ragtime, was not written down. In fact, many jazz musicians including Nick La Rocca, the leader of the Original Dixieland Jazz Band, could neither read nor score music. Until Paul Whiteman started the trend of "composed" jazz in the mid-20s, most jazz musicians used the trial by error method and trusted their own auditory sixth sense.

The most popular dance of the roaring twenties was the Charleston. The original Charleston was a burlesque dance performed by black dockworkers in South Carolina. When the general public was first introduced to this dance during a performance at the Ziegfeld Follies in October 1923, the crowd went wild! To make the Charleston easier for everybody to perform, dance instructors modified the difficult side-kick sequence and added elements lifted from both the two-step and the fox trot. Although the Charleston did not survive for long, its speed and exhilarating liveliness were so infectious that the entire country temporarily went "Charleston-mad."

Two other short-lived dances popular in the era of the flappers and emancipation were the black bottom and the shimmy. Curt Sachs described the black bottom as a "lively mixture of side-turns, stomps, skating-glides, skips and leaps." The shimmy, on the contrary, involved a turning in of the knees and toes, followed with a shake of the rump. Both the black bottom and the shimmy contained suggestive hip movements. In addition, both were performed to energetic, almost frantic, jazz rhythms.

In the 1920s, the Jazz Age was born. Although the origin of the word "jazz" is obscure, Tony Palmer views the word as a corruption of "jezebel," when "jazz belles" was the slang term for prostitute. Many historians suspect that jazz, similar to ragtime, was invented as a form of entertainment popular in brothels.

Although both jazz and ragtime were popular during the 20s, there were a few outstanding differences between these two musical forms. In jazz, the highly syncopated rhythms were set against each other, as the right hand played against the left hand. Jazz also introduced a wider

1930-1940

With the Great Crash of 1929, record sales dropped phenomenally and the word "jazz" began to acquire an old-fashioned ring. The music industry decided to generate enthusiasm by promoting the new sound called swing. In swing, jazz rhythms and improvisations were merged with popular melodies. To perceive the noticeable difference between swing and jazz, compare the music of Benny Goodman, the "King of Swing," with the music of Paul Whiteman, the "King of Jazz." Sometimes the term "boogie-woogie" was substituted for some types of swing music played on the piano. In general, however, swing was less restrained, but more danceable than jazz.

In 1936 the lindy and jitterbug became the most popular swing dances, carried by GIs to all parts of the world during World War II. The jitterbug was basically sensuous, hazardous to perform, and aggressive. In its wildness, the jitterbug was the forerunner of jive and rock dances of the fifties and sixties.

In addition to the lindy and jitterbug, however, there existed a slew of novelty dances, influenced by Latin American rhythms. In the Cuban conga, dancers performed a one-two-three-kick in a long snake-like line. In the rumba, a toned-down version of an erotic dance that combined African with Caribbean rhythms, partners sensuously moved their hips and shoulders. In 1946, however, British dance teachers regularized the pattern for the rumba, turning it into a square or non-progressive box that retained a modified Cuban hip motion.

The samba was another hot dance during the 1930s. Originally created by African slaves and performed at Brazilian carnivals, the samba was introduced at the 1939 New York World's Fair. Popularized in the movies of Carmen Miranda, the samba was jazzed up to become the bossa nova in the early 1960s and restructured to become the two-step (3-count) hustle in the mid-1970s. ♣

BALLROOM DANCERS

1940-1950

In the 1940s the dances became a bit wilder, heavily influenced by Cuban and African rhythms. In 1943, Cuban bandleader, Perez Prado, syncopated the rhythm of the dances performed by the sugarcane cutters and created a unique dance, called the mambo. According to Newsweek, the word "mambo" came from the Nanigo dialect spoken in Cuba, and has no "real" meaning. In the mambo there was one beat in each measure which was "held," as partners performed a series of kicks or crazy wiggles. ♣

MAMBO

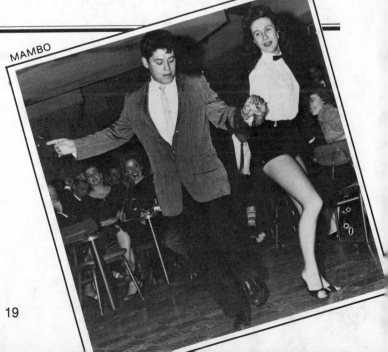

1950-1960

The mambo eventually developed into three distinct forms — single, double, and triple mambo. The third form was modified to produce the cha-cha, a dance popular during the 1950s and revitalized during the 1970s in the guise of the cha-cha hustle. The cha-cha consisted of a rock step (two slow steps), followed with a triple step (by three quick steps). On the triple step many cha-cha dancers preferred to break apart and perform a series of sexy wiggles — a solo technique called ''shining.''

The merengue, another dance popular during the mid-1950s, was performed to music with Latin rhythms and a strong beat. The merengue, imported from the Dominican Republic, contained a unique limp or drag step, nicknamed the ''lame-duck'' style of dance. After the merengue was introduced to the U.S., according to Peter Buckman, ''this 'limp' step was retained and smoothed over; the dance became quite lively, with a step on every beat, plenty of knee action, and that wiggle from side to side that seemed essential to all Latin dances.''

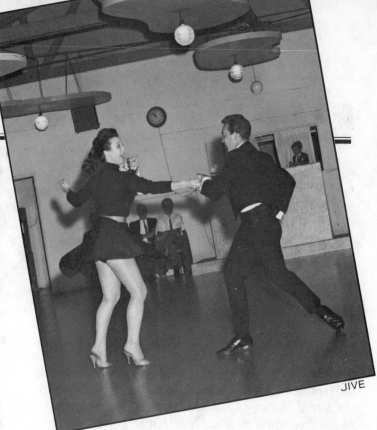
JIVE

By the middle of the 1950s dance bands were rapidly vanishing, replaced by nickel jukeboxes. Moreover, the name ''jive'' was the catch-all phrase for the lindy (with all three of its distinct rhythms) and jitterbug. Jive, however, was a less frenetic version of the jitterbug — a temporary lull before the storm of rock 'n' roll devastated the country in the mid-50s. 🕺

1960-1970

With a little help from television and radio, Bill Haley and His Comets had everyone rocking around the clock in 1957. In his review, ''Telling Rock's Story without Missing a Beat,'' Robert Hilburn explains the impact of mass media on the music scene:

Television and rock 'n' roll once were allies. Dick Clark's ''American Bandstand'' gave millions of teenagers in the 1950s their first glimpses of Chuck Berry and Buddy Holly. Fifty-six million tuned in for Elvis Presley's first appearance on the Ed Sullivan show. The audience was up to 70 million in 1964 for the Beatles' Sullivan performance.

As rock sounds changed, dance forms were forced to change. After sock-hopping and hand-jiving in the 50s, dancers began twisting and shimmying in the 60s. Chubby Checker, an ex-chicken plucker from Philadelphia, gave America the twist during a performance on American Bandstand in 1960. After the twist, the country went wild over such crazy free-style body dances as the hitchhike, the jerk, the shake, the monkey, the swim, the slop, the frug, the hully-gully, and the mashed potato. 🕺

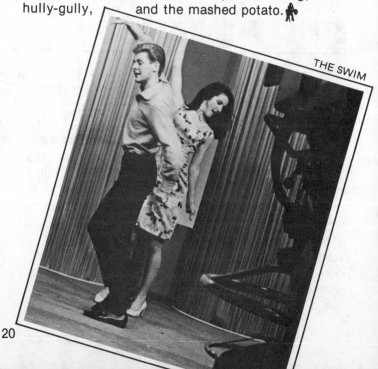
THE SWIM

1970-

After Gloria Gaynor cut ''Never Can Say Goodbye'' in 1974, the first record mixed explicitly for disco, the whole musical and dancing world was turned upside down. It was only a matter of time before Van McCoy's ''Hustle'' touched off a revolutionary type of touch dance that subsequently swept the entire country. In his article, ''The Delerium of Disco,'' Albert Goldman claims that ''the pace is fast, as never before. The beat is literally a gallop. The dancers swing and spin like lindy hoppers, but they slide, clasp and strut with the suave grace and loose hips of Latin lovers.''

''Disco,'' explains Richard A. Peterson, ''is non-stop dance music with a big throbbing beat, topped with crystal-clear, soaring high sounds carried by strings, synthesizers, brass and soprano voices.'' In his article, entitled ''Disco!'' Peterson identifies five types of disco music:

1. *New York (or soft) disco,* "with its uncomplicated and driving two-two beat."("A Taste of Honey" and "If My Friends Could See Me Now")

2. *Disco funk,* with its "fast beat and syncopated counter-rhythms." ("Electrified Funk" and "Macho Man.")

3. *Rhythm and blues disco* "continues the classic blues tradition."

4. *Classical or conceptual disco*, "relying on synthesizers, strings and large choruses, the effect is soft disco music of symphonic dimensions." ("Sphinx," "Supernature," and "Love Trilogy.")

5. *Omnivorous disco* includes "songs taken from other genres and remade with a strong disco beat laid on top." ("MacArthur's Park," "Moonlight Serenade," and "A Whiter Shade of Pale.")

Whether one agrees with Peterson's divisions, it's a known fact that disco spans a perplexing range of danceable music. More important, the music is hot, throbbing with sensual Latin and African rhythms, but cooled with just a touch of blues. So whatever your mood, you're sure to find a disco beat to satisfy your cravings. Whether you prefer to swoon to tunes by Donna Summer, or shimmy and shake to the jangling rhythms of the Village People, there's no show like disco.

Of course, once you've got the need, all you need's the know-how to set you free. And this book teaches you all you'll ever need, if you want to be the hottest dancer on the disco floor. For hip

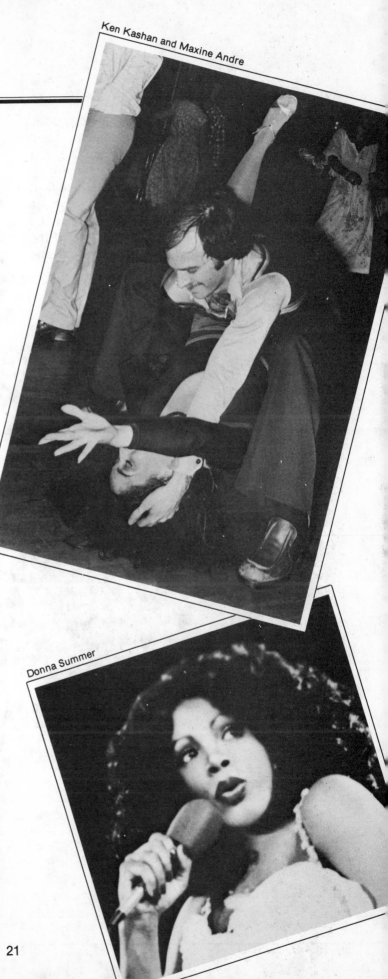

Ken Kashan and Maxine Andre

Donna Summer

21

hugging hustlers, this book gives the inside scoop on all major partner disco dances, from the Latin Hustle and the Cuban Salsa to the Tango Dip. For free-stylers who want to emulate the outstanding, outrageous Lockers, the free-form section tells it like it is. And for those who long for a romantic interlude, there are ballroom dances to melt the hardest of hearts. In fact, after you learn the dances in this book, you will probably be the one to shout: "Okay, everybody — let's dance."

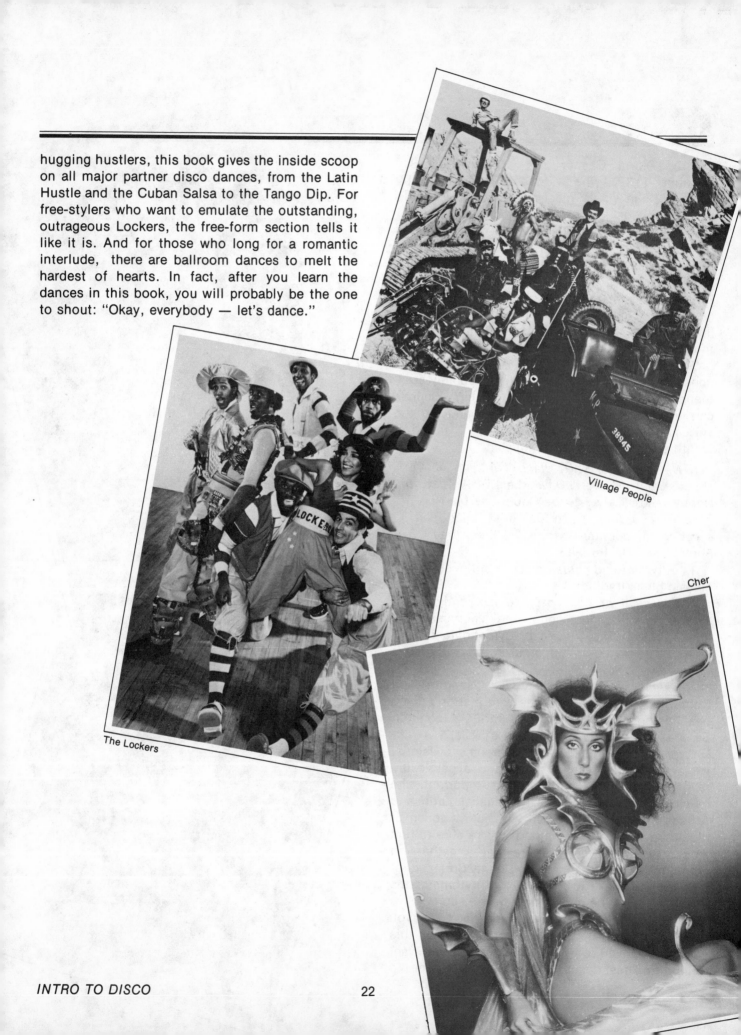

Village People

The Lockers

Cher

CHAPTER 2

DANCE FUNDAMENTALS

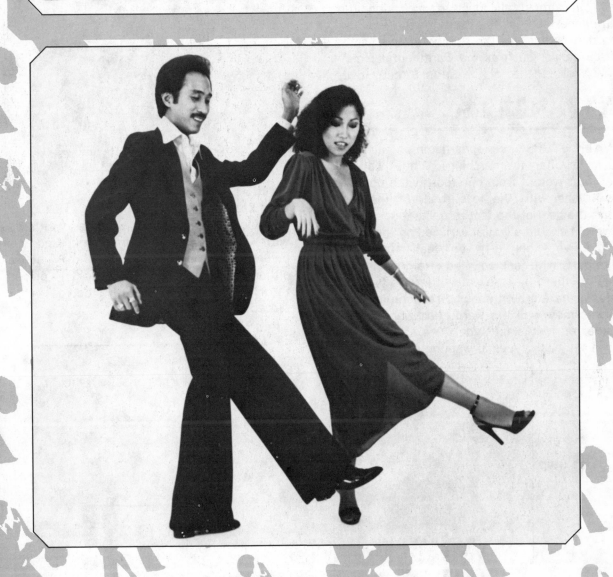

SECTION A:
DANCE STEPS

In dance there are four general types of steps: WALK STEPS, CHASSÉS, ROCK STEPS, and TRIPLE STEPS. A combination of these steps will be used in almost all touch dances, including smooth dances such as the Waltz or the Fox Trot, rhythm dances such as the Rumba or the Samba, and disco dances such as the Continental Hustle, the New York Hustle, or the Latin Street Hustle.

WALK STEPS

In WALK STEPS one step is taken on each beat of music, similar to marching. While walking, transfer your weight from one foot to the opposite foot, but lead with the toes (ball) of the foot. Although the heel of the foot remains touching the floor, weight should always be placed on the ball of the foot. As you walk, keep your feet parallel, but slightly apart, with toes pointing straight ahead.

Although there are several different types of walk steps, there are only four directions in which the dancer may walk: forward, backward, to the right side, or to the left side. The following list describes the basic types of walking steps.

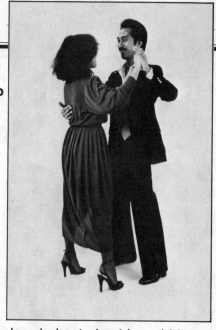

Side Step

b) *Side Step:*
One foot is placed about shoulder width apart, with feet parallel, toes in a line, and weight balanced on one foot. A step may be taken either to the right side, as weight is placed on the right foot, or to the left side, as weight is placed on the left foot.

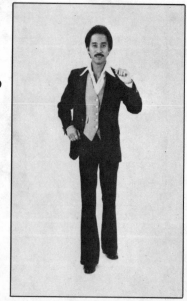

Forward Step

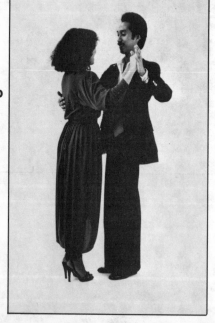

Close Step

a) *Close Step* (Feet Together):
Most step patterns begin and end with feet together in the parallel (close) position, with toes pointing straight ahead.

c) *Forward Step:*
One foot is placed in front of the opposite foot, with feet parallel and toes pointed straight ahead.

d) *Backward Step:*
One foot is placed in back of the opposite foot, with feet parallel and toes pointing straight ahead.

e) Diagonal Step:

A diagonal step, taken forward or backward, is made by placing one foot in front of (or behind) the opposite foot and slightly to the side.

f) Pass Back (Fifth Position) Step:

A pass back or fifth position step is made by crossing one foot behind the opposite foot, as weight is placed on the ball of the foot. Pass back steps enable the dancer to progress across the room in a sideways direction.

h) Step in Place:

A step in place is made by lifting the foot slightly off the floor, then replacing it in the same spot. On the step in place, weight is shifted from one foot to the opposite foot, without changing the direction or placement of the foot.

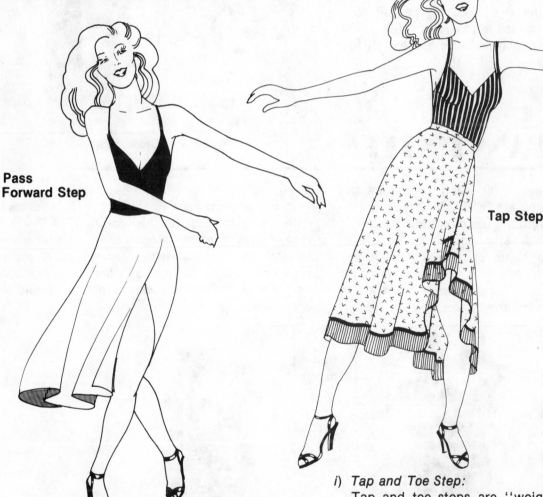

Pass Forward Step

Tap Step

i) Tap and Toe Step:

Tap and toe steps are "weightless" steps in which the ball of one foot touches the floor, but weight remains balanced on the opposite foot. A tap step is made by lightly tapping or touching the ball of one foot against the floor. A toe step is made by pointing the ball of one foot. A tap or a toe step may be taken forward, back, in place, behind the opposite foot, or to either side.

g) Pass Forward Step:

A pass forward step is made by crossing one foot in front of the opposite. Pass forward steps are used for progressing forward in the Promenade Dance Position.

CHASSÉS

Another type of step is called the CHASSE, taken from the French word which means "to chase." A chassé is composed of two steps, completed in two beats of music. On the first beat count, the dancer takes a step to the side. On the second beat count, the dancer draws feet together in the parallel (close) position. In effect, one foot "chases" the opposite foot.

A chassé (side step, followed with a close step) may be taken either to the right or to the left. On a chassé to the left, step to the left side on the left foot, then close the right foot to the left foot. Conversely, on a chassé to the right, step to the right side on the right foot, then close the left foot to the right foot.

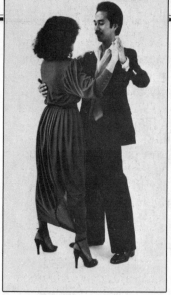

Side Step

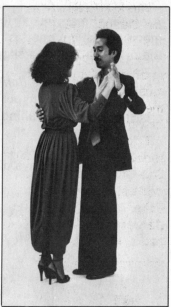

Close Step

ROCK OR BALL-CHANGE STEPS

Some partner dances, including the Samba and the Cha-Cha, incorporate ROCK STEPS or BALL-CHANGE STEPS into the basic pattern. Similar to the chassé, a rock step contains two steps, completed in two beats of music. Unlike the chassé, however, a rock step begins on the first beat count with a step taken forward or back. On the second beat count, the dancer takes a step in place, shifting weight to the opposite foot.

In the *forward rock*, a forward step is followed with a step in place on the back foot. In the *back rock*, however, a back step is followed with a step in place on the forward foot. As weight is shifted from one foot to the opposite foot on the second beat count, a slight rocking motion should be accentuated.

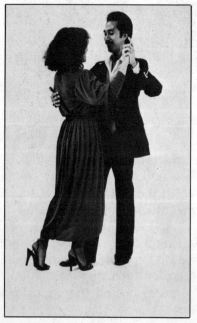

Ball-Change

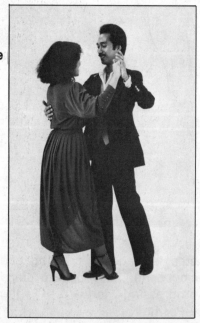

TRIPLE STEPS

The fourth and final type of dance step—used in the Samba, the Cha-Cha, the Two-Step Hustle, and the New York-Latin Hustle, to name just a few—are *triple steps*. Triple steps contain three small steps, completed in two syncopated beats of music. Although triple steps are usually taken to the side, they may also be taken backward, forward, or in place.

Triple steps may be incorporated into a sequence containing another type of step. In the Cha-Cha, for example, rock steps precede the triple step (on beats 4 and 1), which may be taken either to the side (side-together-side) or forward (forward-together-forward) or back (back-together-back). In the Latin Street Hustle, four walk steps precede the triple step (on beats 5 and 6), as partners take two steps back, then one step forward. In the New York-Latin Hustle, on the other hand, the triple step (on beats 3 and 4) is sandwiched in between a tap step, a side step, and two walk steps forward. And finally, there are other dances, such as the Samba and the Two-Step (3-Count) Hustle, which are composed entirely of triple steps.

The order and arrangement of steps in the triple steps, however, will vary widely from dance to dance. In the Samba, for example, partners step side, cross one foot behind the opposite foot, then step in place on the forward foot, repeating the sequence from side to side. In the Two-Step Hustle, on the contrary, partners cross one foot behind the opposite foot, step in place on the forward foot, then step side, repeating the sequence from side to side.

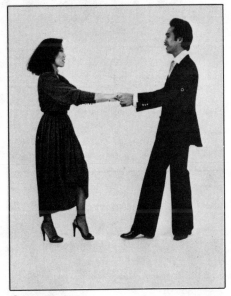

Step Back

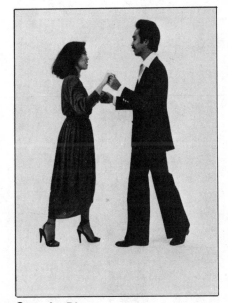

Step in Place

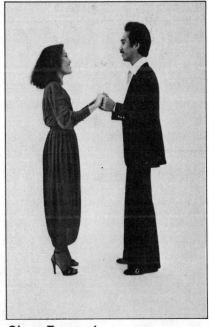

Close Forward

STEP PATTERNS

For most partner dances, particularly ballroom or social dances, the woman's part is the natural opposite of the man's part. Thus, whenever the man steps forward, the woman steps back. Conversely, whenever the man steps back, the woman steps forward. Moreover, most patterns begin as the man steps forward on his left foot, and the woman steps back on her right foot. Although most partner dances follow this general pattern, some disco touch dances, including the New York-Latin Hustle and the Latin Street Hustle, contain their own unique patterns in which the woman's part is *not* the mirror image of the man's part. 💃

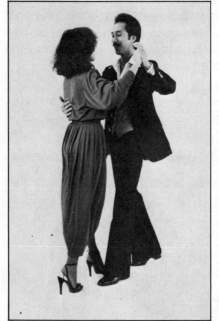

Natural opposite

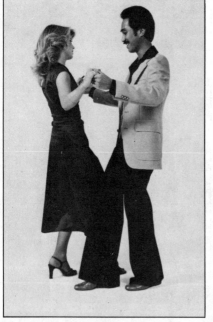

Identical movement

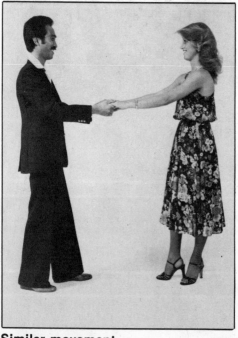

Similar movement

STEP DIAGRAMS

To illustrate the step sequence, most of the partner dances described in this book are accompanied with detailed STEP DIAGRAMS. The black footprint indicates the right foot, and the white footprint indicates the left foot. The woman's footprints, however, are slightly narrower than the man's footprints. Most important, the *number* inside the footprint refers to a particular *step* in the sequence.

Most step diagrams contain *solid footprints*, which indicate that weight should be placed on the foot that steps. Some patterns, however, contain tap or toe steps in which only the ball of the foot lightly touches against the floor, while weight is balanced on the opposite foot. To indicate a toe or tap step, the pattern contains a *partial footprint* in which only the top part of the foot is shown.

In addition, there are other patterns in which one foot is lightly brushed against the opposite foot, but no weight is placed on the foot that brushes. These "weightless" steps are represented with a *jagged footprint*.

To familiarize yourself with reading a step diagram, study the following example. Notice that most patterns begin with feet drawn together in the close position. After learning a basic step sequence, add the rhythm and you'll be ready to get down and boogie!

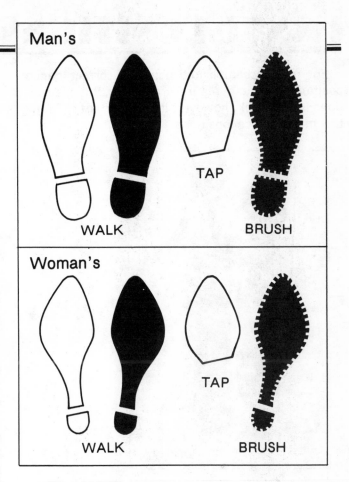

Man's

WALK   TAP   BRUSH

Woman's

WALK   TAP   BRUSH

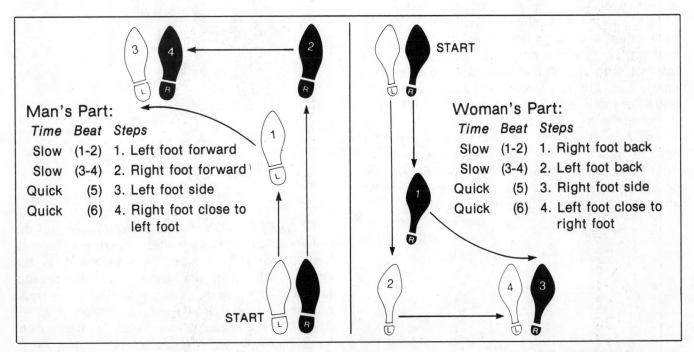

Man's Part:

Time	Beat	Steps
Slow	(1-2)	1. Left foot forward
Slow	(3-4)	2. Right foot forward
Quick	(5)	3. Left foot side
Quick	(6)	4. Right foot close to left foot

Woman's Part:

Time	Beat	Steps
Slow	(1-2)	1. Right foot back
Slow	(3-4)	2. Left foot back
Quick	(5)	3. Right foot side
Quick	(6)	4. Left foot close to right foot

SECTION B:
DANCE POSITIONS

For most accomplished dancers, correct dance position is second nature. To follow the instructions in this book, however, it is important to know the major dance positions.

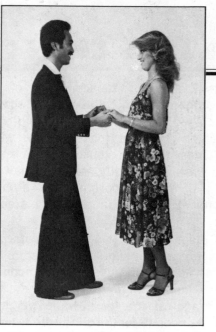

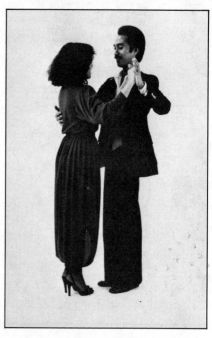

1. *CLOSED DANCE POSITION:* The most frequently used position in both ballroom and disco partner dancing is the Closed Dance Position (also known as Social or Ballroom Dance Position). In the Closed Dance Position partners stand close to each other and face each other in the parallel position, although the woman stands slightly to the man's right. The woman's right hand is placed lightly between the man's left thumb and forefinger, and her left hand is placed slightly behind the man's right shoulder, with her thumb resting on top of his shoulder. The man places his right hand below the woman's shoulder blade, with his right palm pressed firmly against the upper-middle part of the woman's back. Both partners keep their arms relaxed and slightly bent at the elbows.

2. *HOLDING DANCE POSITION:* Many disco partner dances are performed in the Holding Dance Position. In the Holding Dance Position, partners face each other in the parallel position, but stand slightly apart. In addition, partners clasp both pairs of hands in the two-hand or double hand hold. Thus, the woman's right hand is lightly clasped in the man's left hand, and her left hand is lightly clasped in his right hand.

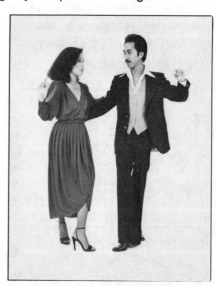

3. *CONVERSATION DANCE POSITION:* In the Conversation Dance Position, partners form a V-shape with their hips. Partners stand in the Open Position, with the woman's left side parallel to the man's right side. In addition, the man releases the woman's right hand from his left hand. The woman's left hand and the man's right hand, however, encircle each other's waist.

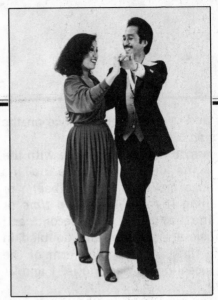

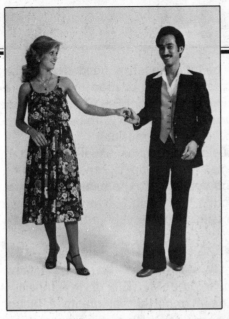

4. *PROMENADE DANCE POSITION:* The Promenade Dance Position is a Closed Position in which partners turn slightly away from each other to face the same forward direction, without releasing their hands. Similar to the Conversation Position, the woman's left hip forms a V-shape with the man's right hip. The Promenade Position is used for variations in which both partners progress in a forward direction, such as in the Tango Hustle or the Merengue Promenade.

6. *LEFT OPEN POSITION:* As the name implies, the Left Open Position is the opposite of the Right Open Position. Although partners face in the same direction, the woman's left side is parallel to the man's right side, similar to the Conversation Position. Moreover, the woman's left hand is held in the man's right hand, although her right hand is released from the man's left hand.

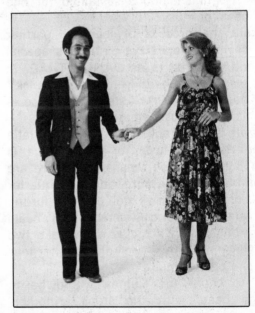

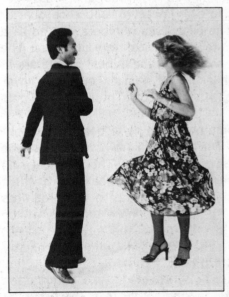

5. *RIGHT OPEN POSITION:* In the Right Open Position, also called an Open Break, partners face in the same direction, and the woman's right side is parallel to the man's left side. In addition, partners are in the Open Position, with the woman's right hand clasped in the man's left hand, although the woman's left hand is released from the man's right hand.

7. *APART DANCE POSITION:* In the Apart Dance Position, also called the Challenge Position, partners stand about an arm's length apart, with all hands released. The Apart Dance Position is used for some Mambo, Cha-Cha, and New York Hustle variations. ♣

Contrary to popular belief, a good dancer may not be able to carry a tune or read music. But all dancers have a strong sense of RHYTHM. The one and only factor that is necessary, therefore, is the ability to keep time to the music.

In dance music, the beat is usually carried by the bass drum. To develop a sense of timing, practice tapping your foot to the beat of the drum. Then walk around the room, taking one step on each beat of music. Voilà — you've got rhythm! ♪

MUSICAL STRUCTURE

For the dancer, the METER of the music is probably the most important element. Although TEMPO is the speed at which a measure of music is played, RHYTHM results from the time value of the notes played in a measure. It is the meter, therefore, which defines the rhythmic element in music.

Except for the Waltz (written in ¾ time) or the Samba and the Two-Step Hustle (written in 2/4 time), the meter for most popular dance music is written in 4/4 time. In 4/4 time, there are four beats of music to each measure, and each quarter note receives one beat. Two numbers written as a fraction constitute the musical time signature. The upper number shows how many beat counts are in one bar or measure of music, but the lower number shows what kind of a musical note gets one count.

In music, some notes are more heavily accented than others. The symbol (>) indicates the primary or strongest beat. The symbol (/) indicates the secondary or light beat count, which means that the secondary beat is accented less than the primary beat, but more than any of the other beats. In 4/4 time the primary accent usually falls on the first beat, with a secondary accent on the third beat.

Music can also be syncopated. Syncopation often refers to a shifting of the accent from the first beat count to another count in the measure. But syncopation may also refer to the continuing of one note, without a new accent, into the ordinarily accented beat. In dance, three steps will usually be taken in two syncopated beats of music. For example, the dancer may kick one foot forward on step 1 (beat 1), then swing the foot back into place on step 2 (beat "and"), then step in place on the opposite foot on step 3 (beat 2).

Moreover, dancers do not always dance with the recurring beat of the music. To spice up the pattern, dancers also move on the "offbeat" or against the prevailing rhythm. In *double time* or the doubling of the basic beat, the second and fourth bars of music are rhythmically doubled in counts, but not in time. A colloquial form of the double time often used in jazz dancing is: 1 and 2/ 3 and 4. ♪

DANCE COUNT AND DANCE TIME

There is, of course, a basic difference between MUSICAL COUNT and DANCE COUNT. Musical count represents the number and sequence of beats to the measure. The dance count, on the contrary, describes the sequence of steps, indicating whether weight should be sustained for one beat or two beats of music.

To facilitate the process of learning partner dances, dance instructors have devised a special timing method, referred to as DANCE TIME. In dance time, steps are defined in terms of "quick" and "slow" beats. The "slow" steps take twice as many beats as the "quick" steps.

To illustrate how dance time works, let's examine the Rumba. Music for the Rumba is written in 4/4 time, which means that there are four beats of music to a measure, and each quarter note receives one beat. But all step patterns for the Rumba contain 6 steps completed in 8 beats (2 measures) of music. Thus, two steps take two beats of music apiece, while each of the other four steps takes one beat of music.

One way to count the Rumba would be to correlate the beats with the steps. Another, simpler way of counting would be to accent the slow and quick steps. In the Rumba, for example, the timing would be: Step 1 (Quick)/ Step 2 (Quick)/ Step 3 (Slow)/ Step 4 (Quick)/ Step 5 (Quick)/ Step 6 (Slow). If all three methods of counting the Rumba were described, the step sequence could be defined in terms of musical count, dance count, and timing. Thus, a complete list would look like the following:

Man's Part:

Musical Count	Dance Count	Timing	Steps
1	1	Quick	1. Left foot side
2	2	Quick	2. Right foot close to left foot
3 - 4	3 - 4	Slow	3. Left foot forward
1	5	Quick	4. Right foot side
2	6	Quick	5. Left foot close to right foot
3 - 4	7 - 8	Slow	6. Right foot back

Woman's Part:

Musical Count	Dance Count	Timing	Steps
1	1	Quick	1. Right foot side
2	2	Quick	2. Left foot close to right foot
3 - 4	3 - 4	Slow	3. Right foot back
1	5	Quick	4. Left foot side
2	6	Quick	5. Right foot close to left foot
3 - 4	7- 8	Slow	6. Left foot forward

Although dance time simplifies many partner dances, this timing technique need not be used for patterns in which a step is taken on each beat of music. In the Waltz, the Tango Hustle, or the Merengue, for example, all the steps are "quick" steps, since one step is taken on each and every beat of music.

In dancing, it is extremely important that each step is taken on the correct beat. Consequently, all of the patterns in this book describe both beat count and step. For instance, a description of the third step in the woman's part of the Merengue would contain both beat count and step: (Beat 3): Step 3: Right foot back. For dances in which dance time is used, timing, beat count, and steps are indicated. A description of the third step in the man's part of the Rumba, for example, would be: Slow (Beats 3-4) Step 3: Left foot forward. 🕺

RHYTHM PATTERNS

Some dance instructors prefer to teach dance in terms of three major types of rhythm patterns: *Single Rhythm, Double Rhythm,* and *Triple Rhythm.*

(a) *Single Rhythm:* In Single Rhythm, one step is taken on two beats of music. A step is taken on beat count one, followed with a tap or toe step, a brush step, a kick, or a "hold" for the second beat count. Single Rhythm Steps are used in many basic partner hustles, as well as in the Fox Trot, the Tango, and Single Swing.

(b) *Double Rhythm:* In Double Rhythm, the dancer steps twice in two beats of music, stepping on every beat similar to marching. In Double Rhythm, the dancer alternates feet, starting with one foot free, but ending with the opposite foot free. Almost all walk steps, in addition to chassés and rock steps, are Double Rhythm Steps. Touch dances that use Double Rhythm Steps include most Salsa variations, the Waltz, and the Merengue.

(c) *Triple Rhythm:* In Triple Rhythm the dancer takes three small steps in two syncopated beats of music. Of course, *all* triple steps can be lumped into this category. In a "Triple Left" the dancer starts on his left foot, then steps on his right foot, and ends on his left foot. In a "Triple Right" the dancer starts on her right foot, then steps on her left foot, and ends on her right foot. Triple Rhythm Steps are used in the Samba, the Cha-Cha, the Two-Step Hustle, the New York-Latin Hustle, and the New York Street Hustle. 🕺

DANCE FUNDAMENTALS

SECTION D:
TURNS

TURN DIRECTION: "THE NOSE KNOWS"

There are two and only two directions in which a dancer may turn. In short, a dancer may turn either right or left. To make a RIGHT TURN, the dancer turns clockwise, traveling in the same direction in which the hands of a clock rotate. Conversely, to make a LEFT TURN, the dancer turns counter-clockwise, traveling opposite to the direction in which the hands of a clock rotate.

A foolproof way to turn correctly is based on the "Nose Knows" principle. In other words, before initiating a turn, the dancer glances over his or her own shoulder, then turns by following the direction in which the nose is pointing. Before starting a right turn, therefore, the dancer glances over his or her right shoulder. Conversely, before starting a left turn, the dancer glances over his or her left shoulder.

TYPES OF TURNS

Most turn variations fall into one of the following six categories: UNDERARM TURNS, HOLDING TURNS, PARALLEL TURNS, ROLLS, FREE SPINS, AND PIVOT TURNS.

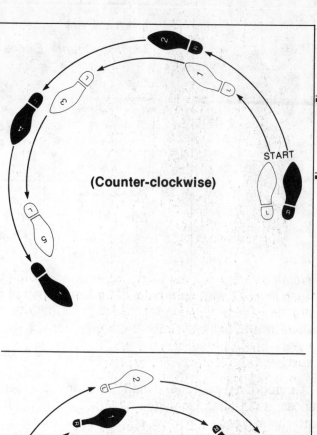

(Counter-clockwise)

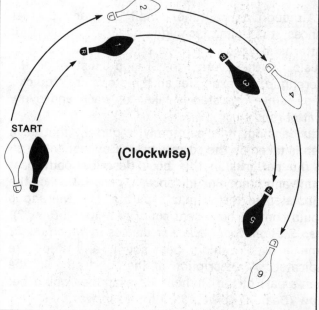

(Clockwise)

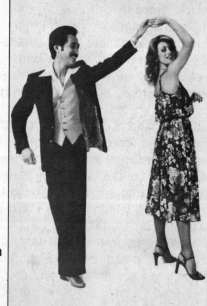

Underarm Turn

a) *Underarm Turns:* Underarm Turns are completed in the Open Position, with a *one-hand hold* (one of the woman's hands uplifted in the man's hand, with opposite hands released). If the Underarm Turn is made to the right, then the uplifted hands rotate clockwise. Conversely, if the Underarm Turn is made to the left, then the uplifted hands rotate counter-clockwise.

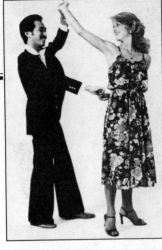

Holding Turn

b) *Holding Turns:* As the name implies, a Holding Turn is made with both pairs of hands clasped in the double or two-hand hold. In some turns, such as the Double Cross Turns, both pairs of hands are uplifted for the turn. Other turns, such as the Cradle, are made with one pair of hands uplifted, while the other pair of hands remain clasped, but held down. Still other turns, such as the Pretzel, are made with one pair of hands uplifted, while the other pair of hands remain held and pinned behind the woman's back.

c) *Parallel Turns:* Parallel Turns are continuous turns, made either to the right (clockwise) or to the left (counter-clockwise). In Parallel Turns both partners turn in the same direction, while they are embraced in the Closed Dance Position.

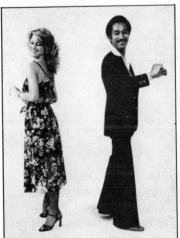

Parallel Turn

Free Spin

d) *Free Spins:* Free Spins are made with all hands released, while partners are standing in the Apart Dance Position. Some spins, such as the Dual Free Spins, contain dual turns in which

both partners make Full Turns in opposite directions. In other spins, such as the Tuck In, only one partner completes a Free Spin, while the other partner completes his basic steps in the Apart Dance Position.

e) *Rolls:* Rolls are made by whipping out towards one side, then whipping back in while hands are clasped in the *one-hand hold.* Although Full Turns will be made on the roll out and the roll in, hands do *not* rotate overhead.

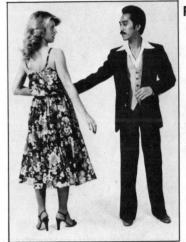

Roll

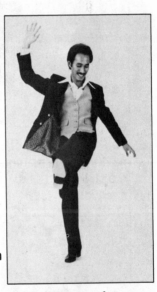

Pivot Turn

f) *Pivot Turns:* The final broad category of turns contains Pivot Turns. As the name implies, a Pivot Turn is made by pivoting around on one foot, while the opposite foot is lifted off the floor. Some Pivot Turns, such as Split Pivots, alternate feet, while the dancer pivots around in a circle. Other Pivot Turns, such as the Pivot Spin, are made by flinging one foot around the opposite foot, as the dancer pivots in a circle on one foot. Other Pivot Turns, such as the ¼ Line Turn, contain partial pivots in which one foot is kicked forward, while the dancer pivots in a ¼ turn on the opposite foot.

DANCE FUNDAMENTALS

TURN DEGREES

Turns may also be defined in terms of degrees. Theoretically, all turn variations form either a partial or a whole circle on the dance floor. Most turns, therefore, fall into one of the following four categories: FULL TURNS, HALF TURNS, QUARTER TURNS, EIGHTH TURNS.

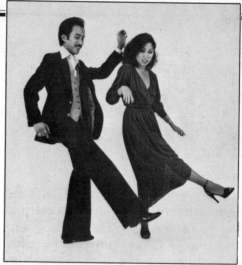

Quarter Turn

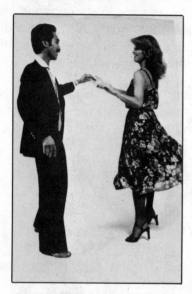

Full Turn

a) *Full Turns;* A Full Turn (360 degrees) is the maximum turn, since the dancer twirls around in a circle and ends up facing the same direction in which he started. Full Turns include Right Underarm Turns; Reverse (Left) Underarm Turns; Pivot Spins; Free Spins; and, Double Cross Turns.

c) *Quarter Turns:* A ¼ turn (90 degrees) is made by turning to face the next wall. Variations that contain ¼ turns include the Fox-Trot Quarter Turns, Cha-Cha Cross-Over Break, and Side Step (Open Break) in the New York Hustle. In addition, all Line Dances conclude with a ¼ Left Line Turn, as dancers kick their right leg forward and pivot 90 degrees counter-clockwise on their left foot.

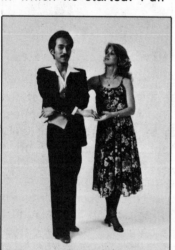

Half Turn

b) *Half Turns:* As the name implies, a Half Turn (180 degrees) is made by turning in a half circle, as the dancer whirls around to face in the opposite direction. Half Turns include: Walk-Around (Cross-Over) Turns; Cradle Turns; Pretzel and Reverse Pretzel Turns.

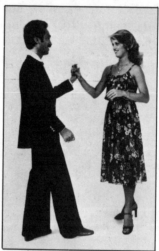

Eighth Turn

d) *Eighth Turns:* A 1/8 turn (45 degrees) is a minimal turn, through which the dancer shifts into a slightly different position. A 1/8 turn is used in the Basic Throw Out (Basic Cross-Body Lead). In addition, slight (1/8) turns are incorporated into "progressive dances," such as the Waltz, Fox Trot, or Tango, since partners follow the Line of Direction by turning gradually to their left (counter-clockwise).

HAND LEADS

Although the man must give the HAND LEAD, it's up to the woman to follow her partner. Some dance experts advocate a push forward and pull back technique: i.e., to lead a right turn, the man gently pushes his left hand forward; conversely, to lead a left turn, the man moves his left hand backward. Other experts argue that a man should never pull the woman's hand; instead, they urge the man to push the woman's hand gently, as he guides her into the turn.

Regardless of how you lead, there are standard types of hand leads. In general, the man gives a hand lead for a right turn by lifting the woman's right hand in his left hand and pushing the woman's right hand *outside* or away from her body. To give a hand lead for a left turn, the man lifts the woman's right hand in his left hand and pushes it *inside* or in front of her face.

More important, the man always gives the woman a hand lead on the *beat count that precedes the turn*. Thus, if the woman is going to turn on beat 2, the man gives a hand lead on beat 1. If the woman is going to turn on beat 5, the man gives a hand lead on beat 4, and so on and so forth.

The type of hand lead varies according to the type of turn. The name, however, refers to the woman's uplifted hand. Moreover, the lead is either a one-hand lead in which only one of the woman's hands is held in the man's hand, or it can be a two-hand lead in which both hands remain clasped in the double or two-hand hold. The most frequently used hand leads include the following:

(a) *right one-hand hold:* The man uplifts the woman's right hand in his left hand, as he releases her left hand from his right hand.

(b) *left one-hand hold:* The man uplifts the woman's left hand in his right hand, as he releases her right hand from his left hand.

(c) *right two-hand hold:* The man uplifts the woman's right hand in his left hand, but continues to hold her left hand in his right hand.

(d) *left two-hand hold:* The man uplifts the woman's left hand in his right hand, but continues to hold her right hand in his left hand. ♟

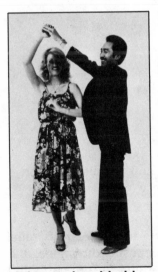

right one-hand hold

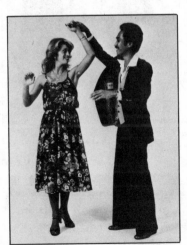

left one-hand hold

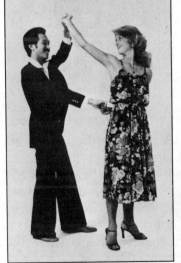

right two-hand hold

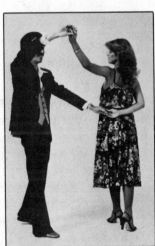

left two-hand hold

DANCE FUNDAMENTALS

TURN POSITION

In addition to the eight basic dance positions, there are four additional positions used to describe turn variations. Notice, however, that the woman's position in relation to the man's position still takes preference. Moreover, these four dance positions may use any hand hold, including a one-hand or two-hand (double) hold.

(a) *Right Side Parallel Position:* In the Right Side Parallel Position partners face in the same direction, although the woman's right side is parallel to the man's left side. The Right Side Parallel Position is used in the Man's Cradle and the Scarecrow.

(*Note:* If partners are standing in the Open Position, with the woman's right hand held in the man's left hand, this position would also be called the Right Open Position.)

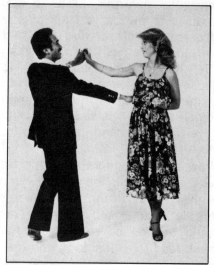

Right Parallel Position

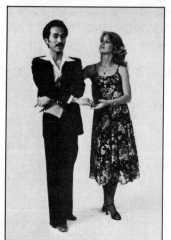

Right Side Parallel Position

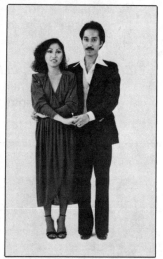

Left Side Parallel Position

(b) *Left Side Parallel Position:* In the Left Side Parallel Position, partners face in the same direction, but the woman's left side is parallel to the man's right side. The Left Side Parallel Position is used in the Woman's Cradle, the Chase, the Whip, and the Boomerang.

(*Note:* If partners are standing in the Open Position, with the woman's left hand held in the man's right hand, this position would also be called the Left Open Position. If, on the other hand, partners are standing in the Open Position, with the woman's right hand and the man's left hand encircling each other's waist, this position would be called the Conversation Dance Position.)

(c) *Right Parallel Position:* In the Right Parallel Position partners face in opposite directions, with the woman's right side parallel to the man's right side. The Right Parallel Position is used in the Pretzel, the Pinwheel, the Handshake, and the Walk Around Right.

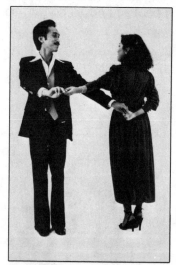

Left Parallel Position

(d) *Left Parallel Position:* In the Left Parallel Position partners face in opposite directions, but the woman's left side is parallel to the man's left side. The Left Parallel Position is used in the Reverse Pretzel, the Reverse Pinwheel, and the Walk Around Left. 🕺

SECTION E:
BODY MOVEMENTS

CONTRABODY

As the name implies, CONTRABODY MOVE-MENT is accomplished by turning the body in the direction that is opposite to the step. Thus, whenever you step forward on your right foot, pull you right shoulder back. Conversely, whenever you step forward on your left foot, pull your left shoulder back.

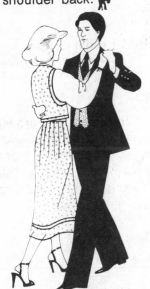

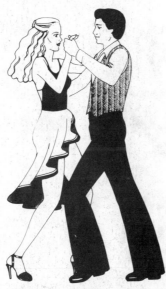

Contrabody Movement   **Cuban Hip Motion**

CUBAN HIP MOTION

The CUBAN OR RUMBA HIP MOTION is fundamental to all Latin or rhythm dances, such as the Rumba, Merengue, Mambo, and the Cha-Cha. In addition, a modified version of the Cuban Hip Motion is used in most disco dances, including Salsa variations, Latin-Street Hustle, and the New York-Latin Hustle. The Cuban motion emphasizes hip movement, but minimizes upper torso movement.

To perform the Cuban Motion correctly, pretend that you are climbing a steep set of stairs. As you step forward on your left foot, bend your left knee, but balance all of your weight on your right foot and keep your right leg straight. While your left knee is bent, your right hip automatically sticks out towards your right side. As you put weight on your left foot, however, your left leg gradually straightens, and the body is once again aligned.

The Cuban Motion is then repeated, using the right foot. As you step forward on your right foot, bend your right knee, but balance all of your weight on your left foot and keep your left leg straight. While your right knee is bent, your left hip automatically sticks out towards your left side. As you put weight on your right foot, your right leg gradually straightens, and the body is once again aligned.

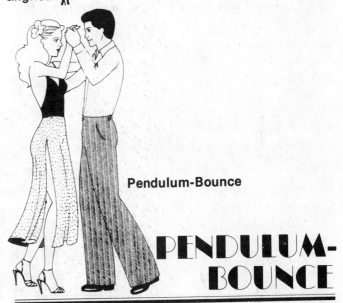

Pendulum-Bounce

PENDULUM-BOUNCE

The PENDULUM-BOUNCE, a motion used in both the Samba and the Two-Step Hustle, contains two basic movements. The subtle flexing of the knees up and down produces the bounce effect. The gentle swaying of the body back and forth produces the pendulum effect. Combining the bounce with the pendulum results in a motion that, according to some dance instructors, resembles the whirling motion of a milk-shake blender.

Although the Pendulum-Bounce is used in both the Samba and the Two-Step Hustle, the motion differs slightly in each dance. In the Samba the body motion is down-up-down (up), with a "down" movement on each whole-numbered count and an "up" movement on each "and" count. In the Two-Step Hustle, on the contrary, the movement is up-down-up (down), with an "up" movement on each whole-numbered count and a "down" movement on each "and" count. For both dances, however, the "down" movement is made by bouncing or sinking down on the knees, while the "up" movement is made by rising up, while straightening the knees.

DANCE FUNDAMENTALS

SECTION F:
LINE OF DIRECTION

Some smooth ballroom dances, particularly Waltz, Fox Trot, and Tango, are progressive dances in which partners move around the dance floor by following the "LINE OF DIRECTION" or "LINE OF DANCE." The Line of Direction is counter-clockwise or opposite to the direction in which the hands of a clock rotate. When the man progresses forward in the Line of Direction, his right hand faces the wall, and his left hand faces the center of the room. Conversely, when the woman progresses backward in the Line of Direction, her left hand faces the wall, and her right hand faces the center of the room. Although most progressive dances follow the Line of Direction, the rhythm dances—including the Rumba, the Samba, the Cha-Cha, and most partner hustles—are non-progressive dances which are performed in one small area of the dance floor.

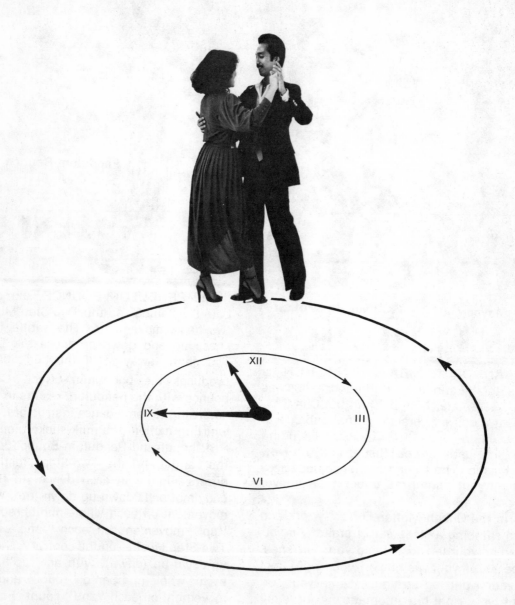

PART II

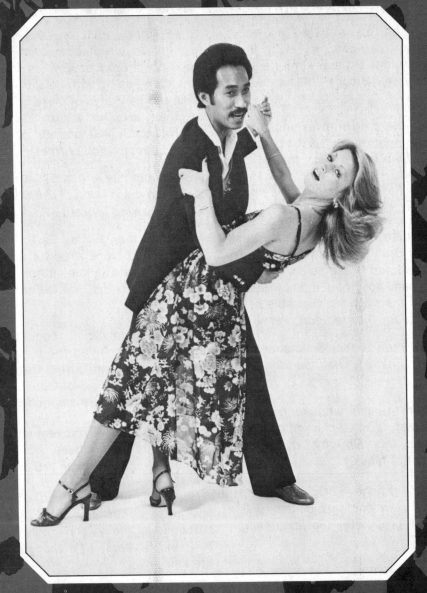

DISCO TOUCH DANCES

DISCO TRIVIA

Most disco clubs operate in the red, because disco dancers have so much fun dancing that they don't have time to get sloshed. (*Of course, Bloody Marys don't count.*)

The "Hustle," the song that exploded the disco fever, was written in 1975 by Van McCoy. (*Van's a man with a short fuse.*)

Perry Bradford, a black man born in 1890 in Atlanta, made up dance steps, worked out tunes and lyrics that explained how to do the steps, and sold them to audiences after his performances. As Bradford himself explains, "The publishers wouldn't take no songs from colored people then, so I had them printed privately and sold them for a nickel apiece in theatres." (*Thanks for the tradition, Perry.*)

There are more than 10,000 discoteques in the U.S. today. (*That's called supply and demand.*)

Chubby Checker, the man who made dance history with his twist, is an ex-chicken plucker from Philadelphia. (*For Chubby, it took a little luck and a lot of pluck.*)

The word "jazz" may have originated from the word "jezebel," when "jazz belles" was the slang term for prostitute. (*So jazz, man, jazz!*)

Donna (Gaines) Summer, the sexy vocalist who skyrocketed to fame via smash hits such as "Love to Love you, Baby," "Last Dance," and "MacArthur Park," started off as a gospel singer who made her singing debut at age 10 in Boston's Grant AME Church. (*Just goes to prove that even God's got soul.*)

Arthur Murray's "Lifetime Executive Course" used to cost $12,000. (*And the price of gold is going up everyday!*)

The disco phenomenon has already spawned a $4 billion dollar industry. (*And you thought canned tuna fish was high!*)

The smoky mist of fake fog that seeps through a discoteque room is made by dropping chunks of dry ice into a machine, then spraying it with jets of hot water that reach temperatures of close to 160 degrees. A fog that lasts for 20 to 30 minutes would require about 400 pounds of dry ice. (*Just think, London's fog is free!*)

Last year more than 37 million Americans danced on disco floors. (*The floor wax industry is also showing a profit.*)

During the 1920s Earl "Snake Hips" Tucker, who wore a tassel on his belt and became known for his slithering gyrations in Harlem nightclubs, was called a freak dancer. (*Freak Out!*)

"Animal dances," popular during the ragtime era, included the crab, the kangaroo dip, the horse trot, the fish tail, and the buzzard lope. (*For obvious reasons, most animal dancers were staunch vegetarians.*)

Discotheques were invented in Paris in the early 1960s as a cheap alternative to live music. (*That, and cheap red wine.*)

Scandals, a $2.5 million dollar restaurant and private bar club in L.A., is the first stupendous Hollywood night palace to be built in 35 years. (*It's the good old country life.*)

Some of the more financially endowed discotheques now feature holograms as part of their fantabulous light shows. In holography, or laser photography, a laser is shot onto a piece of film to create a hologram or three-dimensional image of light. (*Yes, disco will light up your life, if not light your fire!*)

CHAPTER 3

BASIC PARTNER HUSTLES

The seven BASIC PARTNER HUSTLES described in this chapter share two distinguishing features. First and foremost, they all contain basic patterns of 6 steps, completed in 6 beats (1-½ measures) of music. Each step, therefore, is taken on one beat of music. Secondly, most turn variations, which can be performed with any of these hustles, are completed in two steps forward on the last two beats of music (beats 5-6).

In section A of this chapter, there's a complete description of the major types of basic hustles, including the Continental Hustle, American (New York) Hustle, and Lindy Hustle. In Section B there's a thorough discussion on how to make various turns, such as Double Cross Turns, Parallel Turns, and Walk Around Turns. In addition, this section describes a few flashy variations including the Valentino Dip, Disco Dip and the Death Drop.

The difference between disco dancing and rock dancing is a matter of technique and style. Buddy Schwimmer, former rock and disco dance champion of California, makes this distinction: "Rock dancing is up-up. Rock dancers are saying, 'I can do whatever I choose.' Disco dancers, on the other hand, are saying, 'I'm cool. I know what to do.'" Since rock dancers are staunch individualists who prefer to do their own personal type of dancing, it's hard to touch dance with a rocker. Disco dancers, however, know how to spin, twirl, dip and drop without skipping a beat.

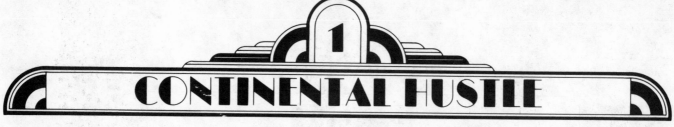

CONTINENTAL HUSTLE

The BASIC FORWARD STEP in the CONTINENTAL HUSTLE, one of the all-time favorite hustles among disco hoofers, contains a basic pattern of 6 steps, completed in 6 beats (1-½ measures) of music. In the Basic Forward Step the pattern begins on beats 1-4 (steps 1-4) with side steps alternated with tap steps. On the odd-numbered beat counts partners transfer their weight to their foot, as they step side. On the even-numbered beat counts, however, partners lightly tap the ball of one foot next to the opposite foot (tap close), without placing any weight on the foot that taps. The Basic Forward Step concludes on beats 5-6 (steps 5-6) with walk steps, as the man takes two steps forward, and the woman takes two steps back. 🕺

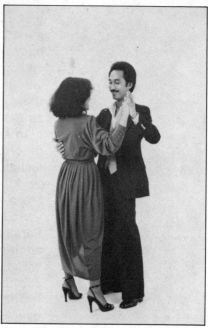

step 3 (beat 3)

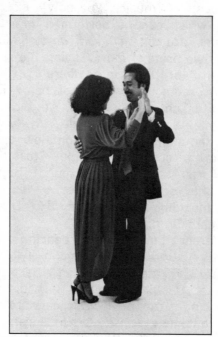

step 2 (beat 2)

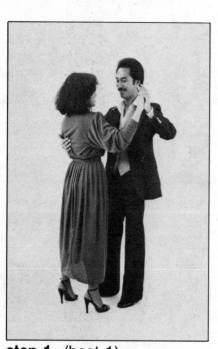

step 1 (beat 1)

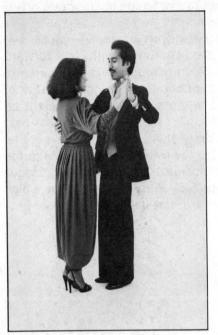

step 4 (beat 4)

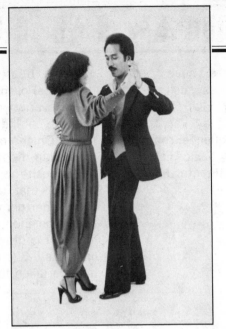

step 5 (beat 5)

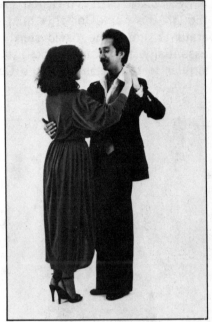

step 6 (beat 6)

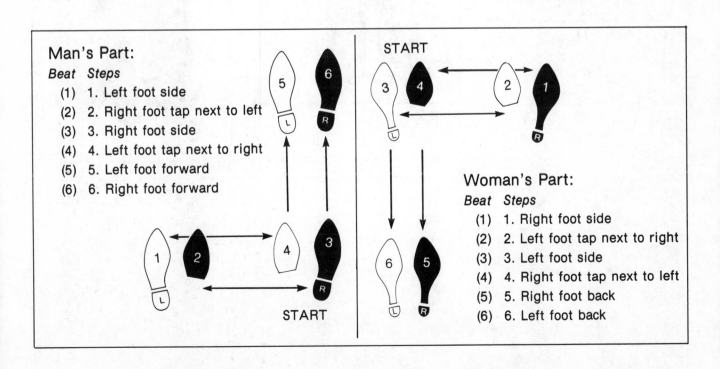

Man's Part:

Beat   Steps

(1)   1. Left foot side
(2)   2. Right foot tap next to left
(3)   3. Right foot side
(4)   4. Left foot tap next to right
(5)   5. Left foot forward
(6)   6. Right foot forward

Woman's Part:

Beat   Steps

(1)   1. Right foot side
(2)   2. Left foot tap next to right
(3)   3. Left foot side
(4)   4. Right foot tap next to left
(5)   5. Right foot back
(6)   6. Left foot back

BASIC PARTNER HUSTLES

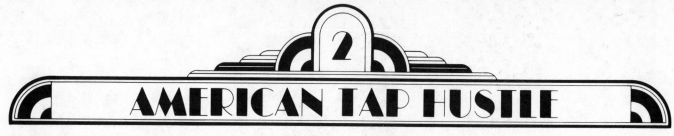

AMERICAN TAP HUSTLE

Several bizarre-sounding names have been tacked onto some disco partner dances, such as the AMERICAN (NEW YORK) TAP HUSTLE. Although the name for this hustle may vary from state to state, the basic step sequence remains essentially the same. Thus, the basic pattern, similar to the pattern for the Continental Hustle, contains 6 steps, completed in 6 beats (1-½ measures) of music.

This variation begins on beats 1-4 (steps 1-4) with tap behind steps alternated with close forward steps. On the odd-numbered beat counts partners lightly tap the ball of one foot behind or in back of the opposite foot, without placing their weight on the foot that taps. On the even-numbered beat counts partners draw their feet into the parallel (close) position, as they transfer their weight to the foot that is drawn forward. This pattern concludes on beats 5-6 (steps 5-6) with two walk steps which may be taken forward, backward, or in place. 🕺

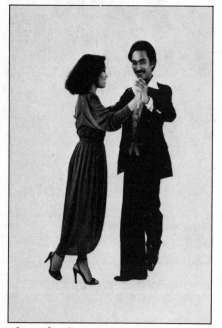

step 1 (beat 1)

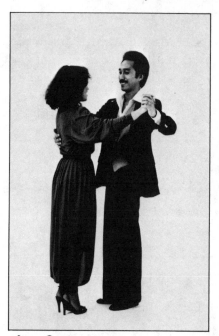

step 2 (beat 2)

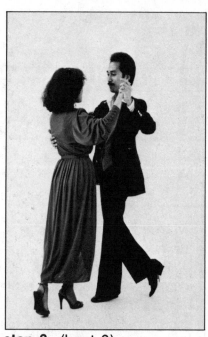

step 3 (beat 3)

Man's Part:
Beat Steps
- (1) 1. Left foot tap behind right
- (2) 2. Left foot close to right
- (3) 3. Right foot tap behind left
- (4) 4. Right foot close to left
- (5) 5. Left foot forward
- (6) 6. Right foot forward

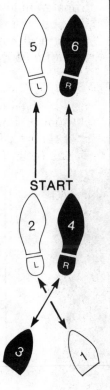

Woman's Part:
Beat Steps
- (1) 1. Right foot tap behind left
- (2) 2. Right foot close to left
- (3) 3. Left foot tap behind right
- (4) 4. Left foot close to right
- (5) 5. Right foot back
- (6) 6. Left foot back

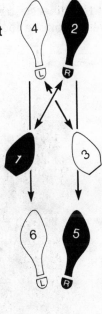

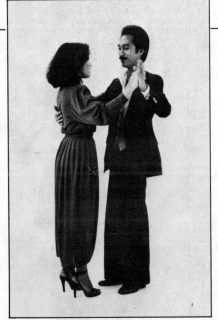

step 4 (beat 4)

47　　　　　　　　　　　　　*BASIC PARTNER HUSTLES*

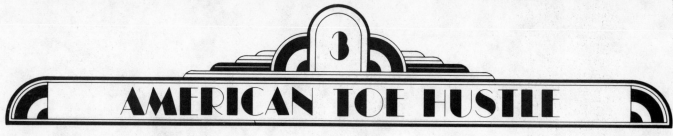

AMERICAN TOE HUSTLE

Except for the substitution of toe (point) steps. for tap steps, the AMERICAN (NEW YORK) TOE HUSTLE closely resembles the Tap Hustle. This variation begins on beats 1-4 (steps 1-4) with toe side steps alternated with close steps. On the odd-numbered beat counts partners toe or point the ball of one foot to the side, without placing any weight on the foot that is pointed. On the even-numbered beat counts partners draw their feet into the parallel (close) position, as they transfer their weight to the foot that is drawn to the opposite foot. This pattern concludes on beats 5-6 (steps 5-6) with two walk steps which may be taken forward, backward, or in place.

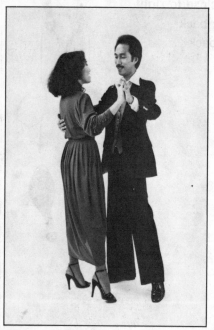

step 1 (beat 1)

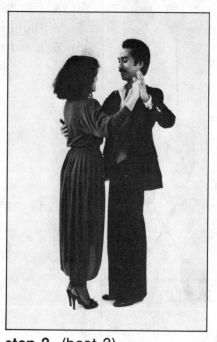

step 2 (beat 2)

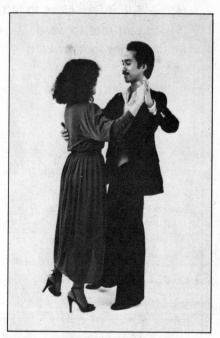

step 3 (beat 3)

Man's Part:

Beat   Steps

(1)   1. Left foot toe side
(2)   2. Left foot close to right foot
(3)   3. Right foot toe side
(4)   4. Right foot close to left foot
(5)   5. Left foot back
(6)   6. Right foot back

Woman's Part:

Beat   Steps

(1)   1. Right foot toe side
(2)   2. Right foot close to left foot
(3)   3. Left foot toe side
(4)   4. Left foot close to right foot
(5)   5. Right foot forward
(6)   6. Left foot forward

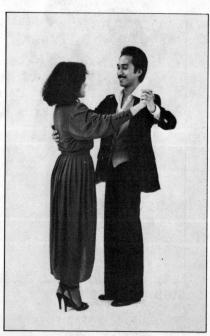

step 4 (beat 4)

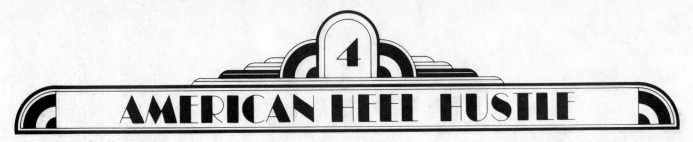

AMERICAN HEEL HUSTLE

Although the pattern for the AMERICAN (NEW YORK) HEEL HUSTLE looks remarkably similar to the previous two variations, this hustle contains heel down steps, instead of tap or toe steps. Thus, this hustle begins on beats 1-4 (steps 1-4) with heel down steps, alternated with close steps. On the odd-numbered beat counts partners place one foot side, with the heel of the foot down, as they lift the ball of their foot off the floor. Although the heel of one foot is down, weight should remain balanced on the opposite foot. On the even-numbered beat counts partners draw their feet together as they transfer their weight to the foot that is drawn into the parallel (close) position. This variation concludes on beats 5-6 (steps 5-6) with two walk steps which can be taken forward, backward, or in place.

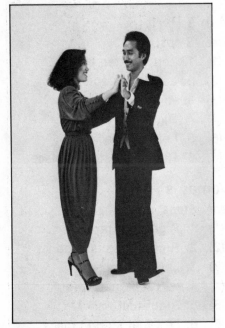

step 1 (beat 1)

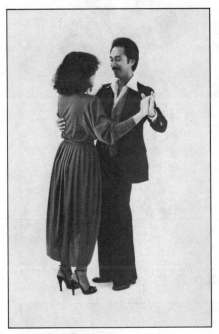

step 2 (beat 2)

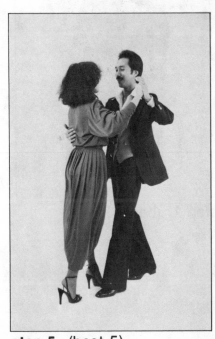

step 5 (beat 5)

Man's Part:
Beat   Steps
- (1)   1. Left foot side, with heel down (toe up)
- (2)   2. Left foot close to right foot
- (3)   3. Right foot side, with heel down (toe up)
- (4)   4. Right foot close to left foot
- (5)   5. Left foot forward
- (6)   6. Right foot forward

Woman's Part:
Beat   Steps
- (1)   1. Right foot side, with heel down (toe up)
- (2)   2. Right foot close to left foot
- (3)   3. Left foot side, with heel down (toe up)
- (4)   4. Left foot close to right foot
- (5)   5. Right foot back
- (6)   6. Left foot back

BASIC PARTNER HUSTLES

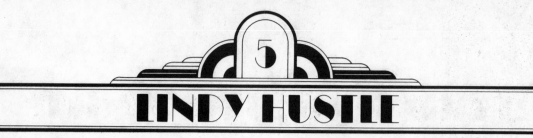

The LINDY HUSTLE, not to be confused with the Lindy Swing Hustle, contains a 6 step pattern, completed in 6 beats (1-½ measures) of music. The pattern begins on beats 1-4 (steps 1-4) with tap side steps alternated with side steps. On odd-numbered beat counts partners tap side, without placing any weight on the foot that taps. On the even-numbered beat counts partners transfer their weight to their foot, as they step side. This variation concludes on beats 5-6 (steps 5-6) with back rock steps. Thus, the man steps back on his left foot, then steps in place on his right foot, as the woman steps back on her right foot, then steps in place on her left foot. A slight rocking motion should be accentuated, as partners shift their weight from their back foot to their forward foot.

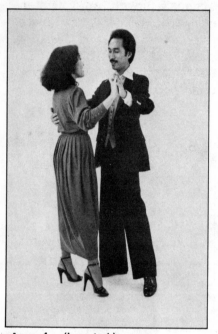

step 1 (beat 1)

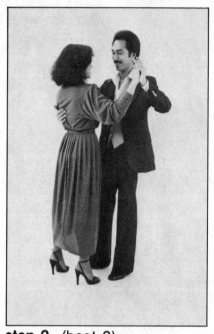

step 2 (beat 2)

Man's Part:
Beat Steps

(1) 1. Left foot tap side
(2) 2. Left foot step side
(3) 3. Right foot tap side
(4) 4. Right foot step side
(5) 5. Left foot back
(6) 6. Right foot step in place

Woman's Part:
Beat Steps

(1) 1. Right foot tap side
(2) 2. Right foot step side
(3) 3. Left foot tap side
(4) 4. Left foot step side
(5) 5. Right foot back
(6) 6. Left foot step in place

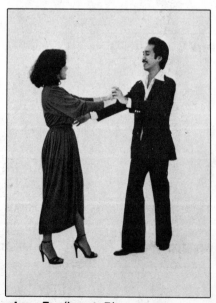

step 5 (beat 5)

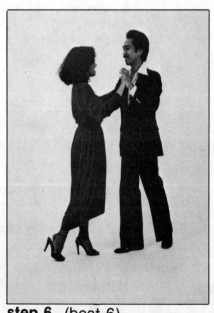

step 6 (beat 6)

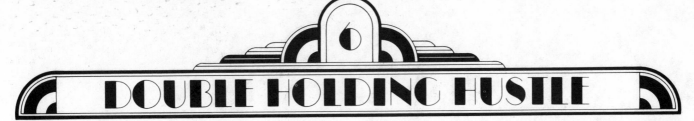

DOUBLE HOLDING HUSTLE

Many turn variations, such as the Walk-Around, are easier to perform with the DOUBLE HOLDING HUSTLE. Similar to the previous six hustles, this hustle contains a 6 step sequence, completed in 6 beats (1-½ measures) of music. Unlike the previous variations which were completed in the Closed Dance Position, this variation is performed in the Holding Dance Position. Consequently, partners face each other and stand slightly apart, as they clasp both pairs of hands in the double or two-hand hold.

This pattern begins on beats 1-4 (steps 1-4) with toe side steps alternated with back steps. On the odd-numbered beat counts partners toe or point the ball of one foot to the side, without placing any weight on the foot that is pointed. On the even-numbered beat counts, partners step back, as the man gently pushes the woman away from him. This variation concludes on beats 5-6 (steps 5-6) with two walk steps forward, as the man gently pulls the woman towards him.

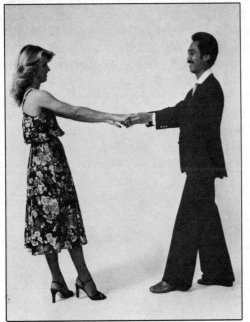

step 4 (beat 4)

Man's Part:

Beat	Steps
(1)	1. Left foot toe side
(2)	2. Left foot back
(3)	3. Right foot toe side
(4)	4. Right foot back
(5)	5. Left foot forward
(6)	6. Right foot forward

Woman's Part:

Beat	Steps
(1)	1. Right foot toe side
(2)	2. Right foot back
(3)	3. Left foot toe side
(4)	4. Left foot back
(5)	5. Right foot forward
(6)	6. Left foot forward

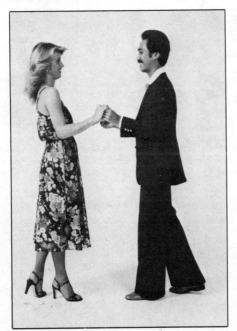

step 5 (beat 5)

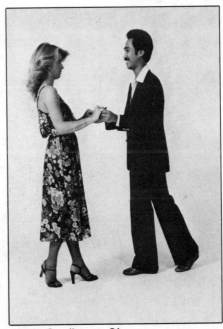

step 6 (beat 6)

BASIC WALK AROUND

The WALK-AROUND, also called a CROSS-OVER, begins with the basic Double Holding Hustle, but concludes with a simple walk rotation. This variation begins on beats 1-4 (steps 1-4) with the Double Holding Hustle in which toe side steps are alternated with walk back steps. On beats 5-6 (steps 5-6), however, partners take two King Kong size steps forward, as they pass each other and reverse positions. Of course, partners may make either a Walk-Around Right or a Walk-Around Left, depending upon the direction of their rotation. Whether partners rotate to their right or to their left, however, they always pass each other, then pivot around to face in the opposite direction.

To perform a Walk-Around Right partners complete the first four steps of the pattern on beats 1-4 (steps 1-4), then they both rotate to their right (clockwise) on the last two beats of music (beats 5-6). On beat 5 (step 5) partners step forward, as they pass each other's right side in the *Right Parallel Position*. On beat 6 (step 6) they continue to step forward, as they complete Dual Half Right Turns in which they both turn 180 degrees clockwise, pivoting around to face in the opposite direction.

Instead of rotating right, many partners prefer to rotate left, as they complete a Walk-Around Left. After completing the first four steps of the pattern on beats 1-4 (steps 1-4), partners rotate counter-clockwise on the last two beats of music (beats 5-6). On beat 5 (step 5) partners step forward, as they pass each other's left side in the *Left Parallel Position*. On beat 6 (step 6) they continue to step forward, as they complete Dual Half Left Turns in which they both turn 180 degrees counter-clockwise, pivoting around to face in the opposite direction.

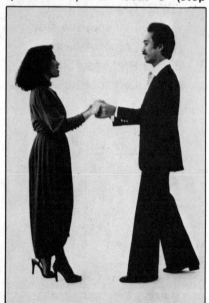 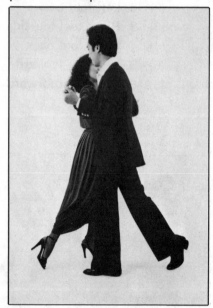 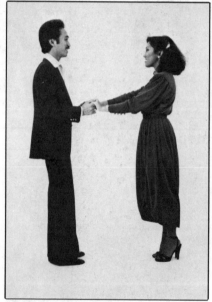

step 4 (beat 4)   **step 5** (beat 5)   **step 6** (beat 6)

Man's Part:

Beat Steps

(1)	1. Left foot toe side	*Complete steps 1-4 in the Holding Dance Position*
(2)	2. Left foot back	
(3)	3. Right foot toe side	
(4)	4. Right foot back	
(5)	5. Left foot forward	*2 steps forward, passing woman's right side and making a Half Right Turn*
(6)	6. Right foot forward	

Woman's Part:

Beat Steps

(1)	1. Right foot toe side	*Complete steps 1-4 in the Holding Dancing Position*
(2)	2. Right foot back	
(3)	3. Left foot toe side	
(4)	4. Left foot back	
(5)	5. Right foot forward	*2 steps forward, passing man's right side and making a Half Right Turn*
(6)	6. Left foot forward	

BASIC PARTNER HUSTLES

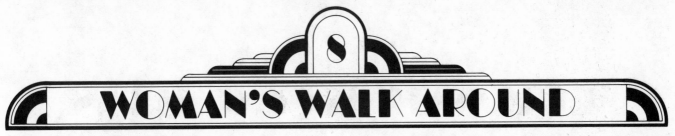

WOMAN'S WALK AROUND

WALK-AROUND (CROSS-OVER) TURNS add a splashy flash to the basic clockwise rotation. This variation begins on beats 1-3 (steps 1-3) with any basic hustle, performed in the Closed Dance Position. For instance, partners may decide to start off with the American (New York) Heel Hustle, which alternates heel down (toe up) steps with close steps.

On beat 4 (step 4), however, the man gives the woman a hand lead for the *right one-hand hold* by lifting the woman's right hand in his left hand, while simultaneously releasing her left hand from his right hand. Moreover, the man gently pushes the woman's right hand inside or in front of her

face, giving the woman a clue that she must turn towards her left.

On beats 5-6 (steps 5-6) partners take two steps forward to pass each other's right side and reverse positions. The man completes his Walk-Around Right, as he passes the woman's right side, then makes a Half Right Turn (180 degrees clockwise), pivoting around to face in the opposite direction. The woman, however, completes her Walk-Around Turn as she makes a Half Left Underarm Turn (180 degrees counter-clockwise) in two steps forward. While the woman is turning, her right hand, uplifted by the man's left hand, rotates counter-clockwise over her head.

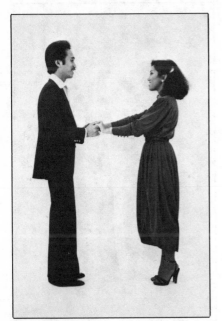

step 4 (beat 4)

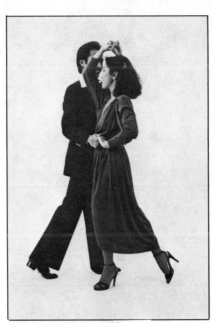

step 5 (beat 5)

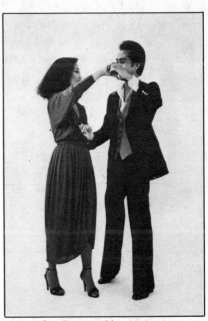

step 6 (beat 6)

Man's Part:

Beat Steps

(1)	1. Left foot side, with heel down (toe up)	
(2)	2. Left foot close to right foot	*Complete steps 1-3 in the Closed Dance Position*
(3)	3. Right foot side, with heel down (toe up)	
(4)	4. Right foot close to left foot, with *right one-hand hold.*	
(5)	5. Left foot forward	*2 steps forward, passing woman's right side, making a Half Right Turn*
(6)	6. Right foot forward	

Woman's Part:

Beat Steps

(1)	1. Right foot side, with heel down (toe up)	
(2)	2. Right foot close to left foot	*Complete steps 1-3 in the Closed Dance Position*
(3)	3. Left foot side, with heel down (toe up)	
(4)	4. Left foot close to right foot, with *right one-hand hold*	
(5)	5. Right foot forward	*2 steps forward, passing man's right side, making a Half Left Underarm Turn*
(6)	6. Left foot forward	

53

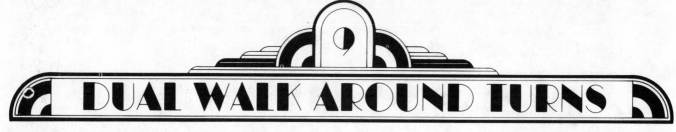

DUAL WALK AROUND TURNS

Now that partners have had the chance to turn separately, they might relish the idea of turning simultaneously in DUAL WALK-AROUND (CROSS-OVER) TURNS. This variation begins on beats 1-3 (steps 1-3) with any basic hustle, performed in the Closed Dance Position. For instance, partners may prefer to begin with the American (New York) Toe Hustle in which toe side steps are alternated with close steps. On beat 4 (step 4) the man gives the woman a hand lead for

the *right one-hand hold*, as he uplifts the woman's right hand with his left hand, but releases her left hand from his right hand.

On beats 5-6 (steps 5-6) partners complete their Dual Walk-Around Turns in two steps forward, as they pass each other's right side and reverse positions. To complete their Dual Walk-Around Turns, both the man and the woman make Half Left Underarm Turns (180 degrees counter-clockwise). As partners turn, the woman's right hand, uplifted in the man's left hand, rotates counter-clockwise.

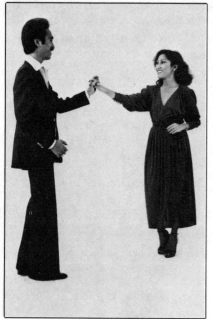

Step 4 (beat 4)

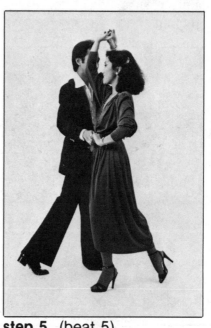

step 5 (beat 5)

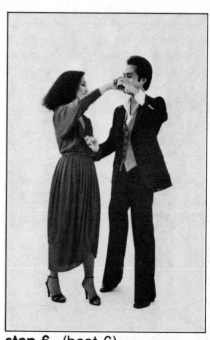

step 6 (beat 6)

Man's Part:

Beat Steps

(1) 1. Left foot toe side

(2) 2. Left foot close to right foot

(3) 3. Right foot toe side

} *Complete Steps 1-3 in the Closed Dance Position*

(4) 4. Right foot close to left foot, with *right one-hand hold*

(5) 5. Left foot forward

(6) 6. Right foot forward

} *2 steps forward, passing woman's right side, and making a Half Left Underarm Turn.*

Woman's Part:

Beat Steps

(1) 1. Right foot toe side

(2) 2. Right foot close to left foot

(3) 3. Left foot toe side

} *Complete steps 1-3 in the Closed Dance Position*

(4) 4. Left foot close to right foot, with *right one-hand hold*

(5) 5. Right foot forward

(6) 6. Left foot forward

} *2 steps forward, passing man's right side, and making a Half Left Underarm Turn*

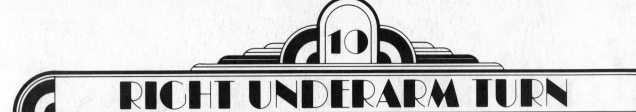

RIGHT UNDERARM TURN

A RIGHT UNDERARM TURN may be performed with most disco or ballroom partner dances. Similar to the Walk-Around Turns, the Right Underarm Turn is preceded on beats 1-4 (steps 1-4) with any basic hustle, completed in the Closed Dance Position. For example, partners may decide to start with the American (New York) Tap Hustle which alternates tap behind steps with close forward steps. On beat 4 (step 4), however, the man gives the woman a hand lead for the *right one-hand hold*, as he lifts the woman's right hand in his left hand, but simultaneously releases her left hand from his right hand. Moreover, the man pushes the woman's right hand outside or away from her face, which prompts the woman to turn right on the next beat count.

On beats 5-6 (steps 5-6), the man continues to keep the woman's right hand uplifted in his left hand, as he takes two steps in place in the Open Position. The woman, on the other hand, makes her Right Underarm Turn in two steps forward, as she turns in a full circle to her right (360 degrees clockwise). As the woman turns, her right hand, loosely clasped in the man's left hand, rotates clockwise over her head.

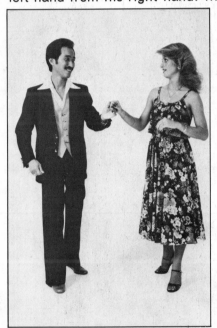

step 4 (beat 4)

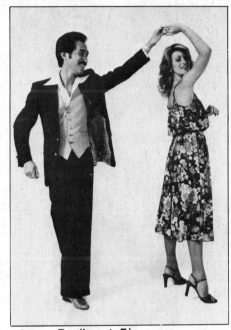

steps 5 (beat 5)

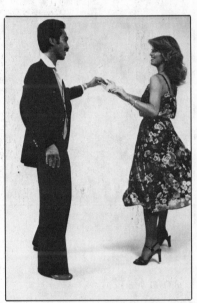

step 6 (beat 6)

Man's Part:

Beat *Steps*

(1) 1. Left foot tap behind right foot

(2) 2. Left foot close to right foot

(3) 3. Right foot tap behind left foot

Complete steps 1-3 in the Closed Dance Position

(4) 4. Right foot close to left foot, with *right one-hand hold*

(5) 5. Left foot step in place

(6) 6. Right foot step in place

2 steps in place in the Open Position

Woman's Part:

Beat *Steps*

(1) 1. Right foot tap behind left foot

(2) 2. Right foot close to left foot

(3) 3. Left foot tap behind right foot

Complete steps 1-3 in the Closed Dance Position

(4) 4. Left foot close to right foot, with *right one-hand hold*

(5) 5. Right foot forward

(6) 6. Left foot forward

2 steps forward, making a Full Right Underarm Turn

For the whirling PARALLEL RIGHT TURNS, partners remain embraced in the Closed Dance Position, as they twirl around the dance floor in a clockwise direction. Although both partners turn towards their right, the man takes 6 small steps forward, but the woman takes 6 small steps backward. To maintain balance throughout these devilishly fast turns, the man centers his right foot between the woman's feet.

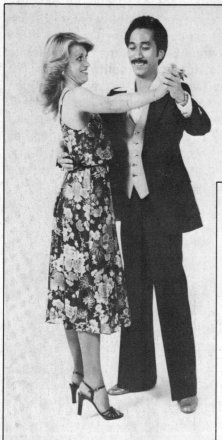

step 1 (beat 1)

Man's Part:

Beat Steps

(1) 1. Left foot forward
(2) 2. Right foot forward
(3) 3. Left foot forward
(4) 4. Right foot forward
(5) 5. Left foot forward
(6) 6. Right foot forward

Woman's Part:

Beat Steps

(1) 1. Right foot back
(2) 2. Left foot back
(3) 3. Right foot back
(4) 4. Left foot back
(5) 5. Right foot back
(6) 6. Left foot back

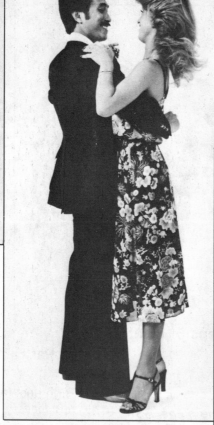

step 2 (beat 2)

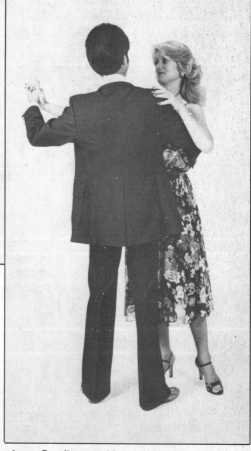

step 3 (beat 3)

BASIC PARTNER HUSTLES

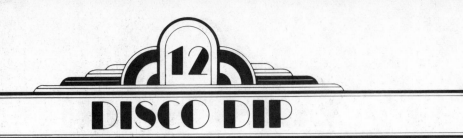

Few hustlers can resist the tempting DISCO DIP. On beat 1 (step 1) partners swing away from each other, as they tap to the side, while completing dual half turns in opposite directions. The man, therefore, taps to his left side with his left foot, as he pivots in a Half Left Turn (180 degrees counter-clockwise). Conversely, the woman taps to her right side with her right foot, as she pivots in a Half Right Turn (180 degrees clockwise).

On beat 2 (step 2) partners begin their Dip. As the man flings the woman into the Dip, he places all of his weight on his left foot, bends his left knee, and supports the woman's back with his right hand. At the same time, the woman pivots towards the man in a Half Left Turn (180 degrees counter-clockwise), as she positions her right foot between the man's feet, then dips back. On beat 3 (step 3) partners hold the dip position, as the man balances his weight on his left foot, and the woman balances her weight on her right foot.

On beat 4 (step 4) partners unwind from the Dip, as they transfer their weight to the opposite foot. The man gently pulls the woman out of the Dip, as he transfers his weight to his right foot. The woman, on the other hand, straightens to an upright position, as she transfers her weight to her left foot. This variation concludes on beats 5-6 (steps 5-6) with two walk steps which may be taken forward, back, or in place.

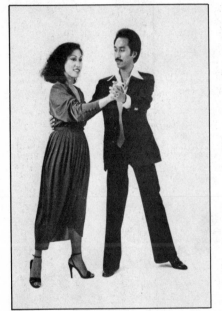

step 1 (beat 1)

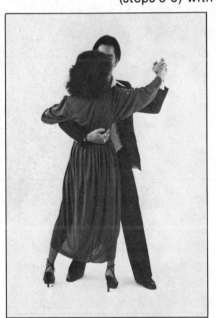

step 2 (beat 2)

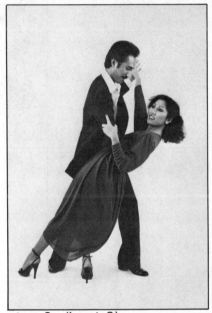

step 3 (beat 3)

Man's Part:

Beat Steps

(1) 1. Left foot tap side, pivoting in a ½ left turn

(2) 2. Left foot step in place, as the man leads the woman into the Dip

(3) 3. Left foot holds the man's weight, as he supports the woman in the Dip

(4) 4. Right foot step in place, as the man lifts the woman out of the Dip

(5) 5. Left foot forward

(6) 6. Right foot forward

Woman's Part:

Beat Steps

(1) 1. Right foot tap side, pivoting in a ½ right turn

(2) 2. Right foot forward, pivoting in a ½ left turn, and dip back

(3) 3. Right foot holds the woman's weight, as she balances in the Dip

(4) 4. Left foot step in place, as woman straightens to an upright position

(5) 5. Right foot back

(6) 6. Left foot back

VALENTINO DIP

For daring dancers, the VALENTINO DIP promises to be devilishly decadent. This variation begins on beats 1-4 (steps 1-4) with the American (New York) Tap Hustle in which tap behind steps are alternated with close forward steps. On beat 5 (step 5) partners prepare for the Dip, as the man steps side on his left foot, and the woman steps back on her right foot. While the woman steps back, she simultaneously turns away from the man by making a ¼ Right Turn (90 degrees clockwise).

On beat 6 (step 6) the man lowers the woman into the Dip, as he bends his right knee and places all of his weight on his right foot. At the same time, the woman leans her torso back, bends both knees, balances her weight on her right foot, and lifts her left foot off the floor. Partners proceed to hold the Valentino Dip for the next four beats (1 measure) of music, then unwind on the last two beat counts.

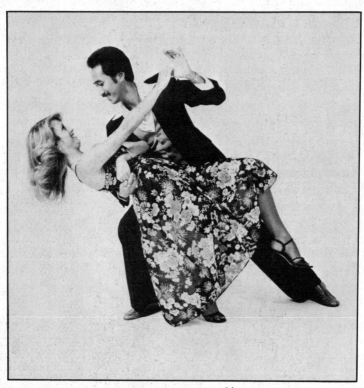

step 6   (beat 6)

Man's Part:
Beat   Steps
  (1) 1. Left foot tap behind right foot
  (2) 2. Left foot close to right foot
  (3) 3. Right foot tap behind left foot
  (4) 4. Right foot close to left foot
  (5) 5. Left foot side
  (6) 6. Right foot step in place, with right knee bent, as man supports the woman in the Dip

Woman's Part:
Beat   Steps
  (1) 1. Right foot tap behind left foot
  (2) 2. Right foot close to left foot
  (3) 3. Left foot tap behind right foot
  (4) 4. Left foot close to right foot
  (5) 5. Right foot back, turning ¼ right
  (6) 6. Right foot holds her weight, as left foot is lifted off the ground, and woman leans her torso back

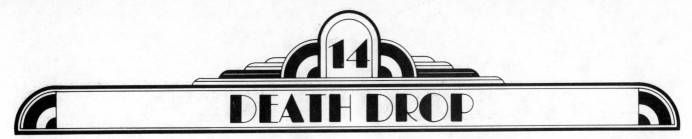

DEATH DROP

The DEATH DROP demands a partner whose machismo is equal to his prowess. This variation begins on beats 1-4 (steps 1-4) with any basic hustle pattern, such as the Continental Hustle which alternates side steps with tap close steps. Then, in two hair-raising seconds on beats 5-6 (steps 5-6), partners perform their death-defying Drop.

On beat 5 (step 5), the man steps side on his left foot, as he grabs both of the woman's wrists in his bare hands and flings her into the Death Drop. As the woman is flung into the Drop, she pivots away from the man by making a ¼ Left Turn (90 degrees counter-clockwise) on her right foot. On beat 6 (step 6) the man continues to hold both of the woman's wrists, as he lowers the woman even further down, until she is barely inches away from the floor. As she is dropped down, the woman balances all of her weight on her right foot, lifts her left foot off the floor, and tilts her head back. Partners continue to hold the Death Drop for the next four beats (1 measure) of music, then unwind on the last two beat counts.

Man's Part:

Beat Steps
- (1) 1. Left foot side
- (2) 2. Right foot tap next to left foot
- (3) 3. Right foot side
- (4) 4. Left foot tap next to right foot
- (5) 5. Left foot side, as he grabs the woman's wrists and flings her into the Death Drop
- (6) 6. Right foot step in place, as he lowers the woman further into the Drop

Woman's Part:

Beat Steps
- (1) 1. Right foot side
- (2) 2. Left foot tap next to right foot
- (3) 3. Left foot side
- (4) 4. Right foot tap next to left foot
- (5) 5. Right foot forward, pivoting ¼ left, as woman is flung into the Death Drop
- (6) 6. Right foot holds her weight, as her left foot is lifted off the floor, and the woman tilts her head back

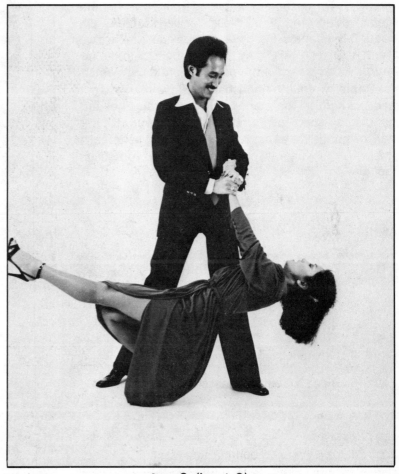

step 6 (beat 6)

DOUBLE CROSS TURNS

DOUBLE CROSS TURNS have been designed for those who hanker after the excitement of elusive danger. Divided into three sections, each part of this variation contains a basic 6 step sequence, completed in 6 beats of music.

Part A begins on beats 1-4 (steps 1-4) with the American (New York) Tap Hustle, but concludes on beats 5-6 (steps 5-6) as partners switch hands into the *double hand cross*. In Part B the woman completes a Double Cross Right Turn. In Part C the woman reverses the direction of her turn, as she completes a Double Cross Left Turn. 🕺

Part A:
HAND CROSS

In Part A partners prepare for the Double Cross Turns by hustling through their basic pattern for the American (New York) Tap Hustle. On beats 1-4 (steps 1-4) partners complete their tap behind steps, alternated with close forward steps. On beats 5-6 (steps 5-6), however, partners take two steps in place, as they switch hands into the *double hand cross*. In the *double hand cross*, which resembles a double handshake, the woman's right hand is held in the man's right hand, and her left hand is clasped in his left hand. Although either pair of hands may rest on top of the opposite pair, this variation begins with right hands crossed on top. 🕺

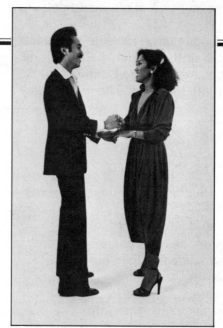

part A **step 5** (beat 5)

Man's Part:
Beat Steps

(1)	1. Left foot tap behind right foot
(2)	2. Left foot close to right foot
(3)	3. Right foot tap behind left foot
(4)	4. Right foot close to left foot

Complete steps 1-4 in the Holding Position, with Hands Crossed

(5)	5. Left foot step in place
(6)	6. Right foot step in place

2 steps in place, while switching hands into the Double Hand Cross

Woman's Part:
Beat Steps

(1)	1. Right foot tap behind left foot
(2)	2. Right foot close to left foot
(3)	3. Left foot tap behind right foot
(4)	4. Left foot close to right foot

Complete steps 1-4 in the Holding Position, with Hands Crossed

(5)	5. Right foot step in place
(6)	6. Left foot step in place

2 steps in place, while switching hands into the Double Hand Cross.

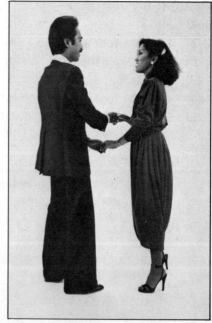

part A **step 6** (beat 6)

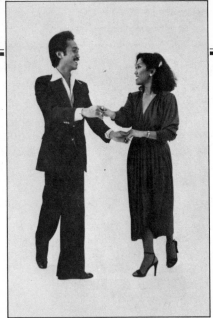

part B **step 3** (beat 3)

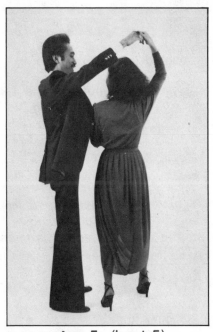

part B **step 5** (beat 5)

Part B:
WOMAN'S DOUBLE CROSS
RIGHT TURN

Part B begins with the American (New York) Tap Hustle, completed in the Holding Position, with hands clasped in the *double hand cross*. On beats 1-4 (steps 1-4) partners complete their tap behind steps, alternated with close forward steps. On beats 5-6 (steps 5-6), however, the man takes two steps in place, while he lifts both of the woman's hands in his hands. At the same time, the woman completes her Double Cross Right Turn, as she turns 360 degrees clockwise in 2 steps forward. While the woman is turning, both pairs of uplifted hands rotate clockwise over her head. Although both pairs of hands circle to her right, they flip-flop in mid-air, until the left hands are crossed on top of the right hands. 🕺

Man's Part:
Beat Steps

(1)	1. Left foot tap behind right foot
(2)	2. Left foot close to right foot
(3)	3. Right foot tap behind left foot
(4)	4. Right foot close to left foot

Complete steps 1-4 in the Holding Position, with Hands Crossed

(5)	5. Left foot step in place
(6)	6. Right foot step in place

2 steps in place, with both hands uplifted, as woman turns

Woman's Part:
Beat Steps

(1)	1. Right foot tap behind left foot
(2)	2. Right foot close to left foot
(3)	3. Left foot tap behind right foot
(4)	4. Left foot close to right foot

Complete steps 1-4 in the Holding Position, with Hands Crossed.

(5)	5. Right foot forward
(6)	6. Left foot forward

Double Cross Right Turn in 2 steps forward, as both hands rotate clockwise

Part C:
WOMAN'S DOUBLE CROSS LEFT TURN

Part C also begins with the American (New York) Tap Hustle, completed in the Holding Position, but this time the left hands are crossed above the right hands. On beats 1-4 (steps 1-4) partners complete their tap behind steps alternated with close forward steps. On beats 5-6 (steps 5-6) the man takes two steps in place, while he lifts both of the woman's hands in his hands. At the same time, the woman completes her Double Cross Left Turn, as she turns 360 degrees counter-clockwise. While the woman is turning, both pairs of uplifted hands rotate counter-clockwise over her head. Although both pairs of hands circle to her left, they flip-flop in mid-air, until the right hands are crossed on top of the left hands.

Partners may continue to repeat these Double Cross Turns, as long as each turn is completed in two steps forward on the last two beats of music (beats 5-6). If the man seeks revenge, then he completes a Double Cross Right Turn, followed with a Double Cross Left Turn. Once partners tire of double-crossing each other, they uncross hands and return to the Closed or Holding Dance Position. 🏃

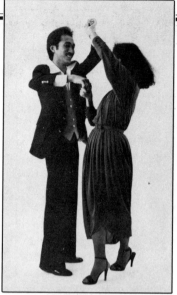

Part C **step 5** (beat 5)

Man's Part:
Beat Steps

(1)	1. Left foot tap behind right foot	
(2)	2. Left foot close to right foot	Complete steps 1-4 in the Holding Position, with Hands Crossed
(3)	3. Right foot tap behind left foot	
(4)	4. Right foot close to left foot	
(5)	5. Left foot step in place	2 steps in place, with both hands uplifted, as woman turns
(6)	6. Right foot step in place	

Woman's Part:
Beat Steps

(1)	1. Right foot tap behind left foot	
(2)	2. Right foot close to left foot	Complete steps 1-4 in the Holding Position, with Hands Crossed
(3)	3. Left foot tap behind right foot	
(4)	4. Left foot close to right foot	
(5)	5. Right foot forward	Double Cross Left Turn in 2 steps forward, as both hands rotate counter-clockwise
(6)	6. Left foot forward	

CHAPTER 4

NEW YORK-LATIN HUSTLE

The NEW YORK-LATIN HUSTLE is, without a doubt, the most popular hustle performed from San Francisco to the Fire Island Shore. Other names for this hustle include L.A. Hustle, West Coast Swing, West Coast Sugarpush, and Latin-Swing Hustle. Regardless of the name, there are several characteristics that make this hustle a sensational disco dance.

First of all, the pattern contains 7 steps, completed in 6 syncopated beats (1-½ measures) of music. The pattern begins on beats 1-2 (steps 1-2) with tap steps, followed with side or close steps. Right smack in the middle, however, is placed a triple step in which three steps (steps 3-5) are taken in two syncopated beats of music (beats 3 and 4). The pattern concludes on beats 5-6 (steps 6-7) with two walk steps which may be taken forward, backward, or in place.

Most turn variations in the New York-Latin Hustle are completed on the last two beats of music (beats 5-6). Thus, the man usually gives the woman a hand lead on beat 4 (step 5). The turn is then completed in two steps forward on beats 5-6 (steps 6-7). Some turns, however, such as the Right Underarm Turn and the Reverse Underarm Turn may also be completed in 3 steps forward or back on the triple step (on beats 3 and 4).

Most important, holding underarm turns, such as the Cradle or the Pretzel, are concocted from two complete sequences of the basic 7 steps. In the first sequence of steps the dancer completes a turn in two steps forward on the last two beats of music (beats 5-6). To unwind in the second sequence of steps, however, the dancer turns in one step forward on beat 2 (step 2).

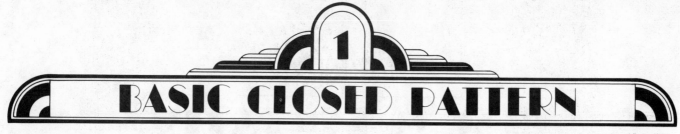

BASIC CLOSED PATTERN

In most ways, the BASIC CLOSED PATTERN for the New York-Latin Hustle is a dead ringer for the American (New York) Tap Hustle described in Chapter 3. Nevertheless, there is one difference which makes the Basic Closed Pattern unique. In short, a triple step is slipped into the basic pattern. As explained in previous chapters, a triple step contains 3 steps, completed in 2 syncopated beats of music. Thus, for the Basic Closed Pattern, partners complete a total of 7 steps in 6 beats (1-½ measures) of music. In addition, partners hustle through all 7 steps, while they are embraced in the Closed Dance Position.

The Basic Closed Pattern begins on beats 1-2 (steps 1-2) with tap behind steps, followed with side steps. On beat 1 (step 1), therefore, the man taps his left foot behind his right foot, but keeps his weight balanced on his right foot; conversely, the woman taps her right foot behind her left foot, but keeps her weight balanced on her left foot. On beat 2 (step 2) partners step side, as the man steps to his left side on his left foot, and the woman steps to her right side on her right foot.

On the triple step, sometimes called the syncopated or coaster step, partners take three small, quick steps (steps 3-5) in two syncopated beats of music (beats 3 and 4). Although these three steps may be taken forward, backward, or in place, the woman's part is still the natural opposite of the man's part. For example, as the man takes two steps forward, then one step back, the woman takes two steps back, then one step forward.

The Basic Closed Pattern concludes on beats 5-6 (steps 6-7) with two walk steps. Although these two walk steps may be taken forward, backward, or in place, the woman's part continues to mirror the man's part. In addition, most turn variations are initiated on these final two walk steps. ♣

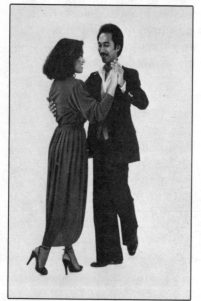

step 1 (beat 1)

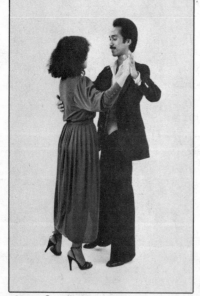

step 2 (beat 2)

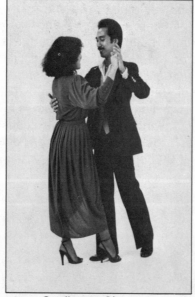

step 3 (beat 3)

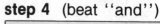

step 4 (beat "and")

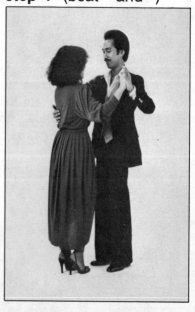

Man's Part:

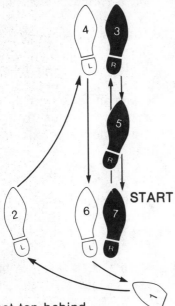

Beat Steps

(1) 1. Left foot tap behind right foot

(2) 2. Left foot side

(3) 3. Right foot forward

(&) 4. Left foot close forward

(4) 5. Right back

(5) 6. Left back

(6) 7. Right foot close back

In the Closed Dance Position, the man completes 7 steps in 6 syncopated beats of music.

Woman's Part:

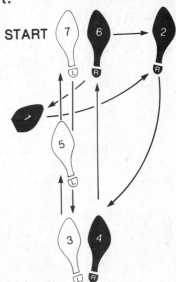

Beat Steps

(1) 1. Right foot tap behind left foot

(2) 2. Right foot side

(3) 3. Left foot back

(&) 4. Right foot close back

(4) 5. Left foot forward

(5) 6. Right foot forward

(6) 7. Left foot close forward

In the Closed Dance Position, the woman completes 7 steps in 6 syncopated beats of music.

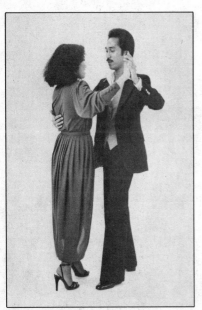

step 5 (beat 4)

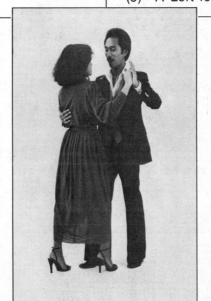

step 6 (beat 5)

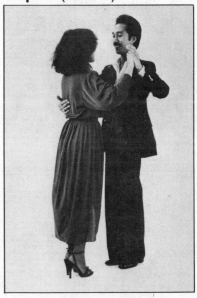

step 7 (beat 6)

NEW YORK-LATIN HUSTLE

The BASIC HOLDING PATTERN for the New York-Latin Hustle is currently the most popular hustle performed on the West Coast. In fact, the Holding variation has acquired so many devoted fans that this hustle is often called the L.A. Hustle, West Coast Sugarpush, or West Coast Swing Hustle. Despite the diverse names, however, the Holding Pattern, similar to the Closed Pattern, contains 7 steps, completed in 6 syncopated beats (1-½ measures) of music. Nevertheless, the Holding Pattern is performed in the Holding Dance Position. Partners, therefore, face each other and clasp both pairs of hands in the double or two-hand hold.

This pattern begins on beats 1-2 (steps 1-2) with tap behind steps followed with close forward steps. Thus, the man taps his left foot behind his right foot, then closes his left foot to his right foot. The woman, on the contrary, taps her right foot behind her left foot, then closes her right foot to her left foot.

On the triple step, completed on beats 3 and 4 (steps 3-5), both the man and the woman take two steps back, then one step forward. As partners step back on step 3 (beat 3), the man gently pushes the woman away from him. On step 4 (beat "and") partners continue to step back, as they draw their feet into the parallel (close) position. On step 5 (beat 4), partners take one small step forward, as the man gently pulls the woman towards him.

Although almost all variations that use the Basic Holding Pattern contain the same triple step (back/ close back/ forward), there are a few exceptions. For instance, whenever a woman makes a Right Underarm Turn on the triple step, she will take 3 steps forward, while turning in a circle to her right (360 degrees clockwise). Nevertheless, the Basic Holding Pattern concludes on beats 5-6 (steps 6-7) with two walk steps forward. Some partners prefer, however, to sneak in another quick triple step (step-ball-change) on the last two beats of music.

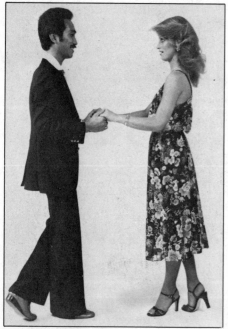

step 1 (beat 1)

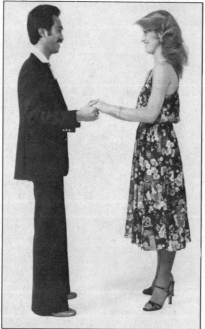

step 2 (beat 2)

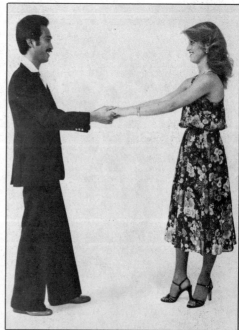

step 3 (beat 3)

Man's Part:

Beat *Steps*

(1) 1. Left foot tap behind right foot

(2) 2. Left foot close forward

(3) 3. Right foot back

(&) 4. Left foot close back

(4) 5. Right foot forward

(5) 6. Left foot forward

(6) 7. Right foot close forward

In the Holding Dance Position, the man completes 7 steps in 6 syncopated beats of music.

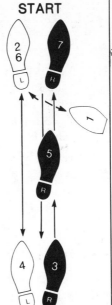

START

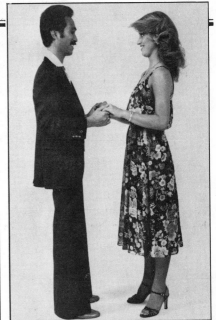

Woman's Part:

Beat *Steps*

(1) 1. Right foot tap behind left foot

(2) 2. Right foot close forward

(3) 3. Left foot back

(&) 4. Right foot close back

(4) 5. Left foot forward

(5) 6. Right foot forward

(6) 7. Left foot close forward

In the Holding Dance Position, the woman completes 7 steps in 6 syncopated beats of music.

START

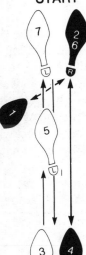

step 7 (beat 6)

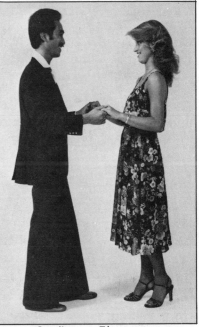

step 6 (beat 5)

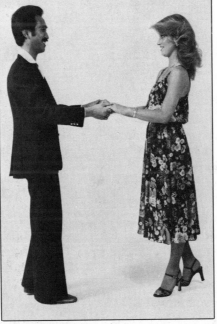

step 5 (beat 4)

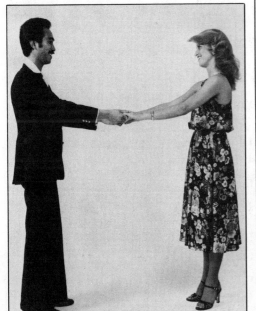

step 4 (beat ''and'')

NEW YORK-LATIN HUSTLE

The BASIC SIDE STEP for the New York-Latin Hustle, often called the OPEN BREAK, combines elements lifted from the Closed Pattern with elements snitched from the Holding Pattern. Similar to the Closed Pattern, the Basic Side Step begins on beats 1-2 (steps 1-2) with tap behind steps, followed with close forward steps, completed in the Closed Dance Position.

On the triple step (on beats 3 and 4) partners take two small steps back, then one small step forward, similar to the triple step used in the Holding Pattern. In the Basic Side Step, however, partners turn *away* from each other, as they break into the Right Open Position. Instead of stepping directly back on step 3, therefore, partners use fifth position or pass back steps, while they make dual ¼ turns in opposite directions. Thus, the man crosses his right foot behind his left foot, as he

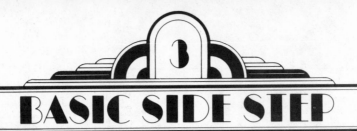

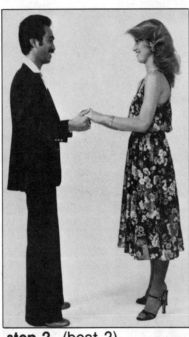

step 1 (beat 1)

step 2 (beat 2)

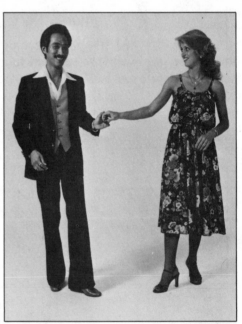

step 3 (beat 3)

Man's Part:

Beat Steps

(1)	1. Left foot tap behind right foot	*Tap, then close forward in Closed Dance Position*
(2)	2. Left foot close forward	
(3)	3. Right foot back, turning ¼ right	*3 steps (triple step) in Right Open Position*
(&)	4. Left foot close back	
(4)	5. Right foot forward	
(5)	6. Left foot, forward, turning ¼ left	*2 steps forward, returning to Closed Position*
(6)	7. Right foot close forward	

Woman's Part:

Beat Steps

(1)	1. Right foot tap behind left foot	*Tap, then close forward in Closed Dance Position*
(2)	2. Right foot close forward	
(3)	3. Left foot back, turning ¼ left	*3 steps (triple step) in Right Open Position*
(&)	4. Right foot close back	
(4)	5. Left foot forward	
(5)	6. Right foot forward, turning ¼ right	*2 steps forward, returning to Closed Position*
(6)	7. Left foot close forward	

makes a ¼ Right Turn (90 degrees clockwise). Conversely, the woman crosses her left foot behind her right foot, as she makes a ¼ Left Turn (90 degrees counter-clockwise). As they complete their cross behind or pass back (fifth position) steps, partners break away from each other and move into the Right Open Position (woman's right side parallel to the man's left side).

The Basic Side Step concludes on beats 5-6 (steps 6-7) with two walk steps forward, as partners return to the Closed Dance Position. On beat 5 (step 6), therefore, partners continue to step forward, as they turn *towards* each other, by making ¼ turns in opposite directions. Thus, the man steps forward on his left foot, as he makes a ¼ Left Turn (90 degrees counter-clockwise). Conversely, the woman steps forward on her right foot, as she makes a ¼ Right Turn (90 degrees clockwise). On beat 6 (step 7) partners take another step forward as they return to the Closed Dance Position. 🕺

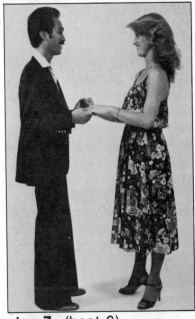

step 7 (beat 6)

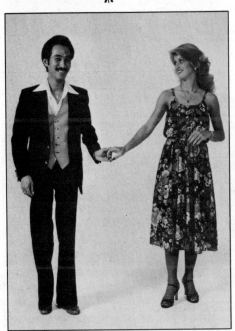

step 4 (beat "and")

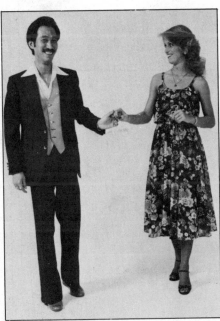

step 5 (beat 4)

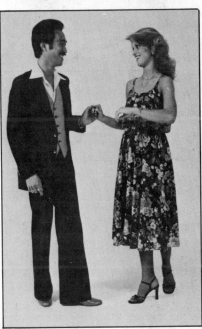

step 6 (beat 5)

NEW YORK-LATIN HUSTLE

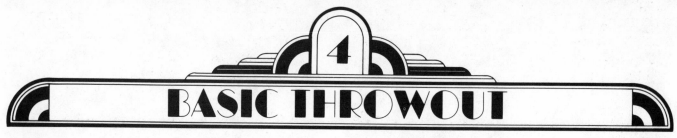

BASIC THROWOUT

The BASIC THROW OUT, sometimes called the BASIC CROSS-BODY LEAD or BASIC OPPOSITION, was a form first popularized in Swing dancing. Although the step pattern still contains 7 steps, completed in 6 syncopated beats (1-½ measures) of music, partners will switch from the Closed Position to the Throw Out Position on the triple step, then return to the Closed Position in two walk steps forward.

The pattern begins in the Closed Dance Position with tap side steps on beat 1 (step 1), as the man taps his left foot to his left side, and the woman taps her right foot to her right side. On beat 2 (step 2), however, partners break into the Throw Out Position, as they step towards their own right side, while making dual 1/8 left turns (45 degrees counter-clockwise). Since both partners rotate left, while stepping towards their right side, the man must complete a fifth position (pass back) step, although the woman merely steps side. Thus, the man crosses his left foot behind his right foot, as he turns 1/8 left. The woman, on the other hand, merely steps towards her right side with her right foot, as she turns 1/8 left. Moreover, as partners make their dual left turns, the man gently pushes the woman into the Throw Out Position. Notice that in the Throw Out Position partners face each other in the Open Position, and their hands are clasped in the *right one-hand hold,* with the woman's right hand clasped in the man's left hand.

Partners complete their triple steps on beats 3 and 4 (steps 3-5) in the Throw Out Position, as they both take two steps back, then one step forward. On beats 5-6 (steps 6-7) partners conclude the pattern with two walk steps forward, as they return to the Closed Dance Position.

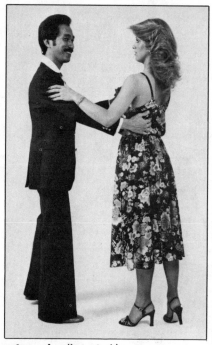

step 1 (beat 1)

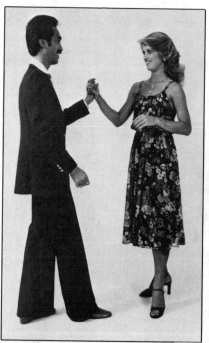

step 2 (beat 2)

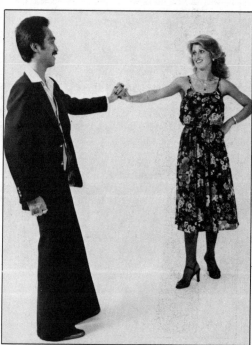

step 3 (beat 3)

Man's Part:

Beat   Steps

(1)   1. Left foot tap side in
   Closed Position

(2)   2. Left foot pass back
   (cross behind right
   foot), turning 1/8
   left, releasing woman
   to Throw Out Position

(3)   3. Right foot back   } *3 steps (triple step)*
(&)   4. Left foot close back   *in Throw Out*
(4)   5. Right foot forward   *Position*

(5)   6. Left foot forward   } *2 steps forward,*
(6)   7. Right foot close   *returning to Closed*
   forward   *Position*

Woman's Part:

Beat   Steps

(1)   1. Right foot tap side
   in Closed Position

(2)   2. Right foot step side,
   turning 1/8 left in
   Throw Out Position

(3)   3. Left foot back   } *3 steps (triple step)*
(&)   4. Right foot close back   *in Throw Out*
(4)   5. Left foot forward   *Position*

(5)   6. Right foot forward   } *2 steps forward,*
(6)   7. Left foot close forward   *returning to*
               Closed Position

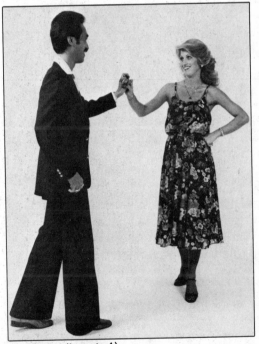

step 5 (beat 4)

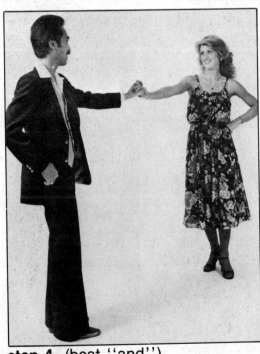

step 4 (beat ''and'')

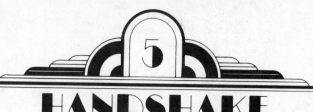

The HANDSHAKE adds pizazz to the Basic Throw Out Pattern. Divided into two sections, each part of this variation contains 7 steps, completed in 6 syncopated beats of music. Part A begins on beats 1-4 (steps 1-5) with the Basic Throw Out Pattern, but concludes on beats 5-6 (steps 6-7) with a Handshake, as partners switch hands and move into the Right Parallel Position. In Part B partners unwind from their Handshake on beat 2 (step 2), then complete their triple step in the Basic Throw Out Position. On beats 5-6 (steps 6-7) partners take two steps forward, returning to the Closed Dance Position. 🚶

Part A: HANDSHAKE

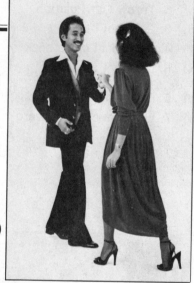

part A
step 5 (beat 4)

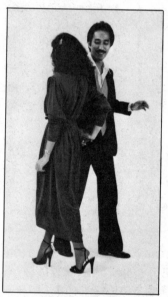

part A
step 6 (beat 5)

Part A begins with the Basic Throw Out for beats 1-4 (steps 1-5), but concludes with the Handshake on beats 5-6 (steps 6-7). On beat 1 (step 1) partners tap to the side in the Closed Dance Position. On beat 2 (step 2) partners step towards their own right side, while making dual 1/8 left turns. Although both partners turn slightly to their left, the man must cross his left foot behind his right foot, as the woman merely steps side on her right foot. While partners are turning left, the man flings the woman into the Throw Out Position, as he releases her left hand from his right hand, but continues to hold her right hand in his left hand in the *right one-hand hold*. Partners then complete their triple step (beats 3 & 4) in the Throw Out Position.

On beats 5-6 (steps 6-7), however, partners do *not* return to the Closed Position. Instead, they take two Godzilla-size steps forward, passing each other's right side. While passing and switching sides, partners simultaneously shake each other's right hand. Part A concludes with partners standing in the Right Parallel Position, with the woman's right side parallel to the man's right side. 🚶

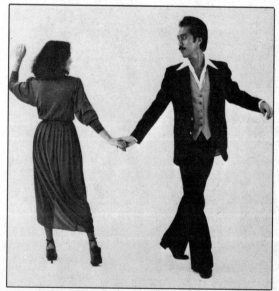

part A **step 7** (beat 6)

Part B:
UNWIND TO CLOSED DANCE POSITION

Part B begins on beat 1 (step 1) with tap steps in the Right Parallel Position. On beat 2 (step 2) partners unwind from their Handshake, as they pass each other's right side and switch hands. Since the man steps to his right side with his left foot, he must cross his left foot behind his right foot. The woman, on the contrary, merely steps towards her right side with her right foot. Moreover, while switching sides, partners simultaneously switch hands, as the man's left hand

clasps the woman's right hand in the *right one-hand hold*. After unwinding, partners complete their triple step (beats 3 & 4) in the Throw Out Position. On beats 5-6 (steps 6-7), partners take two steps forward, as they return to the Closed Dance Position. 🕺

Part B **step 1** (beat 1)

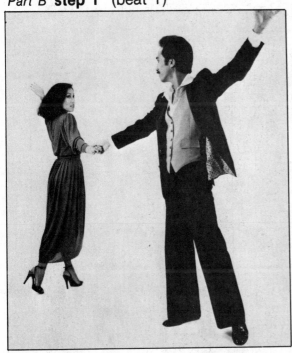

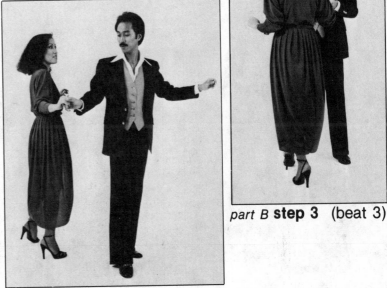

part B **step 3**   (beat 3)

part B **step 2**   (beat 2)

Man's Part:

Beat Steps

(1) 1. Left foot tap side in Closed Position

(2) 2. Left foot pass back (cross behind right foot), turning 1/8 left to Throw Out Position

(3) 3. Right foot back } *3 steps (triple step)*
(&) 4. Left foot close back } *in Throw Out*
(4) 5. Right foot forward } *Position*

(5) 6. Left foot forward } *2 steps forward,*
(6) 7. Right foot forward } *switch hands, and move into the Right Parallel Position*

Woman's Part:

Beat Steps

(1) 1. Right foot tap side in Closed Position

(2) 2. Right foot side, turning 1/8 left to Throw Out Position

(3) 3. Left foot back } *3 steps (triple step)*
(&) 4. Right foot close back } *in Throw Out*
(4) 5. Left foot forward } *Position*

(5) 6. Right foot forward } *2 steps forward,*
(6) 7. Left foot forward } *switch hands, and move into the Right Parallel Position*

NEW YORK-LATIN HUSTLE

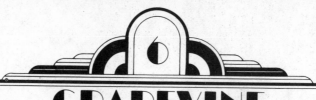

GRAPEVINE

The strutting, sashaying GRAPEVINE is composed of side steps, alternated with pass steps, performed in the Closed Dance Position. All of the steps in this variation are designed to propel partners across the dance floor in a sideways direction. Some side steps, therefore, are followed with pass forward steps in which partners cross one foot in front of the opposite foot. Other side steps, however, are followed with pass back steps in which partners cross one foot behind or in back of the opposite foot. Another name for the pass back step is fifth position step, a term lifted from classical ballet.

Divided into two sections, each part of this variation contains a sequence of 7 steps, completed in 6 syncopated beats of music. In Part A the man travels towards his left side, as the woman travels towards her right side. In Part B, partners fan their feet in half turns, in order to progress sideways in the opposite direction, as the man travels towards his right side, and the woman travels towards her left side. 🕺

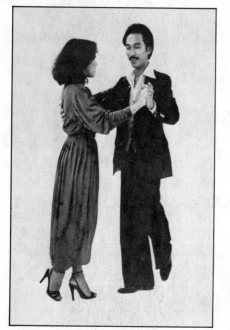

part A **step 1** (beat 1)

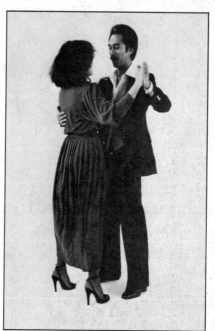

part A **step 2** (beat 2)

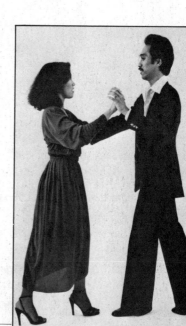

part A **step 3** (beat 3)

Part A:
SASHAY SIDEWAYS

Man's Part

Beat Steps
- (1) 1. Left foot tap behind right foot
- (2) 2. Left foot side
- (3) 3. Right foot pass back
  (cross behind left foot)
- (&) 4. Left foot side
- (4) 5. Right foot pass forward
  (cross in front of left foot)
- (5) 6. Left foot side
- (6) 7. Right foot pass back
  (cross behind left foot)

Woman's Part:

Beat Steps
- (1) 1. Right foot tap behind left foot
- (2) 2. Right foot side
- (3) 3. Left foot pass back
  (cross behind right foot)
- (&) 4. Right foot side
- (4) 5. Left foot pass forward
  (cross in front of right foot)
- (5) 6. Right foot side
- (6) 7. Left foot pass back
  (cross behind right foot)

Part B:
FAN, AND REVERSE DIRECTION

Man's Part:
Beat   *Steps*
- (1)   1. Left foot fan ¼ left
- (2)   2. Left foot fan ¼ left
- (3)   3. Right foot side
- (&)   4. Left foot pass forward
  (cross in front of right foot)
- (4)   5. Right foot side
- (5)   6. Left foot pass back
  (cross behind right foot)
- (6)   7. Right foot side

Woman's Part:
Beat   *Steps*
- (1)   1. Right foot fan ¼ right
- (2)   2. Right foot fan ¼ right
- (3)   3. Left foot side
- (&)   4. Right foot pass forward
  (cross in front of left foot)
- (4)   5. Left foot side
- (5)   6. Right foot pass back
  (cross behind left foot)
- (6)   7. Left foot side

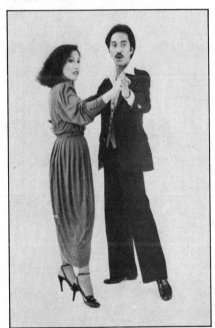

part B **step 1** (beat 1)

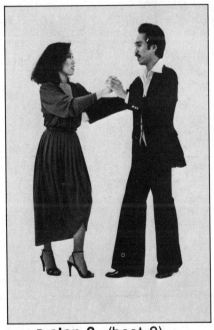

part B **step 2** (beat 2)

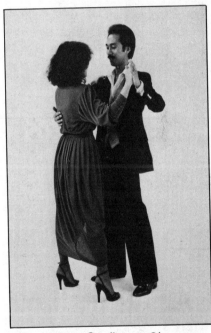

part B **step 3** (beat 3)

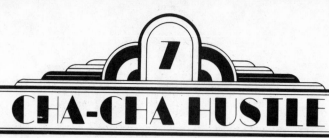

Another hot disco dance, favored by many triple steppers, is the CHA-CHA HUSTLE. Despite the name, the Cha-Cha Hustle shares few affinities with the ballroom version of the Cha-Cha, described in detail in Chapter 18. In the ballroom version, double steps are alternated with triple (cha-cha-cha) steps. In the Cha-Cha Hustle, however, two triple steps are followed by one double step. Thus, the Cha-Cha Hustle contains an 8 step pattern which is completed within 6 beats of syncopated music.

Two triple steps begin the Cha-Cha Hustle in the Closed Dance Position. Although these triple steps may be taken forward, backward, or to either side, partners must move in opposite directions, if they remain embraced in the Closed Dance Position. Thus, if the man steps forward, then the woman must step back; conversely, if the man steps back, the woman must step forward.

The triple (step-ball-change) steps are followed by two walk steps. On beats 5-6 (steps 7-8) partners take two steps in opposite directions, moving either forward or backward. All turn variations for the Cha-Cha Hustle will be completed on these two walk steps.

Although the Cha-Cha Hustle is usually performed in the Closed or Social Dance Position, it can also be done in the Holding Dance Position. In fact, many partners prefer the Holding Position, with both hands held and crossed. In the Holding Crossed Position, partners hold hands in a double handshake, with their held right hands crossed on top of their held left hands. Without releasing their hands from the crossed hold, partners turn to the side on the triple steps, but face each other on the walk steps. 🎵

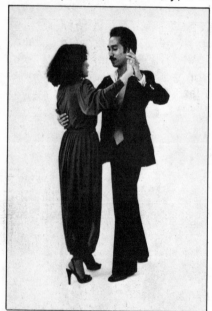 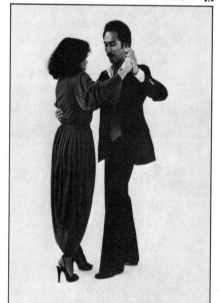 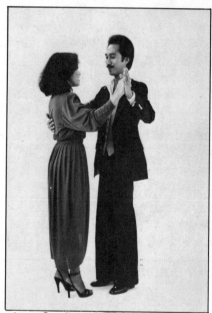

step 1 (beat 1) **step 2** (beat "and") **step 3** (beat 2)

Man's Part:

Beat Steps

(1) 1. Left foot forward

(&) 2. Right foot step in place

(2) 3. Left foot close to right foot

(3) 4. Right foot back

(&) 5. Left foot step in place

(4) 6. Right foot close to left foot

(5) 7. Left foot forward

(6) 8. Right foot close to left foot

Woman's Part:

Beat Steps

(1) 1. Right foot back

(&) 2. Left foot step in place

(2) 3. Right foot close to left foot

(3) 4. Left foot forward

(&) 5. Right foot step in place

(4) 6. Left foot close to right foot

(5) 7. Right foot back

(6) 8. Left foot close to right foot

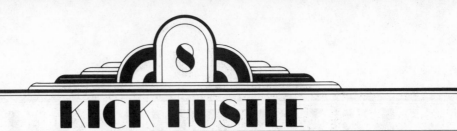

KICK HUSTLE

The KICK HUSTLE is another fast paced disco dance that combines double rhythm with triple rhythm steps, but also sticks in a quick kick. The entire pattern contains a sequence of 8 steps, completed in 6 beats (1-½ measures) of music. Although the pattern begins and ends in the Social (Closed) Dance Position, the four steps completed on the syncopated beats of music are done in the Promenade Dance Position.

The pattern begins tamely enough on beats 1-2 (steps 1-2) with a tap step, followed with a side step. While stepping side, however, partners should point their toes and turn slightly away from each other, as they move into the Promenade Dance Position. The man, therefore, turns slightly left as he steps to his left side, while the woman turns slightly right as she steps to her right side. After partners have completed their side steps, they will be embraced in the Promenade Position, with both facing in the same direction, as the woman's left hip lightly touches against the man's right hip.

On the next four steps, completed in two syncopated beats of music, the fun really begins.

On steps 3-4, partners draw their feet together with a close side step, then step in place with the opposite foot. On step 5, partners swiftly kick one foot forward, while balancing all of their weight on the opposite foot. The man, therefore, kicks his right foot forward, while keeping his weight balanced on his left foot, with his left knee slightly bent; conversely, the woman kicks her left foot forward, while keeping her weight balanced on her right foot, with her right knee slightly bent. As soon as they have kicked one foot forward, partners should swing the same foot back into place on step 6, immediately shifting their weight to the foot that closes back.

The kick pattern concludes on beats 5-6 (steps 7-8) with two walk steps. On beat 5 (step 7), the man takes one step forward, as the woman takes one step back. While partners are taking their walk steps, the man leads the woman back into the Closed Dance Position. On beat 6 (step 8), the man takes one more step forward, as the woman takes another step back. All turn variations, used with the basic pattern for the Kick Hustle, must be completed on these last two walk steps. 💃

Man's Part:

Beat Steps

- (1) 1. Left foot tap side
- (2) 2. Left foot step side
- (3) 3. Right foot close to left foot
- (&) 4. Left foot step in place
- (4) 5. Right foot kick forward
- (&) 6. Right foot close to left foot
- (5) 7. Left foot forward
- (6) 8. Right foot close to left foot

Woman's Part:

Beat Steps

- (1) 1. Right foot tap side
- (2) 2. Right foot step side
- (3) 3. Left foot close to right foot
- (&) 4. Right foot step in place
- (4) 5. Left foot kick forward
- (&) 6. Left foot close to right foot
- (5) 7. Right foot back
- (6) 8. Left foot close to right foot

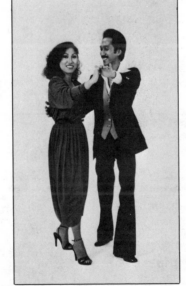

step 2 (beat 2)

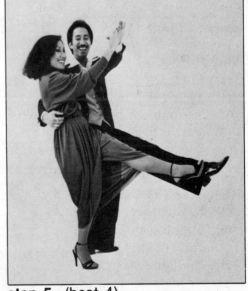

step 5 (beat 4)

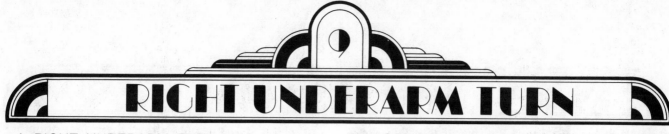

RIGHT UNDERARM TURN

A RIGHT UNDERARM TURN (also called an Outside Turn on "2" in dance lingo) is a Full Right Turn which the woman completes on the triple step. This variation begins on beat 1 (step 1) with tap steps, completed in the Closed Dance Position. On beat 2 (step 2) partners step side as the man gives the woman a hand lead for the *right one-hand hold* by uplifting the woman's right hand in his left hand. To prod the woman into turning right, the man gently swings her right hand outside or away from her face.

On the triple step (beats 3 & 4), the man completes his Basic Side Step (two steps back, then one step forward) in the Open Dance Position, while he keeps the woman's right hand uplifted in his left hand in the *right one-hand hold*. At the same time, the woman completes her Right Underarm Turn, as she turns in a full circle to her right (360 degrees clockwise) in 3 small steps *forward*. While the woman is turning, her right hand rotates clockwise over her head. Partners conclude this variation on beats 5-6 (steps 6-7) with two steps forward, as they walk towards each other and return to the Closed Dance Position. 💃

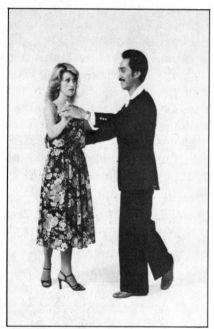

step 1 (beat 1)

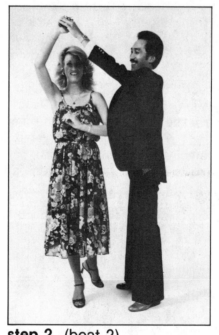

step 2 (beat 2)

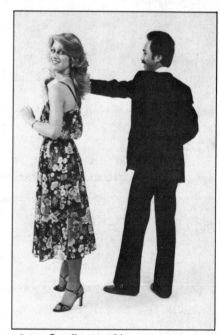

step 3 (beat 3)

Man's Part:

Beat	Steps	Movement
(1)	1. Left foot tap behind right foot	Tap, then step side
(2)	2. Left foot side	
(3)	3. Right foot back, turning ¼ right	3 steps (triple step) in Right Open Position
(&)	4. Left foot close back	
(4)	5. Right foot forward	
(5)	6. Left foot forward, turning ¼ left	2 steps forward, returning to Closed Position
(6)	7. Right foot close forward	

Woman's Part:

Beat	Steps	Movement
(1)	1. Right foot tap behind left foot	Tap, then step side
(2)	2. Right foot side	
(3)	3. Left foot forward	Right Underarm Turn in 3 steps forward
(&)	4. Right foot forward	
(4)	5. Left foot forward	
(5)	6. Right foot forward	2 steps forward, returning to Closed Position
(6)	7. Left foot close forward	

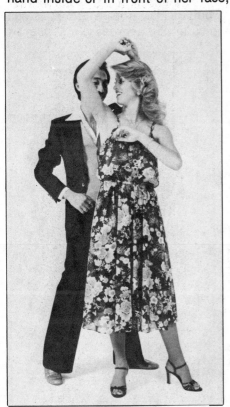 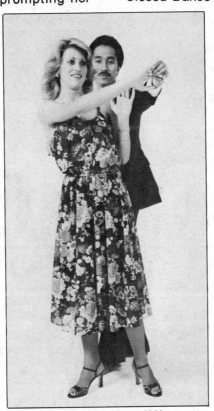 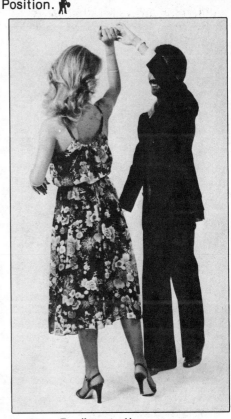

REVERSE UNDERARM TURN

The REVERSE UNDERARM TURN (sometimes called an Inside Turn on "2" in dance jargon) is a Full Left Turn which the woman completes on the triple step. The pattern for the Reverse Underarm Turn begins on beat 1 (step 1) with tap steps, completed in the Closed Dance Position. On beat 2 (step 2) partners step side, as the man gives a hand lead for the *right one-hand hold* by lifting the woman's right hand in his left hand. This time, however, the man gently pushes the woman's right hand inside or in front of her face, prompting her to turn towards her left.

On the triple step (beats 3 & 4) the man completes his Basic Side Step (two steps back, then one step forward) in the Open Dance Position. At the same time, the woman completes her Reverse Underarm Turn, as she turns in a full circle to her left (360 degrees counter-clockwise) in 3 small steps *back*. Partners conclude this variation on beats 5-6 (steps 6-7) with two steps forward, **as** they walk towards each other and resume the Closed Dance Position. 💃

step 3 (beat 3)   **step 4** (beat "and")   **step 5** (beat 4)

Man's Part:

Beat	Steps	Movement
(1)	1. Left foot tap behind right foot	*Tap, then step side*
(2)	2. Left foot side	
(3)	3. Right foot back, turning ¼ right	*3 steps (triple step) in Right Open Position*
(&)	4. Left foot close back	
(4)	5. Right foot forward	
(5)	6. Left foot forward, turning ¼ left	*2 steps forward, returning to Closed Position*
(6)	7. Right foot close forward	

Women's Part:

Beat	Steps	Movement
(1)	1. Right foot tap behind left foot	*Tap, then step side*
(2)	2. Right foot side	
(3)	3. Left foot back	*Reverse Underarm Turn in 3 steps back*
(&)	4. Right foot back	
(4)	5. Left foot back	
(5)	6. Right foot forward	*2 steps forward, returning to Closed Position*
(6)	7. Left foot close forward	

NEW YORK-LATIN HUSTLE

DOUBLE HALF TURNS

As the name implies, the pattern for DOUBLE HALF TURNS (also called an Outside Turn on "4") yokes together two turns. Similar to the Right Underarm Turn, the woman turns outside or to her right. Unlike the Right Underarm Turn, however, the Double Half Turns are completed in two steps forward on the last two beats of music. This pattern begins, therefore, with the Basic Side Step (Open Break) for beats 1-4 (steps 1-5), but concludes with Double Half Turns on beats 5-6 (steps 6-7).

On beats 1-2 (steps 1-2), partners tap behind, then step side in the Closed Dance Position. On the triple step (beats 3 & 4) partners move into the Right Open Position, as they break away from each other by making dual ¼ turns in opposite directions. On beat 4 (step 5), however, the man lifts the woman's right hand in his left hand in the *right one-hand hold*, as he pushes the woman's right hand outside or away from her face. On beats 5-6 (steps 6-7) the man takes two steps forward in the Open Position. The woman, on the other hand, completes her Double Half Turns in 2 steps forward, as she pivots 180 degrees clockwise on each forward step.

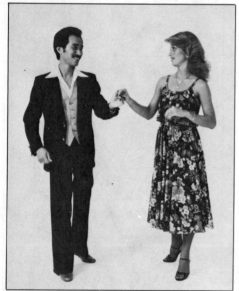

step 5 (beat 4)

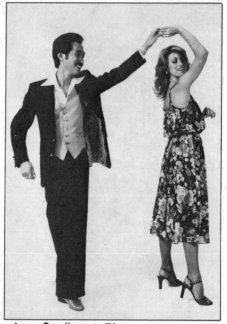

step 6 (beat 5)

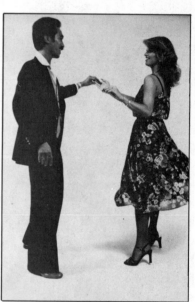

step 7 (beat 6)

Man's Part:

Beat	Steps	Movement
(1)	1. Left foot tap behind right foot	Tap, then step side in Closed Dance Position
(2)	2. Left foot side	
(3)	3. Right foot back, turning ¼ right	3 steps (*triple step*) in Right Open Position
(&)	4. Left foot close back	
(4)	5. Right foot forward	
(5)	6. Left foot forward, turning ¼ left	2 steps forward, returning to Closed Position
(6)	7. Right foot close forward	

Woman's Part:

Beat	Steps	Movement
(1)	1. Right foot tap behind left foot	Tap, then step side in Closed Dance Position
(2)	2. Right foot side	
(3)	3. Left foot back, turning ¼ left	3 steps (*triple step*) in Right Open Position
(&)	4. Right foot close back	
(4)	5. Left foot forward	
(5)	6. Right foot forward	Double Half Turns in 2 steps forward
(6)	7. Left foot forward	

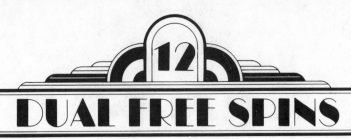

DUAL FREE SPINS

For the DUAL FREE SPINS both partners get the once-a-month chance to make full turns on their triple steps. This variation begins on beats 1-2 (steps 1-2) with tap and side steps, as partners move from the Closed Position to the Apart Position. On the triple step (beats 3 & 4) partners complete their Dual Free Spins in the Apart Position. The man, however, makes a Full Left (Inside) Turn by circling 360 degrees counter-clockwise in 3 small steps back. Conversely, the woman makes a Full Right (Outside) Turn by circling 360 degrees clockwise in 3 small steps forward. After partners complete their Dual Free Spins, they walk towards each other on beats 5-6 (step 6-7) and resume the Closed Dance Position.

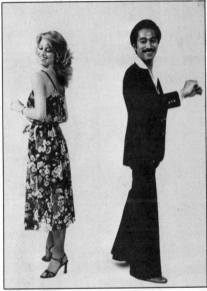

step 3 (beat 3)

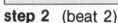

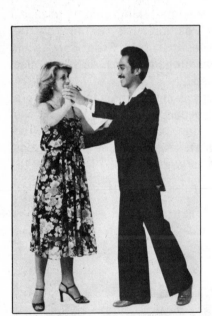

step 2 (beat 2)

step 1 (beat 1)

Man's Part:

Beat   Steps

(1)	1. Left foot tap behind right in Closed Position	
(2)	2. Left foot step side in Apart Position	
(3)	3. Right foot back	*Full Left Turn in 3 steps back in Apart Position*
(&)	4. Left foot back	
(4)	5. Right foot back	
(5)	6. Left foot forward	*2 steps forward, returning to Closed Position*
(6)	7. Right foot forward	

Woman's Part:

Beat   Steps

(1)	1. Right foot tap behind left in Closed Position	
(2)	2. Right foot step side in Apart Position	
(3)	3. Left foot forward	*Full Right Turn in 3 steps forward in Apart Position*
(&)	4. Right foot forward	
(4)	5. Left foot forward	
(5)	6. Right foot forward	*2 steps forward, returning to Closed Position*
(6)	7. Left foot forward	

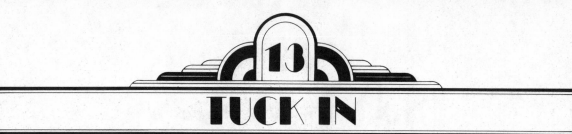
In the TUCK IN the man hustles through his basic step pattern in the Apart Dance Position, while the woman whips through two Free Spins. The Tuck In begins on beat 1 (step 1) with *inside tap steps,* as partners tap one foot in front of the opposite foot. The man, therefore, taps his left foot in front of his right foot, and the woman taps her right foot in front of her left foot. As partners tap

inside, the man swings both pairs of clasped hands inside or towards the woman's left (his right) side.

On beat 2 (step 2) partners unscramble their feet by stepping side. The man, therefore, steps to his left side on his left foot, and the woman steps to her right side on her right foot. As partners step side, the man swings both of their clasped hands outside or towards the woman's right (his left) side. The thrust of the swing in which both pairs of hands are flung outside should be sufficient to propel the woman towards her right.

On the triple step (beats 3 & 4) the man flings the woman into the Apart Dance Position, as partners release both pairs of hands. The man completes his triple step by taking 3 steps in place in the Apart Dance Position. The woman, on the other hand, completes her first Free Spin (Full Right Turn) in 3 small steps forward, as she circles 360 degrees clockwise.

On beats 5-6 (steps 6-7) the man takes 2 more steps in place in the Apart Dance Position. At the same time, the woman completes another Free Spin (Full Right Turn), as she circles 360 degrees clockwise in 2 steps forward. ♣

step 1 (beat 1)

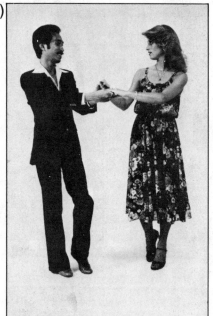

step 2
(beat 2)

step 3 (beat 3)

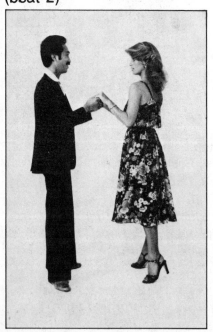

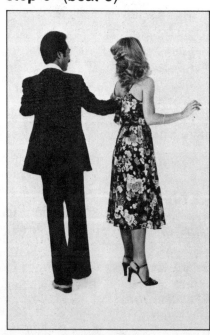

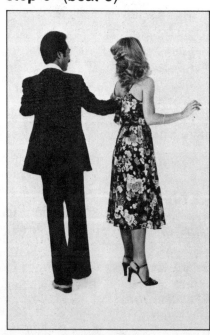

step 4 (beat ''and'')

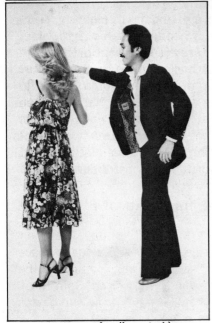

part B **step 1** (beat 1)

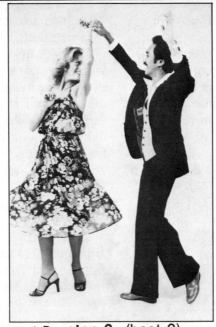

part B **step 2** (beat 2)

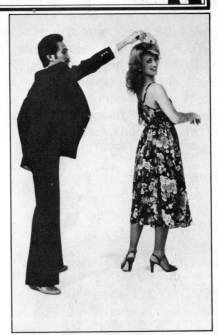

part B **step 5** (beat 5)

As the name implies, SPOT TURNS are made essentially in one spot or place. To make these turns, the dancer stares at one specific spot in the room, which prevents or deters dizziness. Divided into two sections, this variation begins in Part A with the Basic Holding Pattern, as partners complete their basic 7 steps in 6 syncopated beats of music. In Part B, however, the syncopated beats are dropped, as partners complete their Spot Turns in 6 steps forward in 6 beats of music.

To make a smooth transition to the SPOT TURNS, this variation begins in Part A with the Basic Holding Pattern. Partners complete their basic 7 steps in 6 syncopated beats of music. On beat 6 (step 7), however, the man gives the woman a hand lead for the *left one-hand hold,* as he lifts the woman's left hand in his right hand, but simultaneously releases her right hand from his left hand.

In Part B there will be *no* triple steps, since the syncopated beats of music are dropped for the Spot Turns. Thus, on beats 1-6 (steps 1-6) the man takes 6 walk steps forward, as he rotates clockwise around the woman. While sauntering around the twirling woman, the man keeps the woman's left hand uplifted in his right hand in the *left one-hand hold*. The woman, on the other hand, makes two continuous Right Underarm Turns in 6 small steps

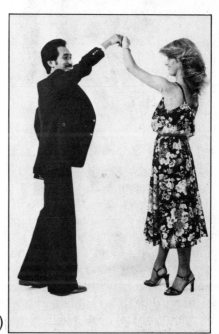

part B
step 6 (beat 6)

forward, as she traces two small right circles on the floor. To prevent dizziness, the woman focuses her eyes on one particular spot in the room. Moreover, as the woman makes each of her Right Underarm Turns by spinning 360 degrees clockwise in 3 small steps forward, her left hand, loosely clasped in the man's right hand, rotates clockwise over her head. 🕺

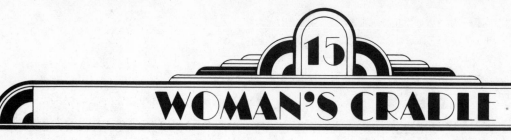
The CRADLE, also called a SWEETHEART or WRAP-AROUND, is a Half Left Holding Underarm Turn. On the one hand, the Cradle resembles a Walk Around (Cross-Over) Turn, because both turns are Half Left (Inside) Turns, which are made by rotating 180 degrees counter-clockwise. On the other hand, the Cradle resembles the Double Cross Turn, because both are Underarm Holding Turns, in which both pairs of hands remain clasped.

Divided into two sections, each part of this variation contains 7 basic steps, completed in 6 syncopated beats of music. In Part A the woman makes her Cradle by rotating 180 degrees counter-clockwise in two steps forward on beats 5-6 (steps 6-7). In Part B the woman unwinds from her Cradle by rotating 180 degrees clockwise in 1 step forward on beat 2 (step 2). 🕺

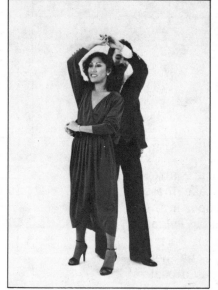

part A
step 6 (beat 5)

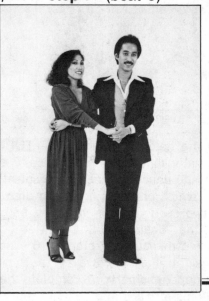

part A **step 7** (beat 6)

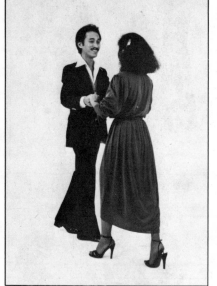

part A **step 5** (beat 4)

Part A:
WOMAN'S CRADLE

Part A begins with the Basic Holding Pattern for beats 1-4 (steps 1-5). On beat 4 (step 5), however, the man gives the woman a hand lead for the *right two-hand hold.* Without releasing hands from the double (two-hand) hold, the man uplifts the woman's right hand in his left hand, but continues to hold her left hand down with his right hand in the *right two-hand hold.* Moreover, he pushes the woman's uplifted right hand across or in front of her face (inside), which prods her to turn left.

On the last two beats of music (beats 5-6), the man takes two steps in place. The woman, however, makes her Cradle (Half Left Holding Underarm Turn) by turning 180 degrees counter-clockwise in 2 steps forward. While the woman is turning, her right hand, uplifted in the man's left hand, rotates counter-clockwise over her head. After the woman completes her Cradle Turn, her right hand drops down, until her right arm is crossed on top of her left arm, straight-jacket style. She then scoots back, until her left side is parallel to the man's right side in the Left Side Parallel Position. 🕺

Man's Part:
Beat   Steps
- (1)   1. Left foot tap behind right foot
- (2)   2. Left foot close forward
- (3)   3. Right foot back
- (&)   4. Left foot close back
- (4)   5. Right foot forward
- (5)   6. Left foot step in place
- (6)   7. Right foot step in place

Woman's Part:
Beat   Steps
- (1)   1. Right foot tap behind
- (2)   2. Right foot close forward
- (3)   3. Left foot back
- (&)   4. Right foot close back
- (4)   5. Left foot forward
- (5)   6. Right foot forward
- (6)   7. Left foot forward

Part B:
UNWIND TO HOLDING POSITION

What winds can also unwind. That may not be a law of physics, but it almost always applies to dance configurations. The unwind is preceded on beat 1 (step 1) with tap steps which both the man and the woman complete, while they are in the Left Side Parallel Position. While they are tapping, the man once again gives the woman a hand lead for the *right two-hand hold* by lifting her right hand in his left hand, without releasing her left hand from his right hand.

On step 2 (beat 2) the man takes one step to the side on his left foot, as the woman unwinds by making a Half Right Holding Underarm Turn (180 degrees clockwise) in one step forward. While the woman is unwinding, her right hand, uplifted in the man's left hand, rotates clockwise over her head. On beats 3-6 (steps 3-7) partners conclude this variation in the Holding Dance Position.

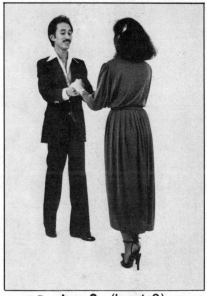

part B **step 3** (beat 3)

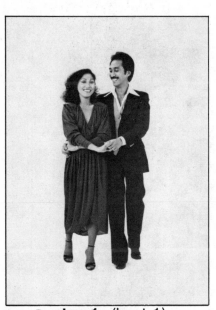

part B **step 1** (beat 1)

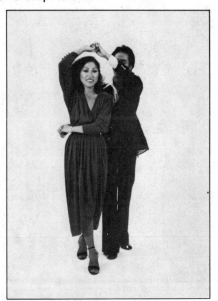

part B **step 2** (beat 2)

Man's Part:
Beat *Steps*
- (1) 1. Left foot tap behind right foot in left side Parallel Position
- (2) 2. Left foot close forward, as woman turns
- (3) 3. Right foot back
- (&) 4. Left foot close back
- (4) 5. Right foot forward
- (5) 6. Left foot forward
- (6) 7. Right foot close forward

Woman's Part:
Beat *Steps*
- (1) 1. Right foot tap behind left foot in Left Side Parallel Position
- (2) 2. Right foot forward, as she makes her Half Right Holding Underarm Turn
- (3) 3. Left foot back
- (&) 4. Right foot close back
- (4) 5. Left foot forward
- (5) 6. Right foot forward
- (6) 7. Left foot close forward

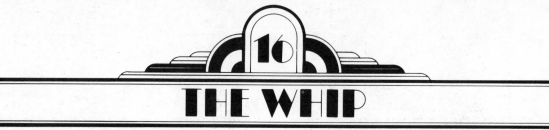
The WHIP, also known as CRADLE ROLLS, adds a mild, but pleasurable form of torture to the Woman's Cradle. This variation, similar to the previous two variations, incorporates two sequences of the basic 7 steps, completed in 6 syncopated beats of music.

In Part A, the woman makes her Cradle in two steps forward on the last two beats of music (beats 5-6). In Part B, the man whips the woman out to the right with a Full Right Turn on the triple step (beats 3 & 4), then whips her back in to the left with a Full Left Turn on the final two beats of music (beats 5-6). 🕺

part A **step 6** (beat 5)

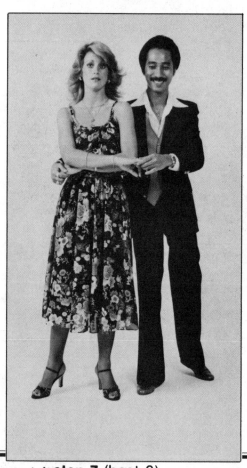

part A **step 7** (beat 6)

Part A:
WOMAN'S CRADLE

This variation begins tamely enough with the Basic Holding Pattern for beats 1-4 (steps 1-5). On beat 4 (step 5) the man gives the woman a hand lead for the *right two-hand hold* by lifting and pushing inside the woman's right hand with his left hand, while holding her left hand down with his right hand. On beats 5-6 (steps 6-7) the man takes two steps in place, as the woman makes her Cradle (Half Left Holding Underarm Turn), by turning 180 degrees counter-clockwise in two steps forward. While the woman is turning, her right hand, uplifted in the man's left hand, rotates counter-clockwise over her head. After the woman completes her turn, her hand drops down, until her right arm is crossed on top of her left arm, straight-jacket style. The woman then scoots back next to the man, until her left side is parallel to the man's right side in the Left Side Parallel Position.

🕺

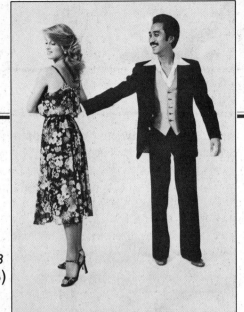

part B
step 3 (beat 3)

Part B:
THE WHIP

Part B begins on beats 1-2 (steps 1-2) with tap steps, followed with side steps in the Left Side Parallel Position. On beat 2 (step 2) the agony of anticipation is momentarily prolonged as the man releases the woman's right hand from his left hand, but continues to hold her left hand in his right hand in the *left one-hand hold.*

On the triple step (beats 3 & 4), the exquisite torture begins as the man whips the woman out towards her right side. The man takes three steps in place in the Left Open Position, as he whips the woman out with a quick flick of his wrist. While rolling away from the man, the woman simultaneously circles around in a Full Right Turn (360 degrees clockwise) in three small steps forward.

On beats 5-6 (steps 6-7) the man takes two steps in place, as he whips the woman back in towards her left side with another sharp snap of his wrist. While rolling towards the man, the woman circles around in a Full Left Turn (360 degrees counterclockwise) in two steps forward. Although the woman's left hand remains clasped in the man's right hand throughout these rolls, her hand does not rotate over her head.

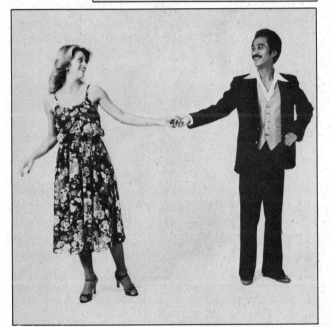

part B
step 5 (beat 4)

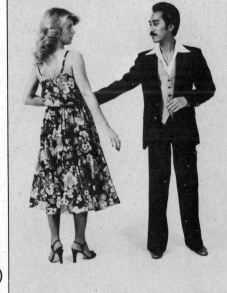

part B
step 6 (beat 5)

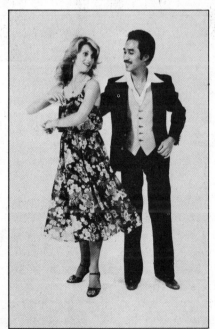

part B **step 7** (beat 6)

NEW YORK-LATIN HUSTLE

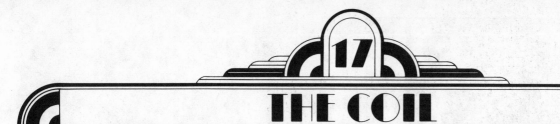

THE COIL

The COIL, another variation that begins with a Woman's Cradle, concludes with two Reverse Underarm Turns. In Part A, the woman completes her Cradle in two steps forward on the last two beats of music (beats 5-6). In Part B, the woman twirls around twice to complete two Reverse (Inside) Underarm Turns.

Part A:
WOMAN'S CRADLE

Similar to the previous variation, Part A begins with the Basic Holding Pattern for beats 1-4 (steps 1-5). On beat 4 (step 5) the man gives the woman a hand lead for the *right two-hand hold*, as he lifts her right hand in his left hand, but holds her left hand down with his right hand. On beats 5-6 (steps 6-7), the man takes two steps in place, while the woman makes her Cradle (Half Left Holding Underarm Turn) in two steps forward. While the woman is turning, her right hand rotates counter-clockwise over her head, then drops down, until her right arm is crossed on top of her left arm. The woman then scoots back next to the man, until her left side is parallel to the man's right side in the Left Side Parallel Position.

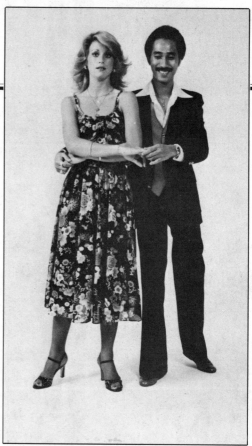

part A **step 7** (beat 6)

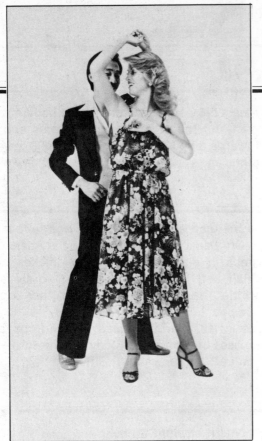

Part B:
REVERSE UNDERARM TURNS

Part B of the Coil begins on beats 1-2 (steps 1-2) with tap steps, followed with side steps in the Left Side Parallel Position. On beat 2 (step 2) the man gives the woman a hand lead for the *right one-hand hold* by lifting her right hand in his left hand, while releasing her left hand from his right hand.

On the triple step (beats 3 & 4) the man takes 3 steps in place, as the woman makes her Reverse Underarm Turn by rotating 360 degrees counter-clockwise in 3 small steps back. On beats 5-6 (steps 6-7) the man takes two additional steps in place, as the woman completes another Reverse Underarm Turn by rotating 360 degrees counter-clockwise in two steps back. While the woman is turning, her right hand, clasped in the man's left hand, rotates counter-clockwise over her head.

part B **step 3** (beat 3)

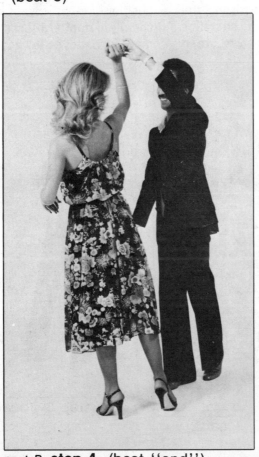

part B **step 4** (beat ''and'')

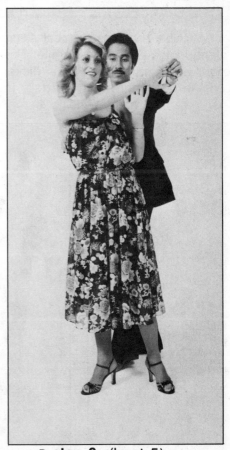

part B **step 6** (beat 5)

NEW YORK-LATIN HUSTLE

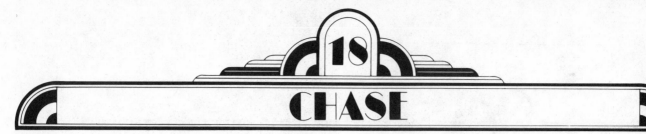

18

CHASE

Before partners scramble through their CHASE of the century, they warm up with a Woman's Cradle. In Part A, the woman makes her Cradle in two steps forward on the last two beats of music (beats 5-6). In Part B the Chase begins as both the man and the woman switch places and fling out towards opposite sides, then walk towards each other and return to the Closed Dance Position. 🕺

Part A:
WOMAN'S CRADLE

To add just a whit of variety, Part A begins on beats 1-4 (steps 1-5) with the Basic Throw Out (Basic Cross-Body Lead). On beat 1 (step 1), partners tap in the Closed Dance Position. On beat 2 (step 2), partners step towards their own right sides, as they concurrently make dual 1/8 Left Turns (45 degrees counter-clockwise). On the triple step (beats 3 & 4) partners break into the Throw Out Position, with the woman's right hand clasped in the man's left hand in the *right one-hand hold*.

On beats 5-6 (steps 6-7), the man takes two steps in place, as the woman makes her Cradle (Half Left Underarm Turn) in two steps forward. While the woman is turning, her right hand, clasped in the man's left hand, rotates counter-clockwise over her head, then drops down and crosses in front of her body, as she scoots back into the Left Side Parallel Position. 🕺

Part B:
THE CHASE

The Chase begins on beat 1 (step 1) with tap steps in the Left Side Parallel Position, with the *right one-hand hold.* For a flicker of flash, the woman does more than just tap: in fact, she slips her free left hand beneath her right arm, then shoots it straight up over her head.

On beat 2 (step 2) partners begin to switch positions with pass forward steps, as they complete dual 1/8 turns in opposite directions. The man, who moves towards his right side, crosses his

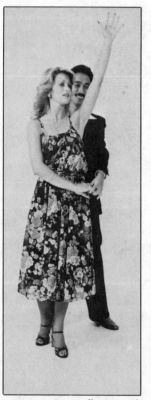

part B **step** (beat 1)

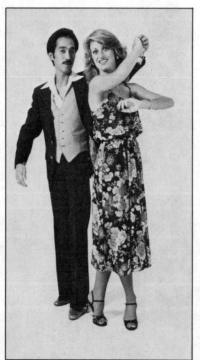

part B **step 2** (beat 2)

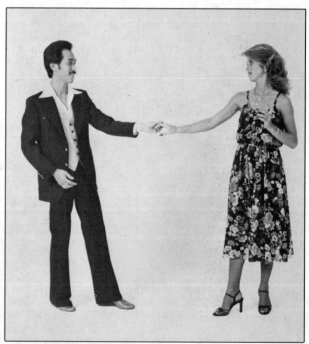

part B **step 3** (beat 3)

left foot in front of his right foot, as he makes a 1/8 Right Turn (45 degrees clockwise). The woman, who moves towards her left side, crosses her right foot in front of her left foot, as she makes a 1/8 Left Turn (45 degrees counter-clockwise).

On the triple steps (beats 3 & 4) partners must extricate themselves from their cross-legged stance. Probably the easiest and certainly the safest method would be to swing the trapped foot around in a ¼ turn. Thus, partners step back as they simultaneously complete dual ¼ turns in opposite directions. On beat 3 (step 3), the man steps back on his right foot, as he makes a ¼ Left Turn (90 degrees counter-clockwise). At the same time, the woman steps back on her left foot, as she makes a ¼ Right Turn (90 degrees clockwise). After partners complete their dual ¼ turns, they should once again be facing each other in the Throw Out Position.

After partners complete steps 4-5 of the triple step in the Throw Out Position, they take two walk steps forward, moving towards each other and returning to the Closed Dance Position. 🕴

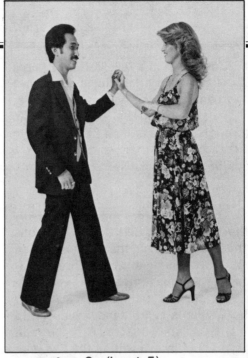

part B **step 6** (beat 5)

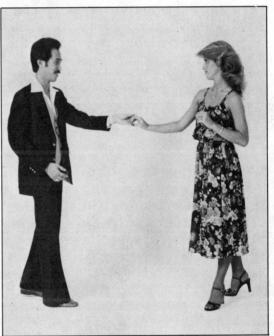

part B **step 5** (beat 4)

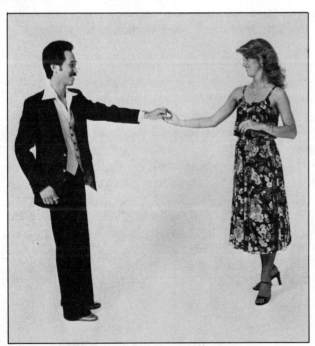

part B **step 4** (beat ''and'')

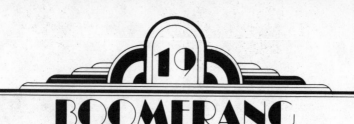

19
BOOMERANG

The BOOMERANG flips in a few Half Left Turns to the basic Chase. This variation starts off in Part A (now don't groan) with the Woman's Cradle, completed on beats 5-6. In Part B, the woman boomerangs through a series of Half Left Turns. In Part C, partners conclude this variation with a Chase sequence. ♣

Part A:
WOMAN'S CRADLE

Similar to the Chase described in the previous variation, partners warm up for the Boomerang on beats 1-4 (steps 1-5) with their Basic Throw Out. On beat 4 (step 5) the man gives the woman a hand lead for the *right one-hand hold,* as he lifts and pushes the woman's right hand inside or in front of her face. On beats 5-6 (steps 6-7) the man takes two steps in place, while the woman completes her Cradle (Half Left Underarm Turn) in two steps forward. While the woman is turning, her right hand, loosely clasped in the man's left hand, rotates counter-clockwise over her head, then drops down and crosses in front of her body. After the woman completes her turn, she wiggles into the Left Side Parallel Position, until her left side is parallel to the man's right side. ♣

Part B:
THE BOOMERANG

Similar to the Chase, the Boomerang begins on beat 1 (step 1) with tap steps in the Left Side Parallel Position. While the woman is tapping, however, she simultaneously flings her free left hand straight up over her head.

On beat 2 (step 2) partners begin to switch positions with pass forward steps, as the man moves towards his right side, and the woman moves towards her left side. Although both partners cross one foot in front of the opposite foot, the man makes a 1/8 Right Turn, and the woman makes a ½ Left Turn. The man, therefore, crosses his left foot in front of his right foot, as he makes a 1/8 Right Turn (45 degrees clockwise). The woman, on the other hand, swings her right foot in front of her left foot, as she makes a ½ Left Turn (180 degrees counter-clockwise).

Despite the minor change evident on the pass forward steps, the triple step (beats 3 & 4) for the Boomerang duplicates the pattern used in the Chase. On beat 3 (step 3) the man swings his right foot back, as he makes a ¼ Left Turn (90 degrees counter-clockwise). Conversely, the woman swings her left foot back, as she makes a ¼ Right Turn

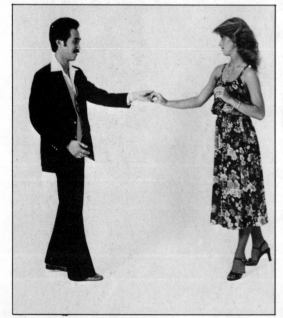

part B **step 5** (beat 4)

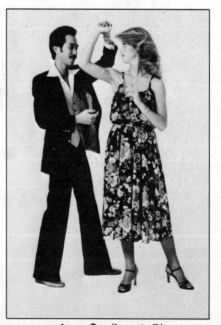

part B **step 6** (beat 5)

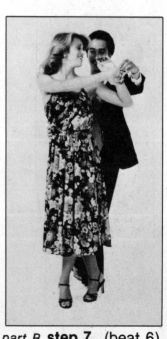

part B **step 7** (beat 6)

(90 degrees clockwise). After making their dual ¼ turns in opposite directions, partners should be facing each other in the Throw Out Position, as they complete steps 4-5 of the triple step.

On beats 5-6 (steps 6-7) partners boomerang back into the Cradle Position in two steps forward. The man, therefore, crosses behind the woman, as he completes a Half Right Turn (180 degrees clockwise). At the same time, the woman crosses in front of the man, as she makes a Half Left Underarm Turn (180 degrees counter-clockwise). Notice that the woman makes an *underarm* turn, as her right hand, which is uplifted by the man's left hand, rotates counter-clockwise over her head. Once partners have completed their dual half turns in opposite directions, they should once again be standing in the Left Side Parallel Position, with the woman's left side parallel to the man's right side.

Part C:
CHASE UNWIND

After boomeranging back and forth, partners unwind with a Chase sequence. On beat 1 (step 1) partners tap in the Left Side Parallel Position, as the woman shoots her free left hand straight up over her head. On beat 2 (step 2) partners begin to switch places, as the man moves towards his right side by crossing his left foot in front of his right foot, and the woman moves towards her left side by crossing her right foot in front of her left foot. On the triple steps (beats 3-4), partners continue to switch places, then turn to face each other in the Throw Out Position. On beats 5-6 (steps 6-7), partners take two steps forward, as they walk towards each other and embrace in the Closed Dance Position.

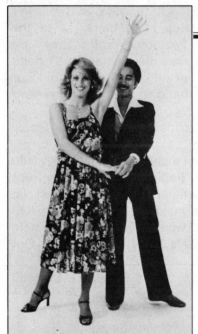

part C
step 1 (beat 1)

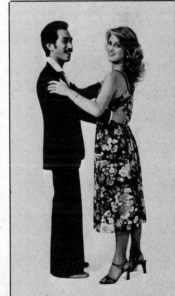

part C **step 7** (beat 6)

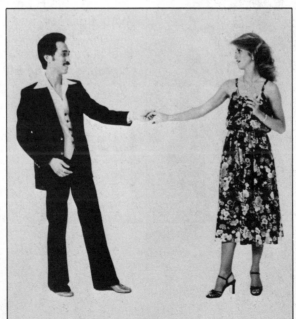

part C **step 3** (beat 3)

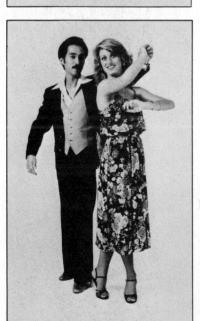

part C **step 2** (beat 2)

NEW YORK-LATIN HUSTLE

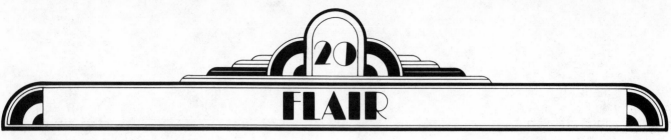

The FLAIR, which lifts tricks from both the Chase and the Boomerang, begins in Part A with the Man's Cradle. In Part B both partners move from the Cradle into the Throw Out Position, but end up back to back in the Flair Position. In Part C partners fly through their Flair. ⚎

Part A:
MAN'S CRADLE

Unlike the previous two variations, Part A of the Flair begins on beats 1-4 (steps 1-5) with the Basic Holding Pattern. In addition, Part A concludes on the last two beats of music with a Man's Cradle. Thus, on beat 4 (step 5) the man gives himself a hand lead for the *left two-hand hold* by lifting the woman's left hand in his right hand, while holding the woman's right hand down with his left hand. On beats 5-6 (steps 6-7) the man completes his Cradle (Half Left Holding Underarm Turn) in two steps forward, while the woman takes two steps in place. As the man turns, his right hand rotates counter-clockwise over his head, then drops down, until his right arm is crossed on top of his left arm. After he completes his turn, the man scoots back, until his left side is parallel to the woman's right side in the Right Side Parallel Position. ⚎

Part B:
CRADLE TO FLAIR

In Part B partners change places three times, as they move from the Cradle to the Throw Out Position, but end up back to back in the Flair Position. On beat 1 (step 1) partners tap in the Right Side Parallel Position. While they are tapping, the man releases the woman's left hand from his right hand, but he continues to hold her right hand in his left hand in the *right one-hand hold.*

On beat 2 (step 2) partners move into the Throw Out Position as they make dual right turns. Although the man must make a ½ Right Turn (180 degrees clockwise) by flinging his left foot in front of his right foot, the woman merely steps back on her right foot, as she makes a 1/8 Left Turn (45 degrees counter-clockwise). Partners complete their triple step (on beats 3 & 4) in the Throw Out Position with the *right one-hand hold.*

On beats 5-6 (steps 6-7) partners release all hands, as they take two steps forward and move into the Flair Position. While stepping forward, both the man and the woman make dual ½ Left Turns (180 degrees counter-clockwise), until they are standing back to back and facing in opposite directions in the Flair Position. ⚎

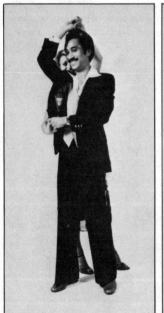

part A
step 6 (beat 5)

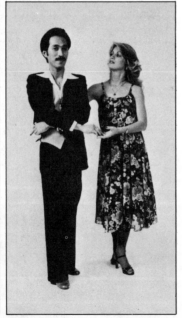

part A
step 7 (beat 6)

Part B:
CRADLE TO FLAIR

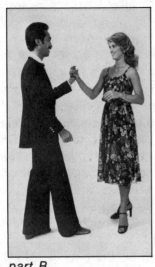

part B
step 2 (beat 2)

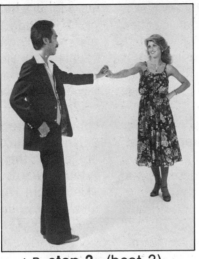

part B **step 3** (beat 3)

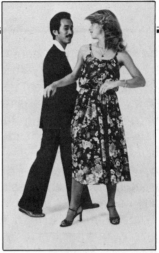

part B **step 6** (beat 5)

Part C:
FLAIR

In Part C partners fling into their Flair. On beat 1 (step 1) partners remain standing back to back, as they tap their feet and flair their hands out to the sides. On beat 2 (step 2) partners make dual ½ Left Turns (180 degrees counter-clockwise) in one step forward. On the triple step (beats 3 & 4) partners turn and face each other in the Apart Dance Position. On beats 5-6 (steps 6-7) partners take two steps forward, as they return to the Flair Position with dual ½ Left Turns.

Whenever partners choose to swing into a different variation, they unwind from the Flair with a Basic Side Step (Open Break).

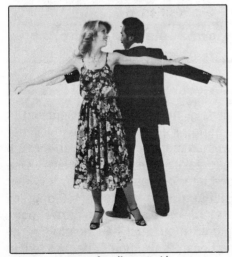

part C **step 1** (beat 1)

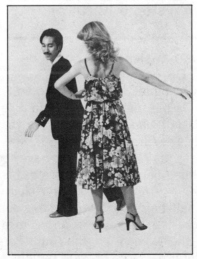

part C **step 2** (beat 2)

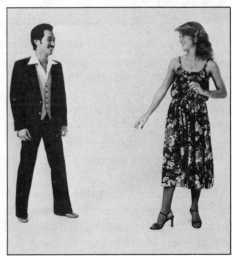

part C **step 3** (beat 3)

95

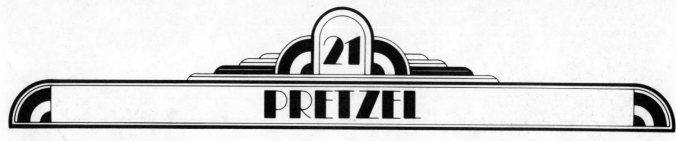

21 PRETZEL

Despite the somewhat silly name, the Pretzel is an epicurean delight. Contrary to popular belief, the Pretzel is not concocted from flour or water. In fact, this low calorie, high energy snack is composed of dual half holding turns, in which partners retain their double hand hold, as they turn in opposite directions.

Similar to Cradle variations, Pretzel variations require two sequences of the basic step pattern, with each part containing 7 steps, completed in 6 syncopated beats of music. In Part A, according to Grandma's pretzel recipe, the man makes a Half Left Holding Turn in one step forward on beat 6 (step 7). The woman, on the other hand, makes a Half Right Holding Underarm Turn in two steps forward on beats 5-6 (steps 6-7). Although the woman makes a holding (two-hand) underarm turn, the man merely pivots around to face in the opposite direction.

In Part B, partners unwind from the Pretzel by reversing the direction of their turns. Thus, in one step forward on beat 2 (step 2) the man makes a Half Right Holding Turn, as the woman makes a Half Left Holding Underarm Turn. 👯

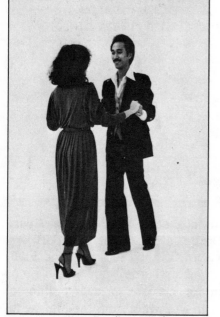

part A **step 5** (beat 4)

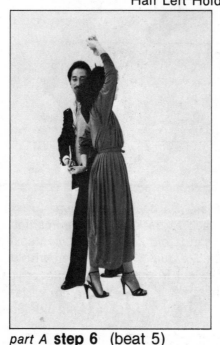

part A **step 6** (beat 5)

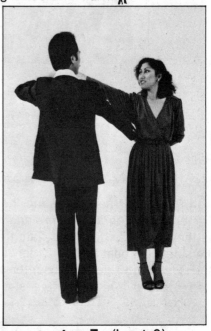

part A **step 7** (beat 6)

Part A: PRETZEL

Part A of the Pretzel begins on beats 1-4 (steps 1-5) with the Basic Holding Pattern. On beat 4 (step 5), however, the man gives the woman a hand lead for the *right two-hand hold*, as the man uplifts the woman's right hand in his left hand, while pushing her right hand outside or away from her face. At the same time, the man uses his right hand to keep the woman's left hand pinned behind her back.

Although both partners make dual half holding turns, the woman turns one beat *before* the man turns. Thus, on beats 5-6 (steps 6-7) the woman makes her Half Right Holding Underarm Turn (180 degrees clockwise) in 2 steps forward. While the woman is turning, her right hand, clenched in the man's left hand, rotates clockwise over her head. As the woman begins her turn on beat 5 (step 6), the man takes one step in place. One microwave second later on beat 6 (step 7), the man completes his Half Left Holding Turn (180 degrees counter-clockwise) in 1 step forward. After partners have completed their dual half holding turns in opposite directions, they should be twisted in the Right Parallel Position, with the woman's right side parallel to the man's right side. 👯

Part B:
UNWIND TO HOLDING
DANCE POSITION

Although most gastronomical mistakes end up in the garbage can, the Pretzel is versatile enough to be undone with dual half turns in the reverse direction. On beat 1 (step 1) partners prepare to unwind by tapping, while they are still twisted in the Right Parallel Position. As they tap, the man gives the woman a hand lead for the *right two-hand hold,* as he lifts the woman's right hand in his left hand, without releasing her left hand from his right hand.

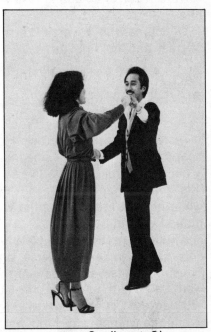

part B **step 3** (beat 3)

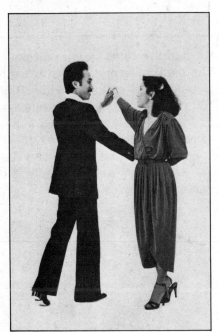

part B **step 1** (beat 1)

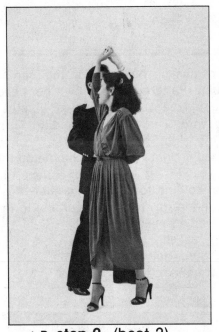

part B **step 2** (beat 2)

On beat 2 (step 2) partners unwind by making dual half holding turns in opposite directions. Of course, both partners now *reverse* the direction of their previous turns. Thus, the man makes a Half Right Holding Turn (180 degrees clockwise) in one step forward. The woman, on the other hand, makes a Half Left Holding Underarm Turn (180 degrees counter-clockwise) in one step forward. While the woman is turning, her left hand, uplifted by the man's right hand, rotates counter-clockwise over her head. After the dancing gormandizers have finished their dual half holding turns, they complete their basic steps on beats 3-6 (steps 3-7) in the Holding Dance Position. 🎵

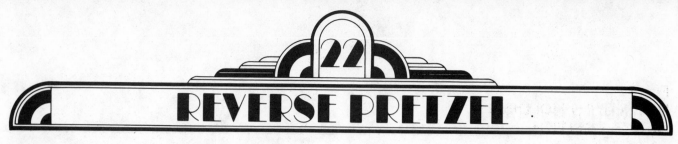

REVERSE PRETZEL

As the name implies the REVERSE PRETZEL is the opposite of a Pretzel. (How original!) Of course, we were tempted to call this variation something bizarre, such as Kamala Keel. Nevertheless, we reluctantly succumbed to plain donkey sense that, regardless of any highfalutin name, the Reverse Pretzel is, and always will be, the flip side of a Pretzel.

Of course, the Reverse Pretzel is also concocted of dual half holding turns. In Part A the woman makes a Half Left Holding Underarm Turn in two steps forward on beats 5-6 (steps 6-7). The man, on the other hand, makes a Half Right Holding Turn in one step forward on beat 6 (step 7). In Part B, partners unwind from the Reverse Pretzel by reversing the direction of their dual turns. Thus, in one step forward on beat 2 (step 2) the woman makes a Half Right Holding Underarm Turn, and the man makes a Half Left Holding Turn. 🕺

Part A:
REVERSE PRETZEL

Part A of the Reverse Pretzel begins on beats 1-4 (steps 1-5) with the Basic Holding Pattern. On beat 4 (step 5), however, the man gives the woman a hand lead for the *left two-hand hold*. The man lifts the woman's left hand in his right hand, while his left hand keeps the woman's right hand pinned behind her back.

Although partners complete dual holding turns, only the woman completes an underarm turn. Thus, on beats 5-6 (steps 6-7) the woman makes a Half Left Holding Underarm Turn, as she turns 180 degrees counter-clockwise in 2 steps forward. While the woman is turning, her left hand, clasped in the man's right hand, rotates counter-clockwise over her head. The man takes one step in place on beat 5 (step 6), before he makes a Half Right Holding Turn (180 degrees clockwise) in one step forward on beat 6 (step 7). After partners have completed their dual half holding turns in opposite directions, they should be twisted in the Left Parallel Position, with the woman's left side parallel to the man's left side. 🕺

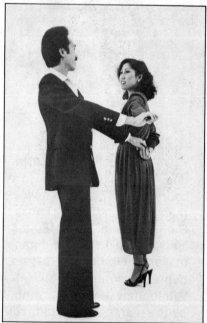

part A **step 7** (beat 6)

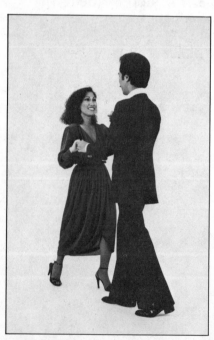

part A **step 5** (beat 4)

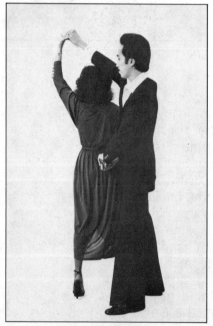

part A **step 6** (beat 5)

Part B:
UNWIND TO HOLDING
DANCE POSITION

It should not take the IQ of an Einstein to figure out how to unwind from a Reverse Pretzel. But, then again, Einstein was probably a lousy dancer. In any case, to unwind, partners reverse the direction of their dual half holding turns. Before unwinding, however, partners tap in the Left Parallel Position. While they are tapping, the man gives the woman a hand lead for the *left two-hand hold* by lifting the woman's left hand in his right hand, but he keeps her right hand pinned down with his left hand.

On beat 2 (step 2) partners unwind with dual half holding turns in opposite directions. This time, the man makes a Half Left Holding Turn, as he pivots 180 degrees counter-clockwise in one step forward. Conversely, the woman makes a Half Right Holding Underarm Turn, as she pivots 180 degrees clockwise in one step forward. While the woman is turning, her left hand, uplifted by the man's right hand, rotates clockwise over her head. After unwinding, partners complete their basic steps on beats 3-6 (steps 3-7) in the Holding Dance Position. 🕺

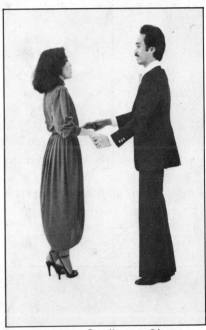

part B **step 3** (beat 3)

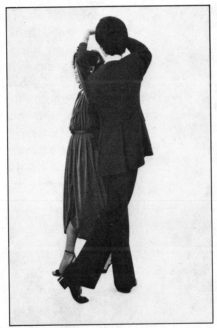

part B **step 2** (beat 2)

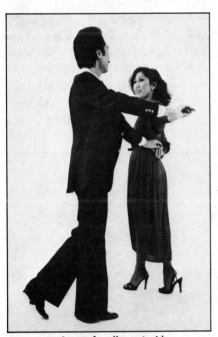

part B **step 1** (beat 1)

The CORKSCREW twists the Pretzel into Reverse Underarm Turns. This variation begins in Part A with the Pretzel in which the man and the woman make dual half holding turns in opposite directions. In Part B this variation concludes with Reverse (Inside) Underarm Turns, as partners move from the Right Parallel Position to the Open Position. 🦶

Part A:
PRETZEL

Part A of the Corkscrew starts off on beats 1-4 (steps 1-5) with the Basic Holding Pattern. On beat 4 (step 5), however, the man gives the woman a hand lead for the *right two-hand hold*. Thus, with his left hand the man lifts and pushes outside the woman's right hand, but he keeps her left hand pinned behind her back with his right hand.

On beats 5-6 (steps 6-7) partners whip into their Pretzel by making dual half holding turns in opposite directions. The woman, of course, starts to turn first, as she completes her Half Right Holding Underarm Turn (180 degrees clockwise) in two steps forward. While the woman is turning, her right hand, uplifted by the man's left hand, rotates clockwise over her head. After the man steps in place on beat 6 (step 7), he makes his Half Left Holding Turn (180 degrees counter-clockwise) in one step forward on beat 6 (step 7). After both partners have completed their turns, they should be twisted into the Right Parallel Position, with the woman's right side parallel to the man's right side. 🦶

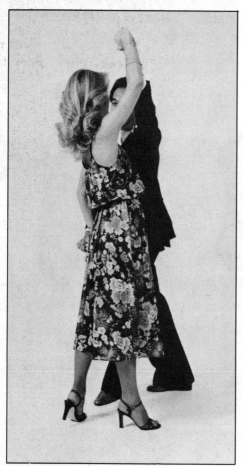

part A **step 6**   (beat 5)

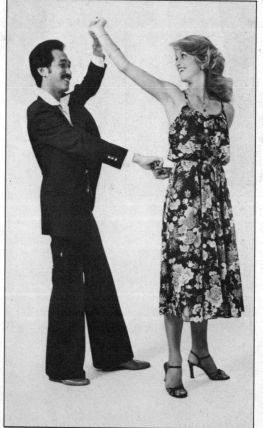

part A
step 7   (beat 6)

Part B:
CORKSCREW (TWO REVERSE UNDERARM TURNS)

In Part B, partners unwind from the Pretzel to the Open Position. On beat 1 (step 1) partners tap, while wrenched in the Right Parallel Position. On beat 2 (step 2) partners step side, as the man gives the woman a hand lead for the *right one-hand hold*. Thus, the man uplifts the woman's right hand in his left hand, as he simultaneously releases her left hand from his right hand.

On the triple step (beats 3 & 4) the man takes two steps back, then one step forward in the Open Position. The woman, on the other hand, zips through a Reverse (Inside) Underarm Turn by circling 360 degrees counter-clockwise in three small steps back. On beats 5-6 (steps 6-7), the man takes two steps forward as the woman twirls through another Reverse (Inside) Underarm Turn by circling 360 degrees counter-clockwise in two steps back. While the woman is turning, her right hand, loosely clasped in the man's left hand, rotates counter-clockwise over her head.

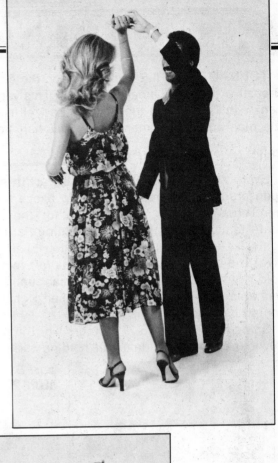

part B **step 3** (beat 3)

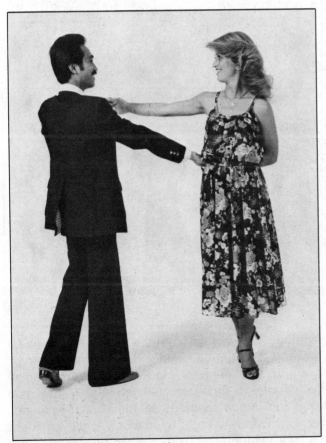

part B **step 1** (beat 1)

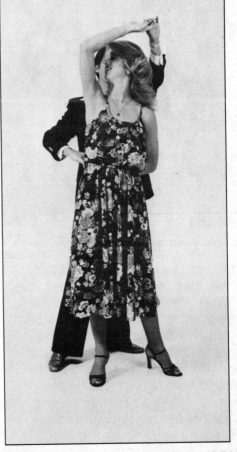

part B
step 2 (beat 2)

NEW YORK-LATIN HUSTLE

TORNADO TWIRLS

TORNADO TWIRLS swirl together the Reverse Pretzel with Right Underarm Turns. This variation begins in Part A with the Reverse Pretzel in which the man and the woman make dual half holding turns in opposite directions. In Part B, however, this variation concludes with two Right (Outside) Underarm Turns, as partners move from the Left Parallel Position into the Open Position. ♣

Part A: REVERSE PRETZEL

Every spring the mythical Disco Earth Festival sponsors a special event, known to dance fans as the Tornado Twirls. To warm up for the event, contestants practice their Basic Holding Pattern on beats 1-4 (steps 1-5). On beat 4 (step 5) the man gives the woman a hand lead for the *left two-hand hold*. With his right hand, the man uplifts the woman's left hand, but he pins her right hand behind her back with his left hand.

On beats 5-6 (steps 6-7) partners whirl into their Reverse Pretzel with dual half holding turns. The woman, of course, starts a beat ahead of the man, as she makes her Half Left Holding Underarm Turn by rotating 180 degrees counter-clockwise in two steps forward. While the woman is turning, her left hand rotates counter-clockwise over her head. Although the man hesitates for one beat of music to step in place on beat 5 (step 6), he makes up for lost time on his Half Right Holding Turn by spinning 180 degrees clockwise in one step forward on beat 6 (step 7). After partners have completed their turns, they should be twisted in the Left Parallel Position, with the woman's left side parallel to the man's left side. ♣

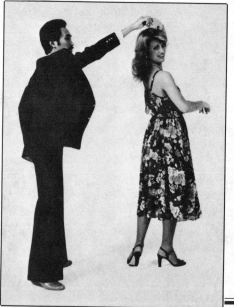

part B **step 2** (beat 2)

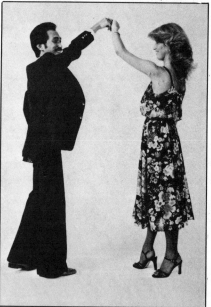

part B **step 3** (beat 3)

part B **step 1** (beat 1)

Part B: TORNADO TWIRLS

Once locked in the Left Parallel Position, contestants tap their feet impatiently on beat 1 (step 1), as they await the referee's whistle. On beat 2 (step 2) they position themselves with side steps, while the man gives the woman a hand lead for the *left one-hand hold*. Thus, the man lifts the woman's left hand in his right hand, but he releases her right hand from his left hand.

On the triple step (beats 3 & 4), the Tornado contest reaches a peak of frenzy, as the man takes two steps back, then one step forward in the Open Position. The woman, on the other hand, twirls through a Right (Outside) Underarm Turn by spinning 360 degrees clockwise in three small steps forward. On beats 5-6 (steps 6-7) the man takes two steps forward, as the woman expends her whirlwind energy by making another Right (Outside) Underarm Turn by spinning 360 degrees clockwise in two steps forward. While the woman is turning, her left hand, loosely clasped in the man's right hand, rotates clockwise over her head. ♣

CHAPTER 5

SALSA VARIATIONS

Although the Spanish word SALSA means "sauce," in dance, the word applies to Latin music of the 1970s which contains Latin rhythms spiced with jazz and disco rhythms. Most dance instructors agree that Salsa was originally the name for a certain type of music, rather than the name for a dance. Nevertheless, there has evolved a group of dances that have been loosely labelled "Salsa" by contemporary dancers.

Skippy Blair has isolated four distinct Salsa styles: *Salsa Valiente, Salsa Picado, Newporter Salsa,* and *Salsa Suave. Salsa Valiente,* known as the "Rope" in street jargon, contains a series of double rhythm or walking steps, with one step taken on each beat of music. Many patterns that fall into this category have also been called Disco Merengue or Merengue Hustle, because the patterns bear a strong resemblance to the Merengue. *Salsa Picado,* on the other hand, contains triple rhythm steps with a rock or break on the "and" count between the beats. Although the *Salsa Picado* resembles the Mambo, there are distinct differences in terms of movement and timing.

In the *Newporter Salsa* and the *Boston Salsa,* commonly called "Disco Swing," double rhythm steps are alternated with triple rhythm steps. *Salsa Suave,* a rarely performed dance, is a stylistic variation of Mambolero or International Rumba. The first three types of Salsa variations are discussed in this chapter. ♠

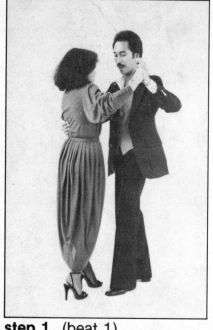

step 1 (beat 1)

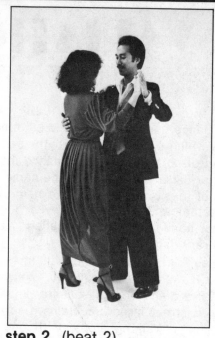

step 2 (beat 2)

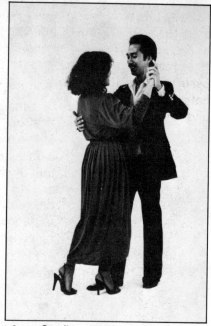

step 3 (beat 3)

One basic Salsa pattern, which is often lumped into the mythical category called "Disco Merengue" or "Merengue Hustle," is the FOUR COUNT HUSTLE. The Four Count Hustle, which can be performed in either the Closed or Holding Dance Position, consists of 4 steps, completed in 4 beats (1 measure) of music. Although the pattern begins sedately enough with a forward or back step, followed with a side step, it concludes with a splash of class through the addition of rock or ball-change steps.

On beat 1 (step 1) the man steps forward on his left foot, as the woman steps back on her right foot. On beat 2 (step 2), the man steps to his right side on his right foot, as the woman steps to her left side on her left foot.

To conclude the pattern, however, the man completes a back rock on beats 3-4 (steps 3-4), as the woman completes a forward rock. On beat 3 (step 3), therefore, the man steps back on his left foot, as the woman steps forward on her right foot. On beat 4 (step 4) partners complete their rock or ball-change steps, as the man steps in place on his right foot, while the woman steps in place on her left foot. Moreover, a slight rocking motion should be emphasized as partners transfer their weight from one foot to the opposite foot.

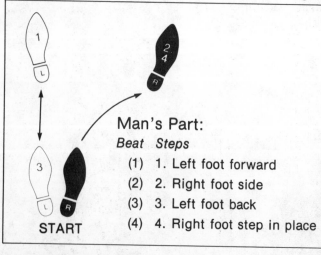

Man's Part:

Beat Steps

(1) 1. Left foot forward

(2) 2. Right foot side

(3) 3. Left foot back

(4) 4. Right foot step in place

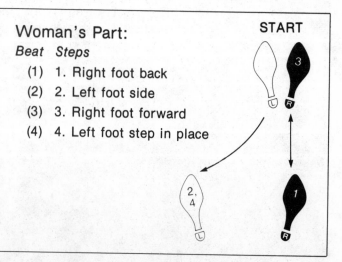

Woman's Part:

Beat Steps

(1) 1. Right foot back

(2) 2. Left foot side

(3) 3. Right foot forward

(4) 4. Left foot step in place

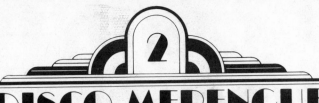

DISCO MERENGUE

One basic Salsa pattern, nicknamed DISCO MERENGUE or MERENGUE HUSTLE, contains a sequence of 4 steps, completed in 4 beats (1 measure) of music. The entire step pattern, performed in the Holding Dance Position, alternates forward and close forward steps with back and close back steps. Notice that after each step taken either forward or backward, feet are drawn into the parallel (close) position.

Moreover, on each forward step, the man gently pulls the woman towards him. Conversely, on each back step, the man gently pushes the woman away from him. This entire pattern, in which one step is taken on each beat of music, may be repeated *ad infinitum.*

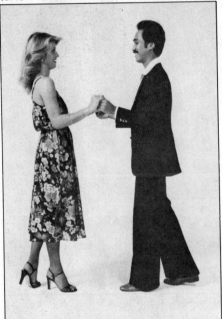

step 1 (beat 1)

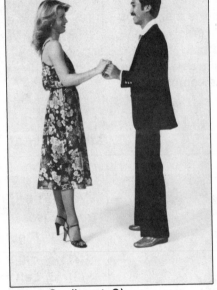

step 2 (beat 2)

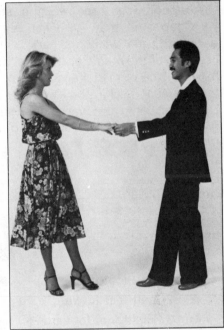

step 3 (beat 3)

Man's Part:

Beat Steps

(1) 1. Left foot forward

(2) 2. Right foot close to left foot

(3) 3. Left foot back

(4) 4. Right foot close to left foot

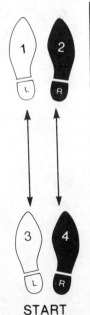

START

Woman's Part:

Beat Steps

(1) 1. Right foot forward

(2) 2. Left foot close to right foot

(3) 3. Right foot back

(4) 4. Left foot close to right foot

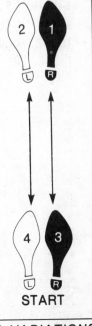

START

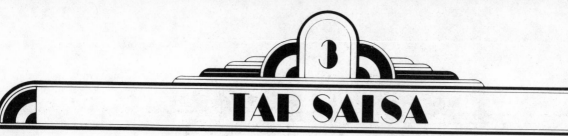

TAP SALSA

The TAP SALSA, another double rhythm variation, starts each measure of music with a tap step, which is followed with three walk steps. Consequently, on the first beat count, partners tap one foot to the side (tap side). Since the foot that taps will be the foot that steps on the next beat of music, this tap step also signals a change in the step direction.

Although the three walking steps that follow each tap step may be taken either forward or backward, the woman's part is still the natural opposite of the man's part. Thus, as the man steps forward, the woman steps back; conversely, as the man steps back, the woman steps forward. Moreover, any turn variations, such as a Cradle (Wrap-Around) or Pretzel, should be completed on the three walk steps.

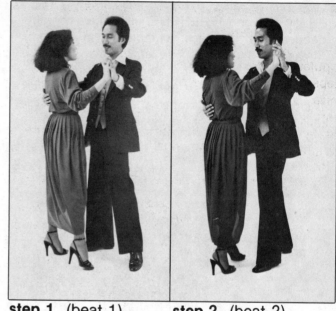

step 1 (beat 1)   **step 2** (beat 2)

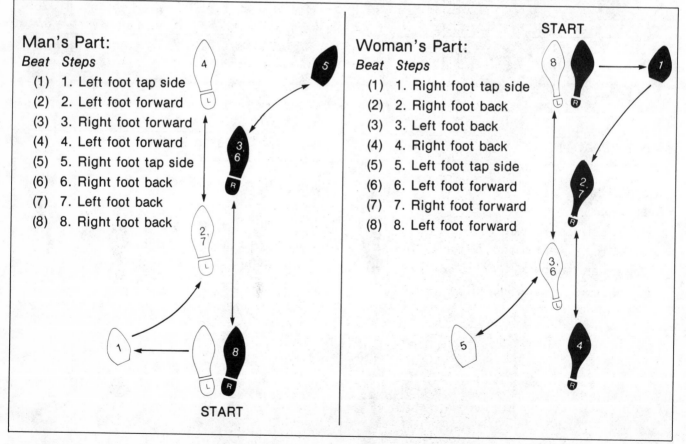

Man's Part:

Beat   Steps

(1)   1. Left foot tap side
(2)   2. Left foot forward
(3)   3. Right foot forward
(4)   4. Left foot forward
(5)   5. Right foot tap side
(6)   6. Right foot back
(7)   7. Left foot back
(8)   8. Right foot back

START

Woman's Part:

Beat   Steps

(1)   1. Right foot tap side
(2)   2. Right foot back
(3)   3. Left foot back
(4)   4. Right foot back
(5)   5. Left foot tap side
(6)   6. Left foot forward
(7)   7. Right foot forward
(8)   8. Left foot forward

START

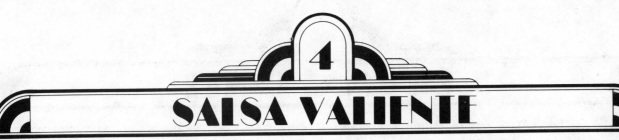

SALSA VALIENTE

SALSA VALIENTE, nicknamed "The Rope," is lifted from a social dance form that has been popular in Mexico for decades. Composed of 8 steps, completed in 8 beats (2 measures) of music, Salsa Valiente consists of double rhythm or marching steps taken forward and backward. Skippy Blair suggests that the dancer imitate "the upright posture of a matador, picking up his feet with every step."

To accentuate the rolling motion of this Salsa variation, partners bend their knees on the first beat count of each measure of music, then gradually straighten their knees on the next three beat counts. Moreover, this Salsa variation has been dubbed "The Rope" because of the unusual arm movements in which partners swing one set of arms out to the side, then swing them in and up from bent elbows, before swinging them down and repeating the movement with the other set of arms.

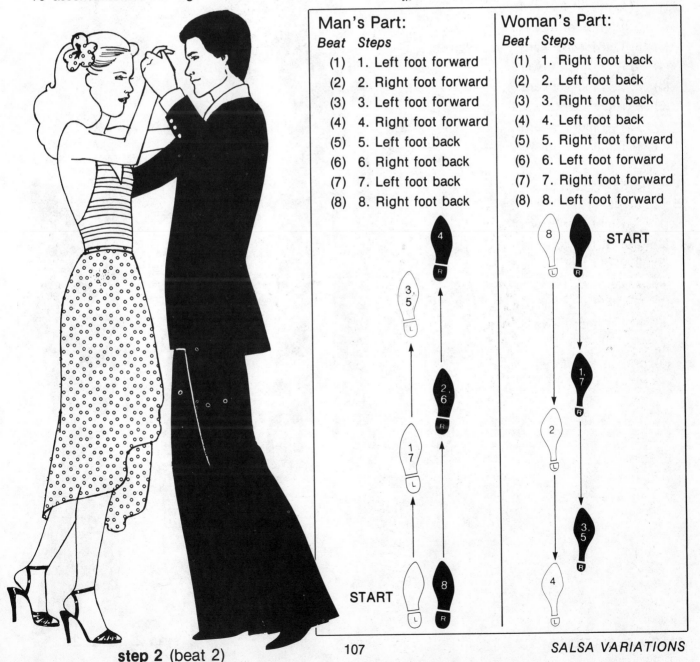

Man's Part:

Beat   *Steps*

(1)   1. Left foot forward
(2)   2. Right foot forward
(3)   3. Left foot forward
(4)   4. Right foot forward
(5)   5. Left foot back
(6)   6. Right foot back
(7)   7. Left foot back
(8)   8. Right foot back

Woman's Part:

Beat   *Steps*

(1)   1. Right foot back
(2)   2. Left foot back
(3)   3. Right foot back
(4)   4. Left foot back
(5)   5. Right foot forward
(6)   6. Left foot forward
(7)   7. Right foot forward
(8)   8. Left foot forward

step 2 (beat 2)

107

SALSA VARIATIONS

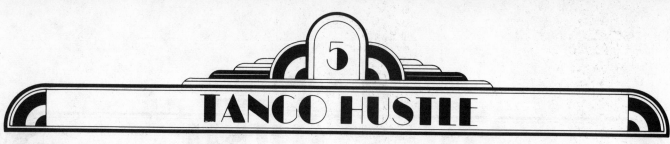

TANGO HUSTLE

The TANGO HUSTLE, another double rhythm Salsa variation, is characterized by a smooth, sensual elegance. Unlike the ballroom version of the Tango, which contains a 5 step pattern, the Tango Hustle contains an 8 step sequence, completed in 8 beats (2 measures) of music. Among dance enthusiasts, such as Buddy Schwimmer, a former rock and disco dance champion, the Tango Hustle has been dubbed "Nightclub Fox Trot." In the basic pattern for the Tango Hustle, both partners progress in a forward (or backward) direction, while they are embraced in the Promenade Dance Position (Closed Position, with the woman's left hip parallel to the man's right hip).

Man's Part:

Beat Steps

- (1) 1. Left foot forward
- (2) 2. Right foot forward
- (3) 3. Left foot forward
- (4) 4. Right foot forward
- (5) 5. Left foot forward
- (6) 6. Right foot forward
- (7) 7. Left foot forward
- (8) 8. Right foot forward

Woman's Part:

Beat Steps

- (1) 1. Right foot forward
- (2) 2. Left foot forward
- (3) 3. Right foot forward
- (4) 4. Left foot forward
- (5) 5. Right foot forward
- (6) 6. Left foot forward
- (7) 7. Right foot forward
- (8) 8. Left foot forward

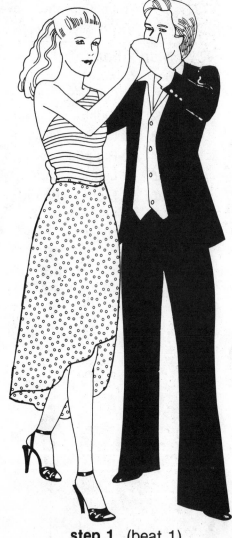

step 1 (beat 1)

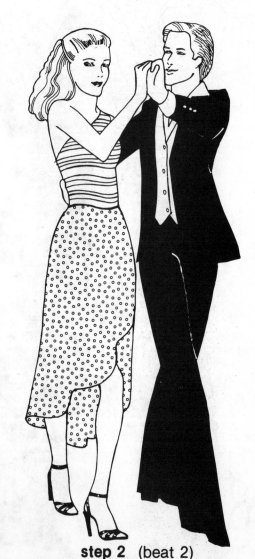

step 2 (beat 2)

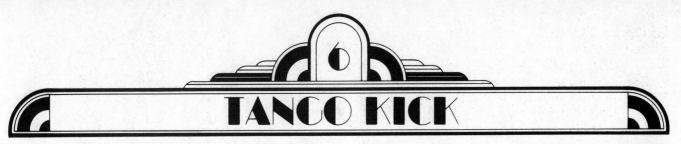

TANGO KICK

The TANGO KICK combines double rhythm (walk) steps with single rhythm (kick) steps in this 10 step pattern, completed in 8 beats (2 measures) of music. To add a dash of class, each partner kicks one foot forward on the last beat count of each measure of music. Thus, the man kicks his right foot forward, as the woman kicks her left foot forward. After kicking forward, then swinging their feet back into the parallel (close) position, partners continue their forward progression in the Promenade Position.

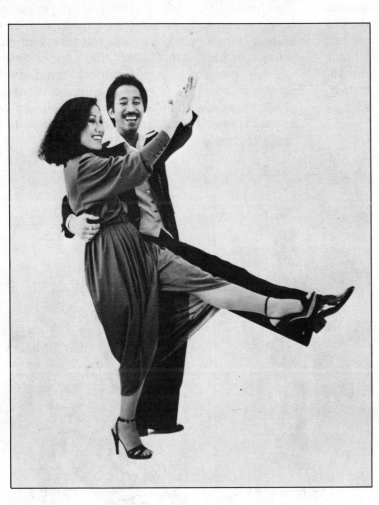

Man's Part:
Beat Steps
- (1) 1. Left foot forward
- (2) 2. Right foot forward
- (3) 3. Left foot forward
- (&) 4. Right foot kick forward
- (4) 5. Right foot swing (close) back
- (5) 6. Left foot forward
- (6) 7. Right foot forward
- (7) 8. Left foot forward
- (&) 9. Right foot kick forward
- (8) 10. Right foot swing (close) back

Woman's Part:
Beat Steps
- (1) 1. Right foot forward
- (2) 2. Left foot forward
- (3) 3. Right foot forward
- (&) 4. Left foot kick forward
- (4) 5. Left foot swing (close) back
- (5) 6. Right foot forward
- (6) 7. Left foot forward
- (7) 8. Right foot forward
- (&) 9. Left foot kick forward
- (8) 10. Left foot swing (close) back

TANGO DIP

Almost all Tango dancers, from Valentino to Travolta, have found the TANGO DIP irresistible. Although the sequence of steps for the Tango Hustle differs slightly from the ballroom version, the movement for the dip remains essentially the same. The pattern begins on beats 1-2 (steps 1-2) with two steps forward for the man, and two steps back for the woman. On beats 3-4 (steps 3-4), the man steps back on his left foot, bends his left knee, and dips or leans his torso back, then holds the dip position for one beat of music. The woman, on the other hand, steps forward on her right foot, bends her right knee, and dips or leans slightly forward, then holds the dip position for one beat of music. Notice that on the dip and "hold," the man's weight is sustained on his left foot, but the woman's weight is sustained on her right foot.

On beats 5-6 (steps 5-6), partners step in place, as they straighten their knees and return to an upright position. Thus, the man steps in place with his right foot and shifts his weight forward, as the woman steps in place with her left foot, and shifts her weight back. After holding the upright position for one beat of music, partners complete the pattern on beats 7-8 (steps 7-8) with a close step in which they draw their feet together, followed with a step in place, as they transfer their weight to the opposite foot.

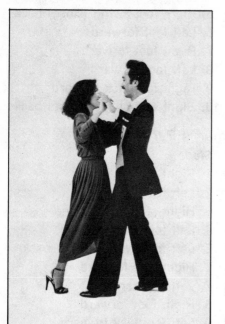

step 1 (beat 1)

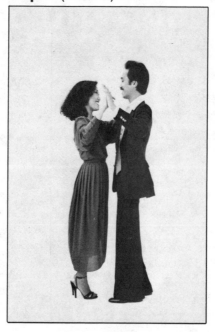

step 2 (beat 2)

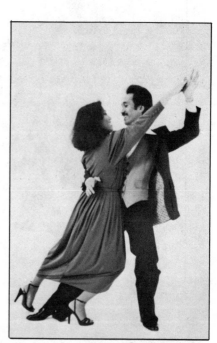

step 3 (beat 3)

Man's Part:
Beat   Steps

(1)   1. Left foot forward
(2)   2. Right foot forward
(3)   3. Left foot back, bend left knee, and dip back
(4)   4. Left foot hold dip position
(5)   5. Right foot step in place, straighten knee and torso
(6)   6. Right foot hold upright position
(7)   7. Left foot close to right foot
(8)   8. Right foot step in place

Woman's Part:

(1)   1. Right foot back
(2)   2. Left foot close to right foot
(3)   3. Right foot forward, bend right knee, and dip forward
(4)   4. Right foot hold dip position
(5)   5. Left foot step in place, straighten knee and torso
(6)   6. Left foot hold upright position
(7)   7. Right foot close to left foot
(8)   8. Left foot step in place

CUBAN SALSA

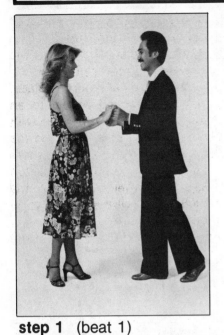

step 1 (beat 1)

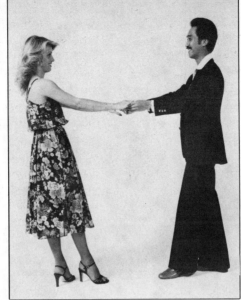

step 3 (beat 3)

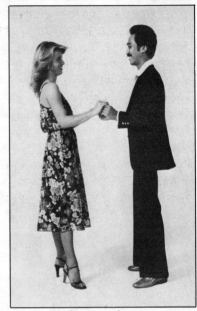

step 5 (beat 4)

The CUBAN SALSA is the current rage in some areas of the country, particularly in Chicago. Moreover, in terms of structure, this Salsa variation bears a vague resemblance to the New York-Latin Hustle. Nevertheless, the Cuban Salsa contains a unique 5 step pattern, completed in 4 syncopated beats (1 measure) of music.

The pattern for the Cuban Salsa begins on beats 1-2 (steps 1-2) with a tap step, followed with a close step. On beat 1 (step 1), the man taps his left foot behind his right foot, but keeps his weight balanced on his right foot; conversely, the woman taps her right foot behind her left foot, but keeps her weight balanced on her left foot. On beat 2 (step 2), the man closes his left foot to his right foot and transfers his weight to his left foot, as the woman closes her right foot to her left foot and

transfers her weight to her right foot.

The Cuban Salsa concludes with a triple step in which three steps (steps 3-5) are completed in two syncopated beats of music (beats 3 and 4). In addition, the triple step begins with a back rock or ball-change steps. Thus, on step 3, the man steps back on his right foot, as the woman steps back on her left foot. On step 4, partners shift their weight to their forward foot, as the man steps in place on his left foot, and the woman steps in place on her right foot. The triple step concludes with a close forward step in which partners draw their feet into the parallel (close) position. The man, therefore, closes his right foot to his left foot and transfers his weight to his right foot, while the woman closes her left foot to her right foot and transfers her weight to her left foot.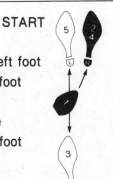

Man's Part:	START
Beat	*Steps*
(1)	1. Left foot tap behind right foot
(2)	2. Left foot close to right foot
(3)	3. Right foot back
(&)	4. Left foot step in place
(4)	5. Right foot close to left foot

Woman's Part:	START
Beat	*Steps*
(1)	1. Right foot tap behind left foot
(2)	2. Right foot close to left foot
(3)	3. Left foot step back
(&)	4. Right foot step in place
(4)	5. Left foot close to right foot

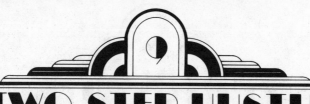

TWO-STEP HUSTLE

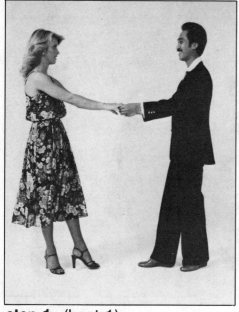

step 1 (beat 1)

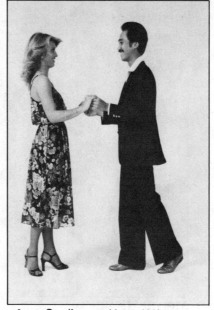

step 2 (beat "and")

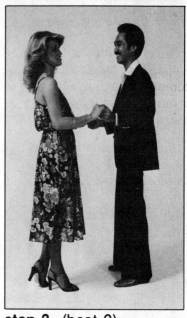

step 3 (beat 2)

The TWO-STEP HUSTLE is a favorite among disco fans who revel in a fast, bouncy dancing style. The name tagged onto this partner dance is taken from the two quick steps of the triple step. A triple step contains three steps, completed in two syncopated beats of music.

In the Two-Step Hustle each triple step begins on the odd-numbered beat counts, with a pass back or fifth position step, as partners cross one foot behind the opposite foot. Each pass back step is followed with a step in place on the forward foot on the syncopated "and" counts. A slight rocking motion should be accented, as partners shift their weight from the back foot to the forward foot. Each triple step concludes on the even-numbered beat counts with a side step. In the Two-Step Hustle, the body motion is up-down-up (down), with an "up" movement on each whole-numbered count, and a "down" movement on each syncopated "and" count.

Man's Part:

Beat	Steps
(1)	1. Left foot cross behind right foot
(&)	2. Right foot step in place
(2)	3. Left foot side
(3)	4. Right foot cross behind left foot
(&)	5. Left foot step in place
(4)	6. Right foot side

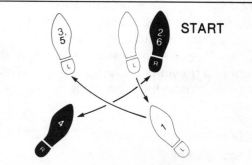

Woman's Part:

Beat	Steps
(1)	1. Right foot cross behind left foot
(&)	2. Left foot step in place
(2)	3. Right foot side
(3)	4. Left foot cross behind right foot
(&)	5. Right foot step in place
(4)	6. Left foot side

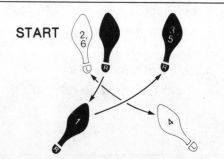

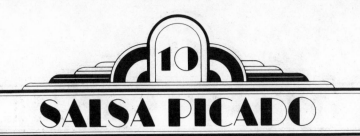

The SALSA PICADO contains a basic pattern of 6 steps, completed in 4 syncopated beats (1 measure) of music. Due to its unusual sequence of steps, the Salsa Picado has, on occasion, been compared to the Mambo, a Cuban dance which combined Latin American and jazz rhythms. Nevertheless, the Salsa Picado retains its own unique movement and timing.

The pattern, according to dance instructor Skippy Blair, contains "triple rhythm units with the 'rock' or 'break' on the 'and' count between the beats." The first triple step of the pattern begins with ball-change steps, as the man completes a forward rock, and the woman completes a back rock. The man, therefore, steps forward with his left foot, then steps in place on his right foot, as the woman steps back on her right foot, then steps in place on her left foot. The triple step concludes as partners draw their feet into the parallel (close) position, then "hold" the position for the "and" count between beats.

In the second half of the pattern, which begins with another triple rhythm step, partners reverse parts. Thus, on the ball-change steps, the man completes a back rock, as the woman completes a forward rock. Consequently, the man steps back on his right foot, then steps in place on his left foot, as the woman steps forward on her left foot, then steps in place on her right foot.

The pattern concludes with a close step in which partners draw their feet into the parallel (close) position, then "hold" the position for the final "and" count between the beats.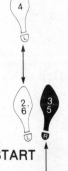

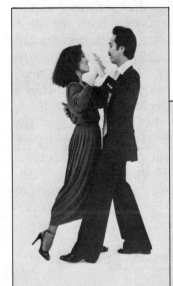

step 4 (beat 3)

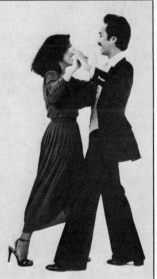

step 5 (beat "and")

Man's Part :

Beat Steps

- (1) 1. Left foot forward
- (&) 2. Right foot step in place
- (2) 3. Left foot close to right foot
- (3) 4. Right foot back
- (&) 5. Left foot step in place
- (4) 6. Right foot close to left foot

Woman's Part:

Beat Steps

- (1) 1. Right foot back
- (&) 2. Left foot step in place
- (2) 3. Right foot close to left foot
- (3) 4. Left foot forward
- (&) 5. Right foot step in place
- (4) 6. Left foot close to right foot

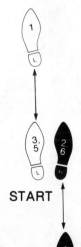

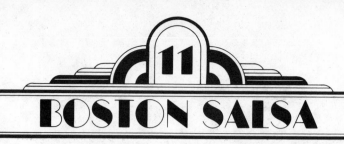

BOSTON SALSA

The BOSTON SALSA is, for the most part, a mirror image of the Newporter Salsa. Although developed in opposite areas of the country, both of these disco dances have acquired the informal street name, ''Disco Swing.'' Moreover, both of these dances contain 10 step patterns completed in 8 syncopated beats of music. Both patterns alternate double rhythm steps with triple rhythm steps. Both contain slightly different step sequences for the Closed and Holding Dance Positions. In fact, the only major difference between the Newporter Salsa and the Boston Salsa is the order in which the double steps are alternated with triple steps. Unlike the Newporter Salsa, the Boston Salsa begins with a triple step. The basic pattern for the Boston Salsa, therefore, alternates triple rhythm steps with double rhythm

steps. The change in step pattern corresponds, of course, to a reversal in the rhythm pattern.

The triple steps, completed on beats 1 and 2 (steps 1-3) and beats 5 and 6 (steps 6-8), may be taken either to the side (side, pass back, step in place) for the Closed Pattern or in the same direction (back, back, forward) for the Holding Pattern. The double steps, completed on beats 3-4 (steps 4-5) and beats 7-8 (steps 9-10) are walk steps which may be taken in opposite directions for the Closed Pattern or forward for the Holding Pattern. For all three patterns, completed in the Closed, Holding, or Open Dance Position, turn variations must be completed on the double rhythm walk steps. For suggestions on turn variations, glance at the chapter on the New York - Latin Hustle (Chapter 4). Notice that most turns, including Cradle, Pretzel, and Underarm Turns, can be done with the basic pattern for the Boston Salsa. 🕴

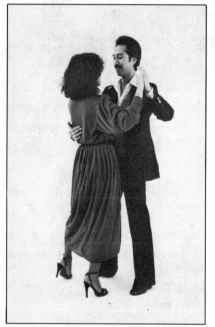

step 1 (beat 1)

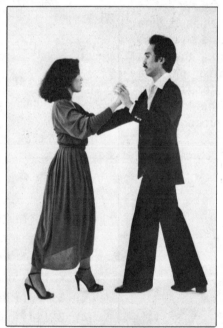

step 2 (beat ''and'')

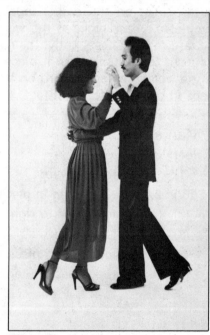

step 3 (beat 2)

Man's Part:

Beat *Steps*

- (1) 1. Left foot side
- (&) 2. Right foot pass back
  (cross behind left foot)
- (2) 3. Left foot step in place
- (3) 4. Right foot forward
- (4) 5. Left foot close to right foot
- (5) 6. Right foot side
- (&) 7. Left foot pass back
  (cross behind right foot)
- (6) 8. Right foot step in place
- (7) 9. Left foot back
- (8) 10. Right foot close to left foot

Woman's Part:

Beat *Steps*

- (1) 1. Right foot side
- (&) 2. Left foot pass back
  (cross behind right foot)
- (2) 3. Right foot step in place
- (3) 4. Left foot back
- (4) 5. Right foot close to left foot
- (5) 6. Left foot side
- (&) 7. Right foot pass back
  (cross behind left foot)
- (6) 8. Left foot step in place
- (7) 9. Right foot forward
- (8) 10. Left foot close to right foot

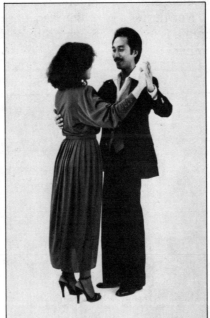

step 5 (beat 4)

step 4 (beat 3)

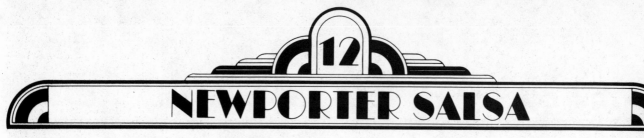

NEWPORTER SALSA

NEWPORTER SALSA is the West Coast version of a disco pattern quite similar to the Boston Salsa. Local legend insists that Bob and Sharon Bois first introduced this partner dance at the Newporter in Newport Beach. Similar to the Boston Salsa, the Newporter Salsa alternates double and triple rhythm steps. Unlike the Boston version, however, the Newporter Salsa begins with double rhythm steps, followed by triple rhythm steps. This is the one and only difference between the Boston Salsa and the Newporter Salsa. Thus, the Newporter Salsa, with its 10 step pattern, completed in 8 beats (2 measures) of music, is another blood relative, belonging to the street family called Disco Swing.

In the Newporter Salsa, all turn variations must be made on either the first or last set of walk steps, completed on beats 1-2 (steps 1-2) or on beats 5-6 (steps 6-7). Moreover, each turn variation should conclude with a triple step sequence. For suggestions on turn variations, glance at the chapter on the New York-Latin Hustle (Chapter 4), which contains a slew of turns which can easily be adapted to fit the Newporter Salsa pattern.

NEWPORTER SALSA IN CLOSED DANCE POSITION

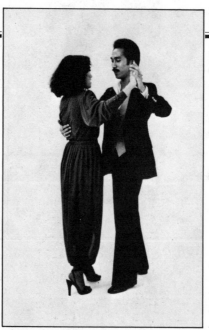

step 1 (beat 1)

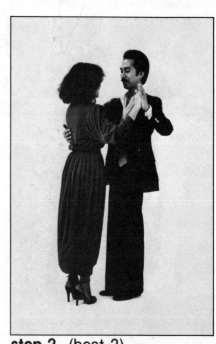

step 2 (beat 2)

The pattern for the NEWPORTER SALSA done in the Closed Dance Position alternates double rhythm with triple rhythm steps. On these double rhythm walk steps, taken on beats 1-2 (steps 1-2) and beats 5-6 (steps 6-7), partners either step in place or walk in opposite directions. If the man walks forward, therefore, the woman must walk back; conversely, if the man walks back, then the woman must walk forward. Alternated with the double steps are the triple steps, completed on beats 3 and 4 (steps 3-5) and beats 7 and 8 (steps 8-10). These triple steps begin with a side step, followed with a pass back (cross behind or fifth position) step, and conclude with a step in place on the forward foot.

Man's Part:

Beat Steps

(1) 1. Left foot forward

(2) 2. Right foot close to left foot

(3) 3. Left foot side

(&) 4. Right foot pass back
     (cross behind left foot)

(4) 5. Left foot step in place

(5) 6. Right foot back

(6) 7. Left foot close to right foot

(7) 8. Right foot side

(&) 9. Left foot pass back
     (cross behind right foot)

(8) 10. Right foot step in place

Woman's Part:

Beat Steps

(1) 1. Right foot back

(2) 2. Left foot close to right foot

(3) 3. Right foot side

(&) 4. Left foot pass back
     (cross behind right foot)

(4) 5. Right foot step in place

(5) 6. Left foot forward

(6) 7. Right foot close to left foot

(7) 8. Left foot side

(&) 9. Right foot pass back
     (cross behind left foot)

(8) 10. Left foot step in place

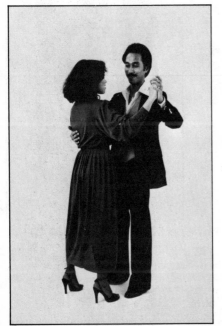

step 3 (beat 3)

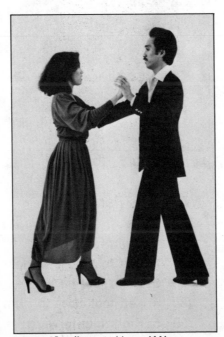

step 4 (beat "and")

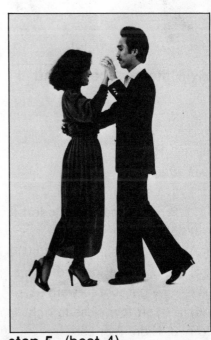

step 5 (beat 4)

SALSA VARIATIONS

Part B
NEWPORTER SALSA IN THE HOLDING DANCE POSITION

In most ways, the HOLDING PATTERN for the NEWPORTER SALSA is identical to the pattern completed in the Dance Position. Both contain 10 steps completed in 8 beats (2 measures) of music, alternating double rhythm with triple rhythm steps. Both contain walk steps on beats 1-2 (steps 1-2) and on beats 5-6 (steps 6-7), interspersed with triple steps on beats 3 and 4 (steps 3-5) and beats 7 and 8 (steps 8-10). Both patterns incorporate turn variations on the double rhythm walk steps.

Unlike the Closed Pattern, however, the Holding Pattern uses a different step sequence for both the double and triple rhythm steps. On the double rhythm walk steps, the man and the woman move in the same direction, although they begin stepping with opposite feet. On the two walk steps forward, therefore, partners walk towards each other. On the triple steps, both the man and the woman take two small steps back, then one small step forward, in two syncopated beats of music. On the two backward steps, the man gently pushes the woman away from him, then pulls her towards him on the forward step.

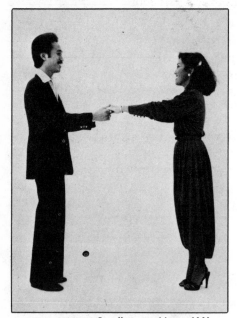

part B **step 4** (beat "and")

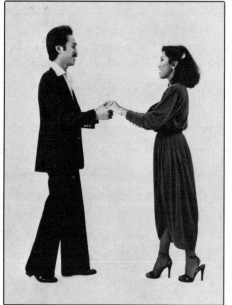

part B **step 5** (beat 4)

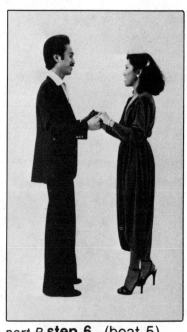

part B **step 6** (beat 5)

Man's Part:

Beat Steps

(1) 1. Left foot forward
(2) 2. Right foot close to left foot
(3) 3. Left foot back
(&) 4. Right foot close to left foot
(4) 5. Left foot forward
(5) 6. Right foot forward
(6) 7. Left foot close to right foot
(7) 8. Right foot back
(&) 9. Left foot close to right foot
(8) 10. Right foot forward

Woman's Part:

Beat Steps

(1) 1. Right foot forward
(2) 2. Left foot close to right foot
(3) 3. Right foot back
(&) 4. Left foot close to right foot
(4) 5. Right foot forward
(5) 6. Left foot forward
(6) 7. Right foot close to left foot
(7) 8. Left foot back
(&) 9. Right foot close to left foot
(8) 10. Left foot forward

CHAPTER 6

LATIN STREET HUSTLE

And now for something completely new and different — THE LATIN STREET HUSTLE. Unlike most other hustles which are, more or less, bowdlerized versions of social (ballroom) dances, the Latin Street Hustle is a genuine disco creation. The unique steps, the stomp, the hip swaying sensuality are all unique creations invented by disco dancers who snubbed conventional dance standards.

Who specifically created this original hustle? Nobody knows for sure (except maybe her hairdresser). Perhaps a strutter in LA, or a bopper in Philly, or a bumper in NYC, or a space cadet on Mars all met one dark, mysterious night and hustled their way into a never-before-seen dance. Somehow, somewhere, perhaps through the disco underground, the Latin Street Hustle hit Main Street USA.

While it popularized touch-dancing, it also introduced a unique step pattern that concluded with a triple (syncopated) step. In addition, it dropped the faint-hearted tap step, and added a foot-stomping stamp step. On top of it all, it adapted the hip swaying, knee bending, undulating Cuban motion to make this dance a sensual, as well as sensuous, experience. In short, the Latin Street Hustle ignited the fuse that fired today's disco explosion!

There is one important fact, however, that should be stored in the "little grey matter" that vegetates someplace upstairs: all turn variations made with the Latin Street Hustle must be completed on the first three beats of music (on beats 1-3). Ergo, you will make or break your turns on the first three steps (steps 1-3). Except for rare exceptions, such as Spot Turns, this rule will not change. 🕺

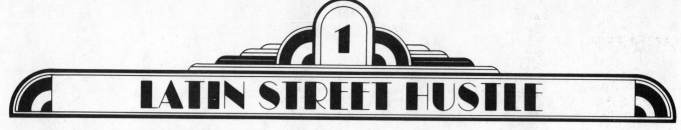

LATIN STREET HUSTLE

The LATIN STREET HUSTLE, similar to many other triple step hustles, contains 7 steps, completed in 6 beats of syncopated music. But there the same begins and ends, because the Latin Street Hustle is truly a unique experience. Unlike other triple step hustles, such as the New York-L.A. Hustle, the Latin Street Hustle contains an unusual sequence of steps in which the triple step is tacked onto the end (beats 5 & 6), rather than squashed into the middle of the pattern.

In addition, the basic sequence of steps barely resembles any other step pattern, past or present, at least in terms of other twentieth century partner dances. On the first 3 steps, completed in the first 3 beats of music (beats 1-3), the pattern begins tamely enough with two steps taken in place, followed by one walk forward step, turning 1/8 right (45 degrees clockwise). On step 4 (beat 4), however, a stamp forward step is slapped into the pattern.

Similar to the tap or toe step, the stamp forward step is made while the body weight is balanced on the opposite foot. Unlike the dainty

tap or toe steps in which the tip of the foot lightly brushes against the floor, the stamp forward step is made by stomping the sole of the right foot against the floor, although the left foot still holds the weight of the body. In addition, the stamp forward step is made while partners are standing in the right parallel position (right side by right side, and facing in opposite directions). Consequently, both the man and the woman will have to turn slightly to the right (about 1/8 right or 45 degrees clockwise), then stamp forward in the right parallel position.

Not surprisingly, the basic pattern concludes with a triple step (back/ back/ forward), completed in 2 beats of music (on beats 5 & 6). What is perhaps not so predictable, however, is the fact that the triple step begins with the right foot back: i.e., the foot that stamps forward is the same foot that steps back on the next beat of music. In addition, each of the two back steps is made while turning 1/8 left (45 degrees counter-clockwise), until partners have returned to their starting positions. The triple step concludes, therefore, with one small step forward in the Holding Position, with partners staring into each other's

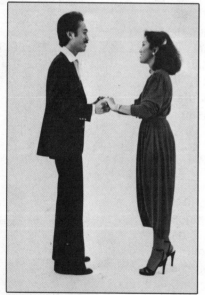

step 1 (beat 1)

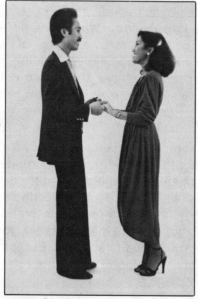

step 2 (beat 2)

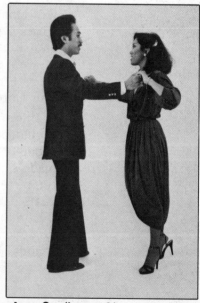

step 3 (beat 3)

Beat	Steps		Beat	Steps
(1)	1. Left foot step in place		(1)	1. Left foot step in place
(2)	2. Right foot step in place		(2)	2. Right foot step in place
(3)	3. Left foot forward, turning right		(3)	3. Left foot forward, turning right
(4)	4. Right foot stamp forward in Right Parallel Position		(4)	4. Right foot stamp forward in Right Parallel Position
(5)	5. Right foot back, turning left		(5)	5. Right foot back, turning left
(&)	6. Left foot close to right foot		(&)	6. Left foot close to right foot
(6)	7. Right foot forward		(6)	7. Right foot forward

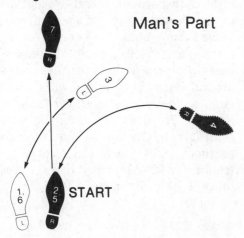

Man's Part

Woman's Part

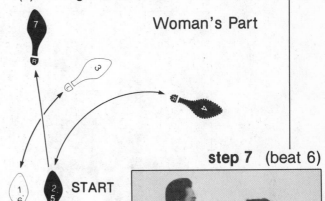

step 7 (beat 6)

fiery eyes.

Another fascinating, yet characteristic feature of the basic step pattern is that the woman's part duplicates the man's part. Although in most traditional touch dances, the woman's part is the natural opposite of the man's part, this is simply not true for the Latin Street Hustle. In fact, the woman's part duplicates the man's part, step for step, and movement for movement. 🕺

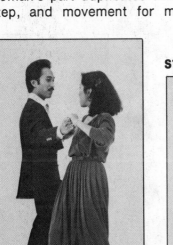

step 4 (beat 4)

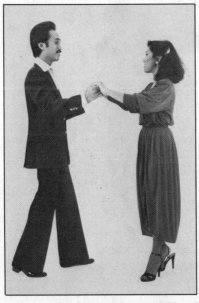

step 5 (beat 5)

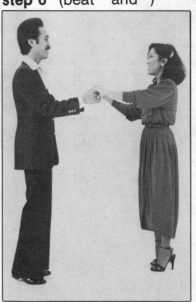

step 6 (beat "and")

121

The WALK AROUND RIGHT practically duplicates the step pattern used for the Basic Step: 7 steps, completed in 6 beats of music, with a triple step tacked onto the end of the pattern. In addition, the man will lead the woman into the Walk Around Right by gently pulling on her left hand with his right hand, without releasing either hand from the *two-hand hold*. The only major difference between these two patterns is that, for the Walk Around Right, each of the first 3 *walking steps*, completed on beats 1-3, is taken while turning right (clockwise). While walking forward, therefore, the man and the woman will rotate around each other and switch places. On beat 4 (step 4) they will still stamp forward in the Right Parallel Position (woman's right side by man's right side). On the triple step (beats 5 & 6) partners take two steps back, rotating left (counter-clockwise), then one step forward, moving towards each other.

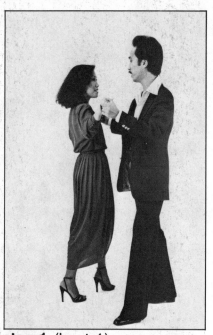

step 1 (beat 1)

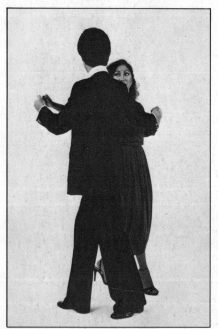

step 2 (beat 2)

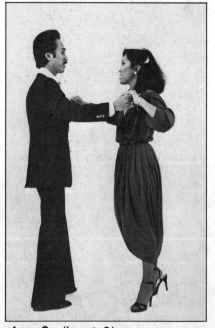

step 3 (beat 3)

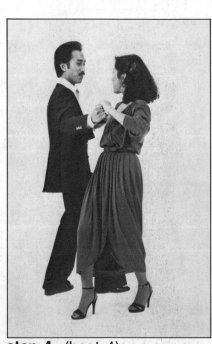

step 4 (beat 4)

Beat	Steps
(1)	1. Left foot forward, turning right
(2)	2. Right foot forward, turning right
(3)	3. Left foot forward, turning right
(4)	4. Right foot stamp forward in Right Parallel Position
(5)	5. Right foot back, turning left
(&)	6. Left foot close to right foot
(6)	7. Right foot forward

Man's Part:

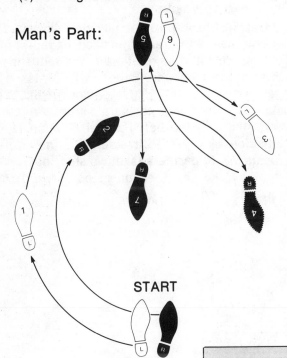

Beat	Steps
(1)	1. Left foot forward, turning right
(2)	2. Right foot forward, turning right
(3)	3. Left foot forward, turning right
(4)	4. Right foot stamp forward in Right Parallel Position
(5)	5. Right foot back, turning left
(&)	6. Left foot close to right foot
(6)	7. Right foot forward

Woman's Part:

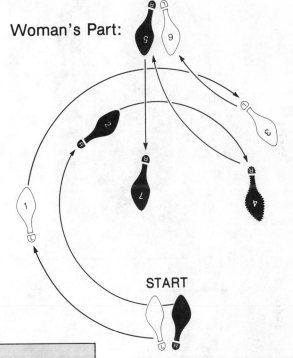

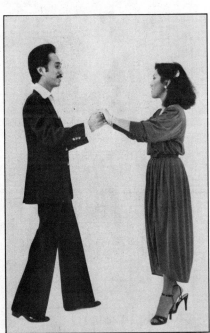

step 5 (beat 5)

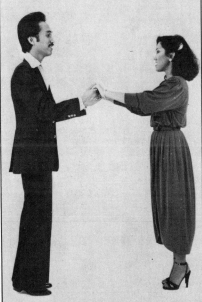

step 6 (beat ''and'')

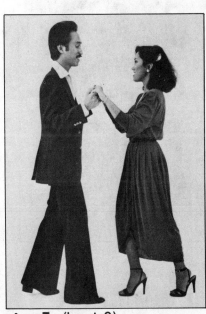

step 7 (beat 6)

LATIN STREET HUSTLE

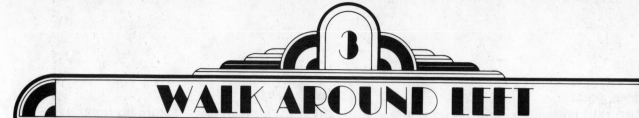

WALK AROUND LEFT

The WALK AROUND LEFT in the Latin Street Hustle is almost, but not quite, the same as the Walk Around Right. Yes, there will still be 7 steps,

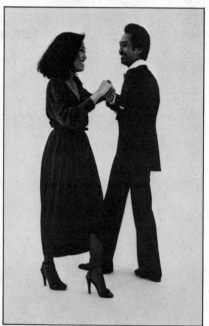

step 1 (beat 1)

completed in 6 beats of music. Yes, the sequence of steps, starting with the left foot forward, will stay the same: 3 steps forward (on beats 1-3); right foot stamp forward (on beat 4); triple step back/ back/ forward (on beats 5 & 6). Yes, partners will switch sides with each other, ending up in the position that is directly opposite from their starting positions.

Despite these three similarities, however, there is one major difference: instead of rotating right, the couple will now rotate *left*. Consequently, each of the three forward steps will be taken while partners turn left (counter-clockwise). On the stamp forward step partners continue rotating left and stamp in the Left Parallel Position (woman's left side by man's left side). On the triple step (beats 5 & 6) partners take two steps back, rotating right (clockwise), then one step forward, moving towards each other.

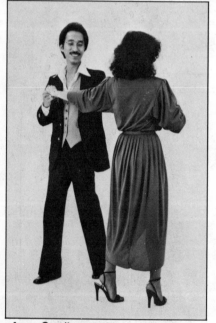

step 2 (beat 2)

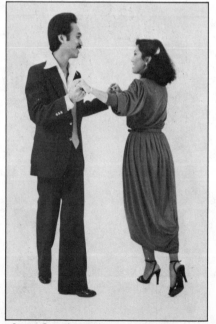

step 3 (beat 3)

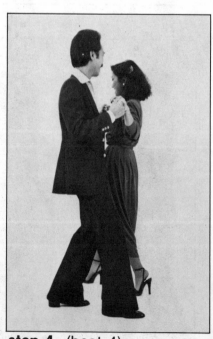

step 4 (beat 4)

Beat *Steps*

(1) 1. Left foot forward, turning left
(2) 2. Right foot forward, turning left
(3) 3. Left foot forward, turning left
(4) 4. Right foot stamp forward in Left Parallel Position
(5) 5. Right foot back, turning right
(&) 6. Left foot close to right foot
(6) 7. Right foot forward

Man's Part:

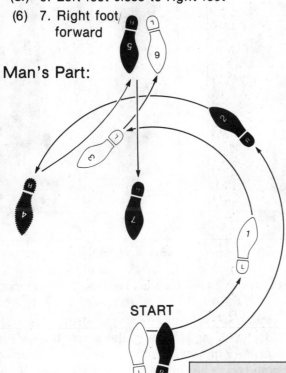

Beat *Steps*

(1) 1. Left foot forward, turning left
(2) 2. Right foot forward, turning left
(3) 3. Left foot forward, turning left
(4) 4. Right foot stamp forward in Left Parallel Position
(5) 5. Right foot back, turning right
(&) 6. Left foot close to right foot
(6) 7. Right foot forward

Woman's Part:

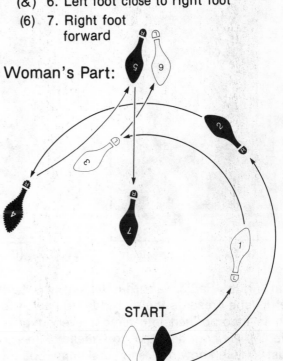

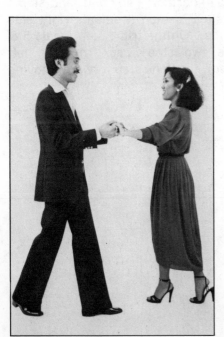

step 5 (beat 5)

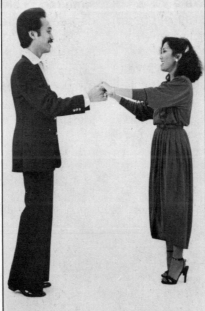

step 6 (beat "and")

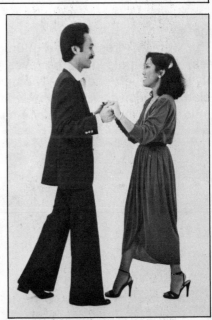

step 7 (beat 6)

125

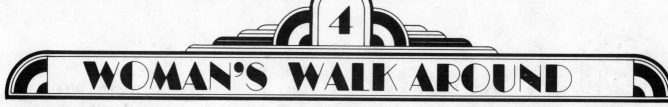

WOMAN'S WALK AROUND

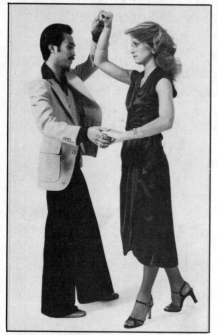

step 1 (beat 1)

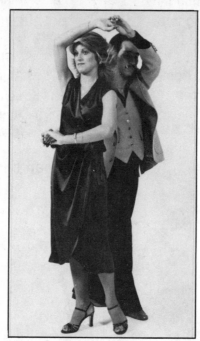

step 2 (beat 2)

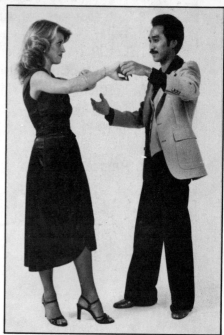

step 3 (beat 3)

That's right, ladies and gentlemen, the Latin Street Hustle presents the old under-the-arm trick which is incorporated into almost every type of hustle. We are confident that you already know (or at least should know, unless you skimmed blindly through the last fifty pages) how to make a WALK AROUND TURN. In case it momentarily slipped your mind, however, we will briefly reset the stage.

The woman, dressed in a midnight blue velvet dress, stands poised, as her eyes glance expectantly over her left shoulder. The man, sumptuously clad in black velvet, lifts the woman's left hand in his right hand (*right one-hand hold*). On

beats 1-3 the music reaches a crescendo, the curtain rises, and the woman glides into her Walk Around Turn, while the man struts past her right side. In 3 steps forward, therefore, they will switch places with each other, but the woman will simultaneously make her Walk Around Turn (180 degrees counter-clockwise).

On beat 4 (step 4) partners join hands and stamp in the Right Parallel Position (woman's right side by man's right side). On the triple step (beats 5 & 6) partners take two steps back, rotating left (counter-clockwise), then one step forward, moving towards each other. 💃

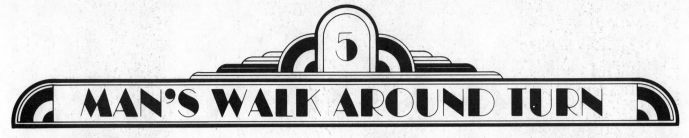

MAN'S WALK AROUND TURN

If the woman can turn, so can the dancing man. So no more excuses gentlemen — it's time to show your spinning stuff. Similar to the turn just described, the MAN'S WALK AROUND TURN is a Half Left Underarm Turn, completed on beats 1-3 (on steps 1-3), while he passes the woman's right side. More important, the man will turn under his *left* (the woman's right) hand. In other words, the *right one-hand hold* will still be used for the Man's Walk Around Turn, although his *left* hand will be pushed *away* from his left side.

While the man turns, the woman continues to walk around the man's right side in 3 steps forward. By step 3, therefore, the man and the woman will have switched places with each other. On step 4 (beat 4), they join hands and stamp in the Right Parallel Position (right side by right side, and facing in opposite directions). To conclude this variation, they take 2 steps back, rotating left, then 1 step forward to complete the triple step (on beats 5 & 6).

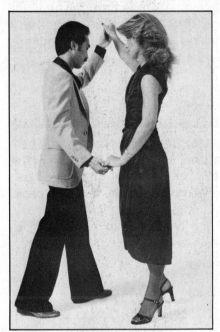

step 1   (beat 1)

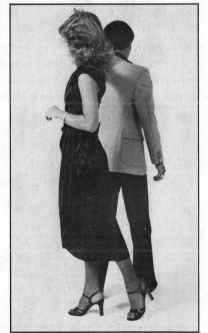

step 2   (beat 2)

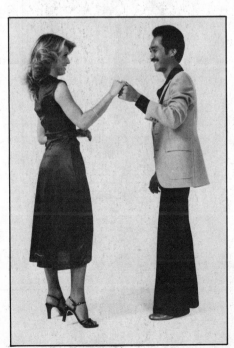

step 3   (beat 3)

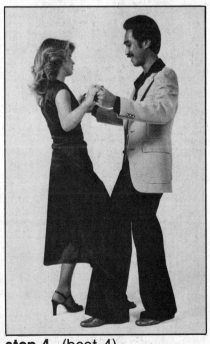

step 4   (beat 4)

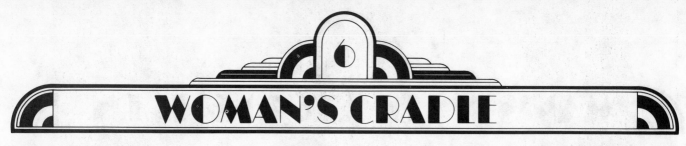

WOMAN'S CRADLE

After the lengthy harangue in Chapter Four (*variations 15-21*), if you don't know how to make a WOMAN'S CRADLE (WRAP-AROUND OR SWEETHEART TURN), you are going to be drawn and quartered! In Part A the woman makes her Cradle (Half Left Holding Underarm Turn) in 3 steps forward. In Part B the woman unwinds from the Cradle by making a Half Right Holding Underarm Turn in 3 steps forward. ♣

Part A:
WOMAN'S CRADLE

In Part A the man takes 3 steps in place on beats 1-3 (steps 1-3), while the woman makes her Cradle (Half Left Holding Underarm Turn) in 3 steps forward. As the woman turns, her right hand, uplifted in the man's left hand in the *right two-hand hold,* rotates counter-clockwise over her head. After the woman completes her turn, her right arm drops down and crosses straight-jacket style on top of her left arm, as she wiggles back next to the man's right side. Both partners complete steps 4-7 (on beats 4-6) in the Left Side Parallel Position. ♣

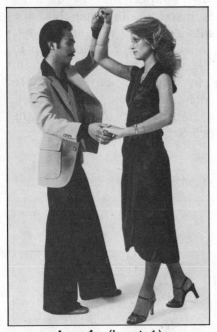

part A **step 1** (beat 1)

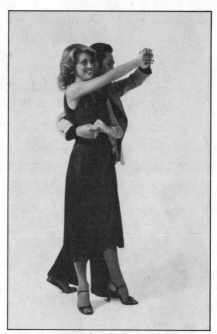

part A **step 2** (beat 2)

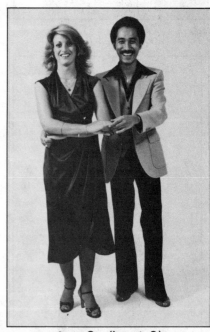

part A **step 3** (beat 3)

Part B:
UNWIND

To unwind from the Cradle in Part B, the woman makes a Half Right Holding Underarm Turn (180 degrees clockwise) in 3 steps forward on beats 1-3 (step 1-3) while the man takes 3 steps in place. As the woman turns, her right hand, uplifted in the man's left hand in the right *two-hand hold*, rotates clockwise over her head. After the woman unwinds, both partners conclude this variation with steps 4-7 (on beats 4-6) in the Holding Dance Position. 👣

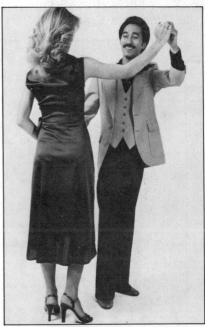

part B **step 2** (beat 2)

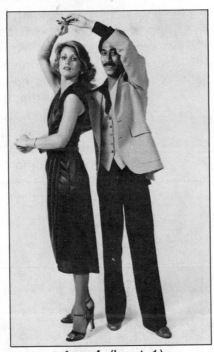

part B **step 1** (beat 1)

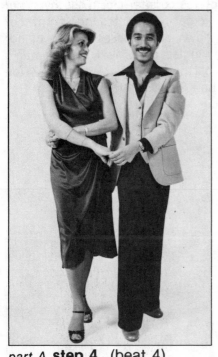

part A **step 4** (beat 4)

LATIN STREET HUSTLE

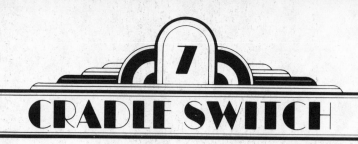

CRADLE SWITCH

In the CRADLE SWITCH partners switch places with each other, while wrapped in the Cradle. Divided into four parts, with each section containing the basic 7 steps completed in 6 syncopated beats of music, this variation begins in Part A with the Woman's Cradle. In Part B partners switch places, as they move into the Right Side Parallel Position. In Part C, partners again switch places, as they return to the Left Side Parallel Position. In Part D the woman unwinds by making a Half Right Holding Underarm Turn. 🕺

Part A: WOMAN'S CRADLE

In Part A the woman makes her Cradle (Half Left Holding Underarm Turn) in 3 steps forward on beats 1-3 (steps 1-3), while the man takes 3 steps in place. As the woman turns, her right hand, uplifted in the man's left hand in the *right two-hand hold,* rotates counter-clockwise over her head. After the woman completes her turn, her right hand drops down and crosses on top of her left arm, as she wiggles back next to the man's right side. Both partners complete steps 4-7 (on beats 4-6) in the Left Side Parallel Position. 🕺

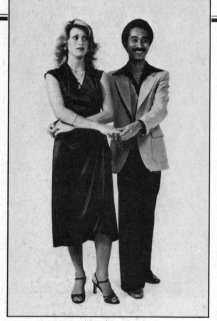

part A **step 1** (beat 1)

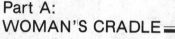

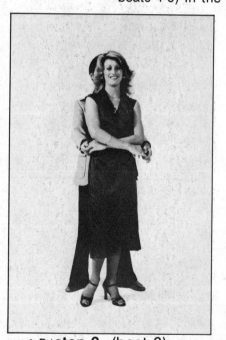

part B **step 2** (beat 2)

Part B: SWITCH POSITIONS

In Part B partners switch places with each other, as they take 3 steps to opposite sides on beats 1-3 (steps 1-3). The man, passing behind the woman, takes 3 steps towards his *right* side, as the woman takes 3 steps towards her *left* side. After switching places, both partners complete steps 4-7 (on beats 4-6) in the Right Side Parallel Position.

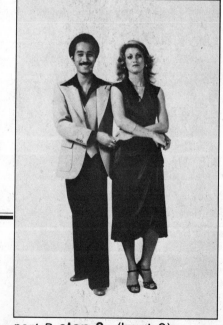

part B **step 3** (beat 3)

Part C:
SWITCH POSITIONS

In Part C partners once again switch places, as they take 3 steps to opposite sides on beats 1-3 (steps 1-3). The man, passing behind the woman, takes 3 steps towards his *left* side, as the woman takes 3 steps towards her *right* side. After switching places, both partners complete steps 4-7 (on beats 4-6) in the Left Side Parallel Position. 🕺

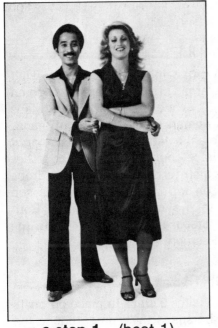

part C **step 1** (beat 1)

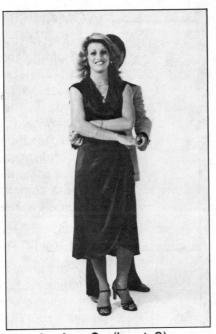

part C **step 2** (beat 2)

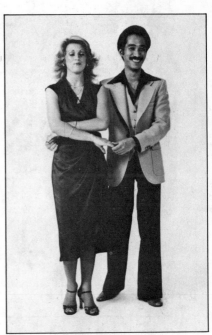

part C **step 3** (beat 3)

Part D:
UNWIND

Whenever partners lose interest in the double switch, the woman unwinds by making a Half Right Holding Underarm Turn (180 degrees clockwise) in 3 steps forward on beats 1-3 (steps 1-3), while the man takes 3 steps in place. As the woman turns, her right hand, uplifted in the man's left hand in the *right two-hand hold*, rotates clockwise over her head. After the woman unwinds, both partners conclude this variation with steps 4-7 (on beats 4-6) in the Holding Dance Position. 🕺

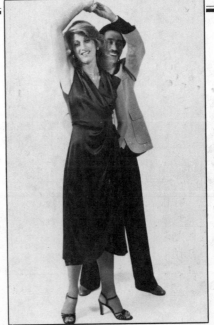

part D
step 1 (beat 1)

LATIN STREET HUSTLE

CRADLE ROLLS

CRADLE ROLLS form a snappy variation that begins in Part A with the Woman's Cradle. In Part B the man whips the woman out to the right, then snaps her back in to the left in Part C. In this variation, which contains three sequences of the basic 7 steps, the woman completes each roll by making a Full Turn in 3 steps forward.

Part A:
WOMAN'S CRADLE

In Part A the woman makes her Cradle (Half Left Holding Underarm Turn) in 3 steps forward on beats 1-3 (steps 1-3), while the man takes 3 steps in place. As the woman turns, her right hand, uplifted in the man's left hand in the *right two-hand hold*, rotates counter-clockwise over her head. After the woman turns, her right arm drops down and crosses on top of her left arm, as she scoots back next to the man's right side. Both partners complete steps 4-7 (on beats 4-6) in the Left Side Parallel Position.

Part B:
ROLL OUT RIGHT

In Part B the man takes 3 steps in place on beats 1-3 (steps 1-3), as he snaps the woman out to the right. As the woman rolls away from the man, she makes a Full Right Turn (360 degrees clockwise) in 3 steps forward. After the woman completes her roll, both partners conclude steps 4-7 (on beats 4-6) in the Left Open Position.

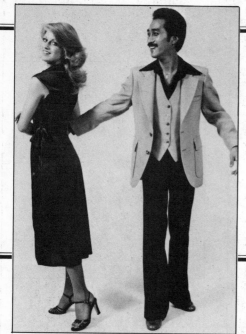

part B **step 2**   (beat 2)

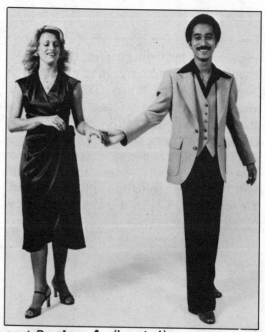

part B **step 4**   (beat 4)

part B **step 3**   (beat 3)

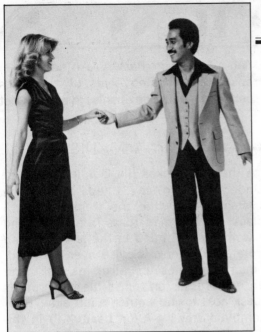

part C **step 1** (beat 1)

Part C:
ROLL IN LEFT

In Part C the man takes 3 steps in place, as he snaps the woman back in to the left on beats 1-3 (steps 1-3). As the woman rolls toward the man, she makes a Full Left Turn (360 degrees counter-clockwise) in 3 steps forward. After the woman completes her roll, both partners conclude steps 4-7 (on beats 4-6) in the Left Side Parallel Position.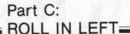

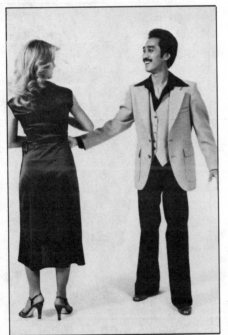

part C **step 2** (beat 2)

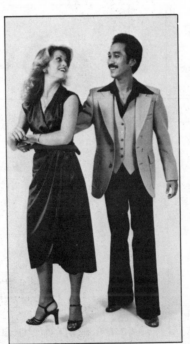

part C **step 3** (beat 3)

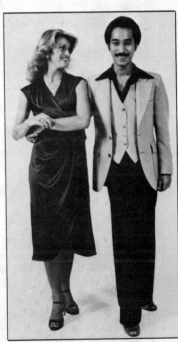

part C **step 4** (beat 4)

This tricky variation, called CRADLE TO SPOT TURNS, is guaranteed to add some whirling excitement to your life. Since you must be sick to death of the Woman's Cradle, you will now have the chance (or forever hold your peace) to start with the Man's Cradle in Part A. As an encore, Part B drops all syncopated beats of music, as partners perform their devilishly daring Spot Turns. 👯

Part A: MAN'S CRADLE

In Part A the man makes his Cradle (Half Left Holding Underarm Turn) in 3 steps forward on beats 1-3 (steps 1-3), while the woman takes 3 steps in place. As the man turns, his right hand uplifts the woman's left hand in the *left two-hand hold* and rotates counter-clockwise over his head. After the man completes his turn, his right arm drops down and crosses on top of his left arm, as he scoots back next to the women's left side. Both partners complete steps 4-7 (on beats 4-6) in the Right Side Parallel Position. 👯

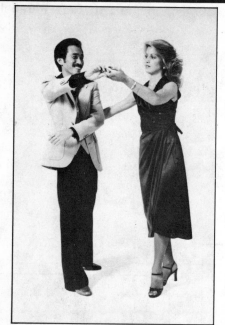

part A **step 1** (beat 1)

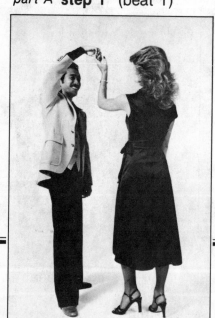

part A **step 2** (beat 2)

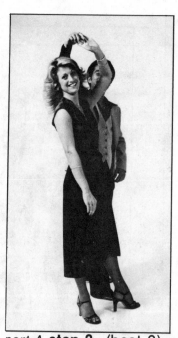

part A **step 3** (beat 3)

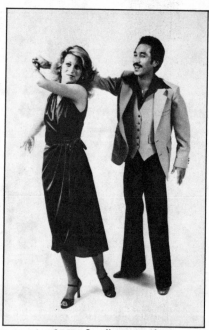

part A **step 4** (beat 4)

Part B: SPOT TURNS

In Part B there will be *no* triple step, since the syncopated beats of music are temporarily dropped for the Spot Turns. Thus, on beats 1-6 (steps 1-6) the man takes 6 walk steps forward and saunters around the twirling woman. While walking around the woman, the man keeps the woman's left hand uplifted in his right hand in the *left one-hand hold*. The woman, of course, makes two continuous Right Underarm Turns in 6 small steps forward. 👯

In most ways, the SHADOW duplicates the movement for the Woman's Cradle. Now don't groan, because the Shadow does necessitate a slight change in body and hand positions. In Part A the woman makes her Shadow (Half Left Holding Underarm Turn) with both pairs of her hands uplifted in both of the man's hands in the *two-hand stack*. In Part B the woman unwinds from the Shadow by making a Half Right Holding Underarm Turn.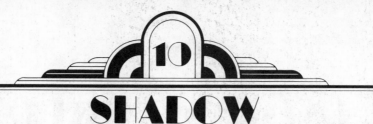

Part A:
SHADOW

In Part A the man takes 3 steps in place on beats 1-3 (steps 1-3), while the woman makes her Shadow (Half Left Holding Underarm Turn) in 3 steps forward. As the woman turns, both of her hands are uplifted and grabbed by both of the man's hands in the *two-hand stack*. After the woman completes her turn, she does *not* scoot back next to the man. Instead, she stands in front of him, with her back facing his stomach. Both partners complete steps 4-7 (on beats 4-6) in the Shadow Position with the *two-hand stack*.

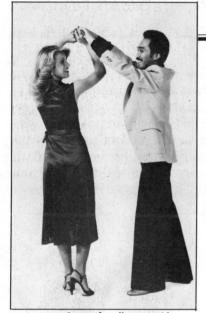

part A **step 1** (beat 1)

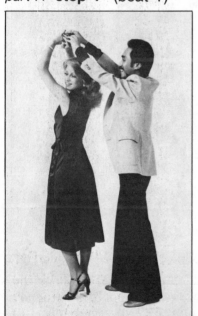

part A **step 2** (beat 2)

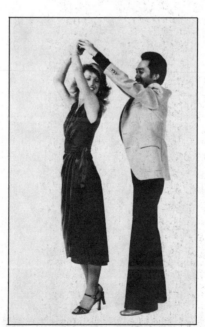

part A **step 3** (beat 3)

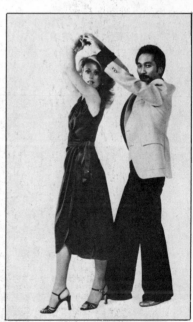

part A **step 4** (beat 4)

Part B: UNWIND

To unwind from the Shadow in Part B, the woman makes a Half Right Holding Underarm Turn (180 degrees clockwise) in 3 steps forward on beats 1-3 (steps 1-3), while the man takes 3 steps in place. As the woman turns, both of her hands rotate clockwise over her head. After the woman unwinds, both partners join hands in the two-hand hold and complete steps 4-7 (on beats 4-6) in the Holding Dance Position.

LATIN STREET HUSTLE

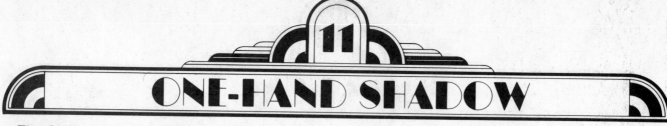

ONE-HAND SHADOW

The ONE-HAND SHADOW is performed in the Shadow Position, with both of the woman's hands clasped in the man's right hand in the *one-hand stack*. In Part A the woman makes her Shadow (Half Left Holding Underarm Turn) with both of her hands uplifted and held in one of the man's hands. In Part B the woman unwinds from the Shadow by making a Half Right Holding Underarm Turn.

Part A:
ONE-HAND SHADOW

In Part A the man takes 3 steps in place on beats 1-3 (steps 1-3), while the woman makes her Shadow (Half Left Holding Underarm Turn) in 3 steps forward. As the woman turns, both of her hands are uplifted and grabbed by the man's right hand in the *one-hand stack.* After the woman completes her turn, she stands directly in front of the man. This time, however, the man places his left hand on the woman's left shoulder, but continues to keep both of the woman's hands uplifted in his right hand. Partners complete steps 4-7 (on beats 4-6) in the Shadow Position with the *one-hand stack.*

Part B:
UNWIND

To unwind from the Shadow in Part B, the woman makes a Half Right Holding Underarm Turn (180 degrees clockwise) in 3 steps forward on beats 1-3 (steps 1-3), while the man takes 3 steps in place. As the woman turns, both of her hands, clasped in the man's hands, rotate clockwise. After the woman unwinds, both partners join hands in the two-hand hold and complete steps 4-7 (on beats 4-6) in the Holding Dance Position.

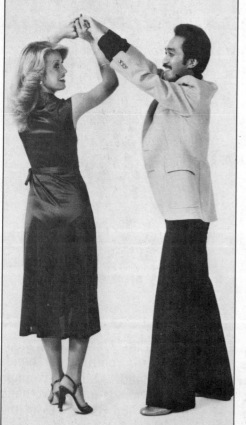

part A **step 1** (beat 1)

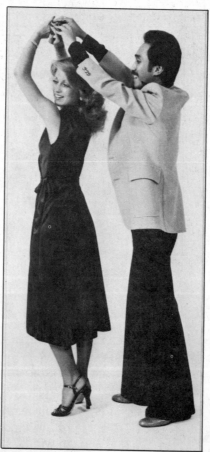

part A **step 2** (beat 2)

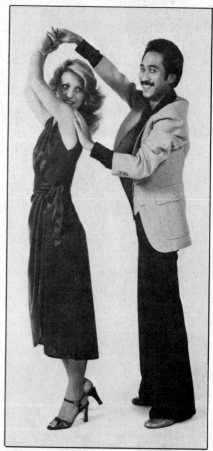

part A **step 3** (beat 3)

12
PRETZEL

As you may recall from our discussion in Chapter Four (*variations 21-24*), the PRETZEL is concocted from dual half holding turns in which partners turn in opposite directions. In Part A partners twist themselves into the Pretzel, as the woman makes a Half Right Holding Underarm Turn, and the man makes a Half Left Holding Turn. To unwind from the Pretzel in Part B, partners reverse the direction of their dual holding turns, as the woman makes a Half Left Holding Underarm Turn, and the man makes a Half Right Holding Turn. Of course, the Pretzel is made with both pairs of hands clasped in the double hold. Thus, as the woman turns, her right hand uplifted in the man's left hand in the *right two-hand hold* rotates over her head. ⚊

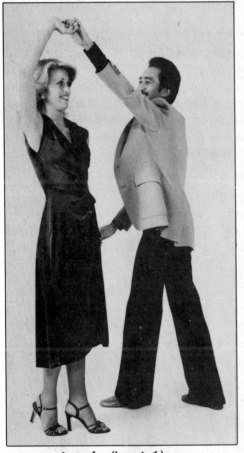

part A **step 1** (beat 1)

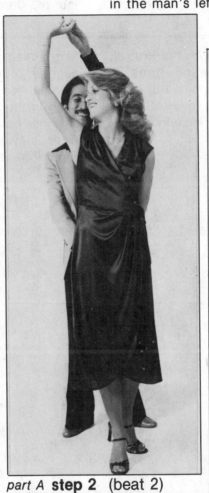

part A **step 2** (beat 2)

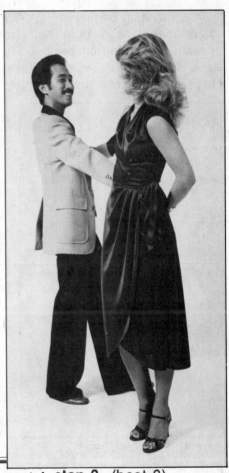

part A **step 3** (beat 3)

Part A: PRETZEL

In Part A partners twist themselves into the Pretzel by making dual half holding turns in opposite directions on beats 1-3 (steps 1-3). In 3 steps forward, therefore, the woman makes a Half Right Holding Underarm Turn (180 degrees clockwise), as the man makes a Half Left Holding Turn (180 degrees counter-clockwise). While the woman is turning, her right hand, uplifted in the man's left hand rotates clockwise, while her left hand, held in the man's right hand, remains pinned behind her back. After partners complete their dual turns, they conclude steps 4-7 (on beats 4-6) in the Right Parallel Position. ⚊

Part B: UNWIND

Once wrapped in the Pretzel, partners continue to repeat their Basic Step as long as their insatiable hearts desire. Whenever they begin to feel like a twisted piece of dough, however, they unwind on beats 1-3 (steps 1-3) by making dual half holding turns in the reverse direction. In 3 steps forward the woman makes a Half Left Holding Underarm Turn, as the man makes a Half Right Holding Turn. After partners unwind, they complete steps 4-7 (on beats 4-6) in the Holding Dance Position. ⚊

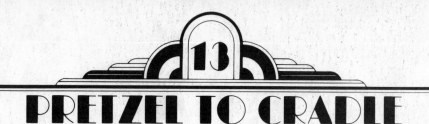

PRETZEL TO CRADLE

For all you die-hard kids, the PRETZEL TO CRADLE, sometimes called TRIPLE DECKER TURNS, offers a unique taste treat. Layered into three sections, each part of this variation contains the same basic 7 steps completed in 6 syncopated beats of music, with all changes made on the first 3 beats of music. In Part A partners twist themselves into the Pretzel by making dual half holding turns in opposite directions. In Part B partners unscramble themselves from the Pretzel, before cuddling into the Woman's Cradle. In Part C partners unwind from the Cradle. (Although this variation begins with the Pretzel, feel free to start off with the Reverse Pretzel, before wrapping into the Cradle). 💃

Part A: PRETZEL

This variation begins in Part A with the Pretzel, as partners make dual half holding turns in opposite directions on beats 1-3 (steps 1-3). In 3 steps forward the woman makes a Half Right Holding Underarm Turn (180 degrees clockwise), as the man makes a Half Left Holding Turn (180 degrees counter-clockwise). While the woman is turning, her right hand, uplifted in the man's left hand in the *right two-hand hold* rotates clockwise over her head. After partners complete their dual turns, they conclude steps 4-7 (on beats 4-6) in the Right Parallel Position.

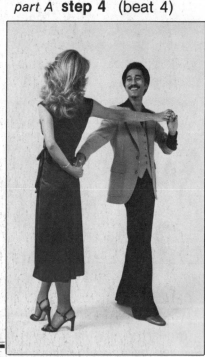

part A **step 4** (beat 4)

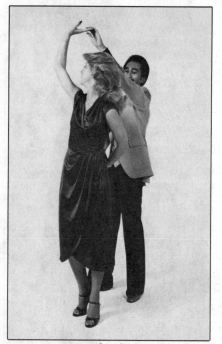

part A **step 2** (beat 2)

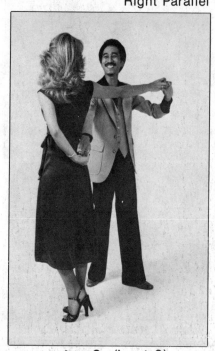

part A **step 3** (beat 3)

Part B: PRETZEL TO CRADLE

In Part B both partners zip out of the Pretzel, before the woman spins into her Cradle. On beat 1 (step 1) partners make dual half holding turns in opposite directions in one step forward, as the woman makes a Half Left Holding Underarm Turn (180 degrees counter-clockwise), and the man makes a Half Right Holding Turn (180 degrees clockwise). While the woman is turning, her right hand uplifted in the man's left hand in the *right two-hand hold*, rotates clockwise over her head. On beat 2 (step 2) partners face each other in the Holding Dance Position. On beat 3 (step 3) the woman makes her Cradle (Half Left Holding Underarm Turn), as her right hand, still uplifted in the man's left hand, rotates counter-clockwise over her head. After the woman completes her turn, she scoots back next to the man, then both partners conclude steps 4-7 (on beats 4-6) in the Left Side Parallel Position. 💃

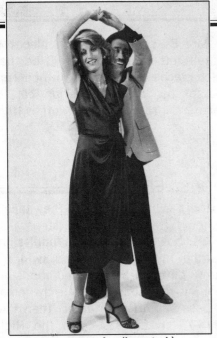

part B **step 1** (beat 1)

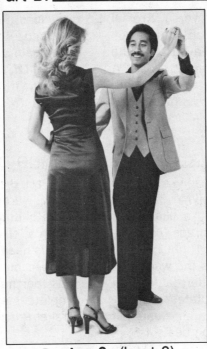

part B **step 2** (beat 2)

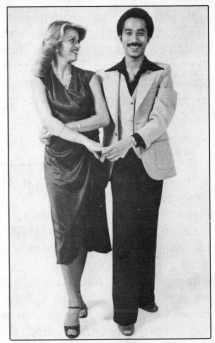

part B **step 4** (beat 4)

Part C:
UNWIND

To unwind from the Cradle, the woman makes a Half Right Holding Underarm Turn (180 degrees clockwise) in 3 steps forward, while the man takes 3 steps in place. As the woman turns, her right hand, uplifted in the man's left hand in the *right two-hand hold,* rotates clockwise over her head. After the woman completes her turn, both partners conclude steps 4-7 (on beats 4-6) in the Holding Dance Position.

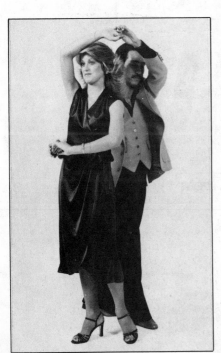

part C **step 1** (beat 1)

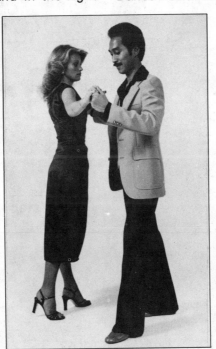

part C **step 3** (beat 3)

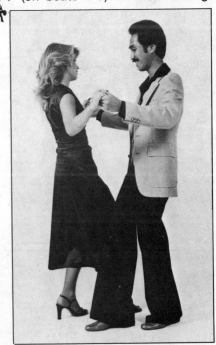

part C **step 4** (beat 4)

139

LATIN STREET HUSTLE

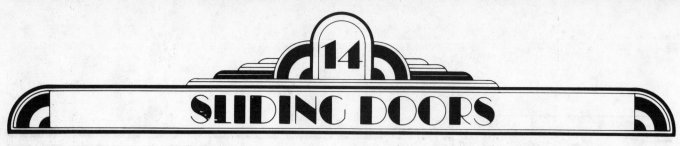
If you tried to perform the Reverse Pretzel described in the previous variation, then you should be ready to start slip sliding away with the SLIDING DOORS. Divided into three parts, Part A starts off with the Reverse Pretzel, as both partners make dual half holding turns in opposite directions. In Part B, partners switch places as they slide to their left sides. In Part C partners once again switch places as they slide to their right sides. (Of course this entire variation can be flopped, if partners prefer to start off with a Pretzel). 🕺

Part A:
REVERSE PRETZEL

In Part A partners bring themselves into a Reverse Pretzel on beats 1-3 (steps 1-3). In 3 steps forward, the woman makes a Half Left Holding Underarm Turn (180 degrees counter-clockwise), as the man makes a Half Right Holding Turn (180 degrees clockwise). While the woman is turning, her left hand, uplifted in the man's right hand in the *left two-hand hold*, rotates counter-clockwise over her. After making their dual half turns, partners complete steps 4-7 (on beats 4-6) in the Left Parallel Position. 🕺

Part B:
SLIDING DOORS LEFT

In Part B partners switch places as they take 3 steps towards their left on beats 1-3 (steps 1-3). Before sliding left, however, the man uplifts the woman's left hand in his right hand and swings it over his head, until both pairs of clasped hands are extended out behind their backs. While switching sides, partners pass *behind* each other, then they complete steps 4-7 (on beats 4-6) in the Right Parallel Position. 🕺

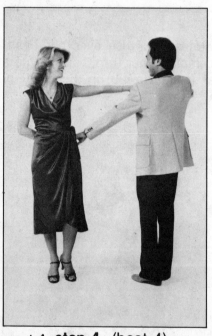

part A **step 4** (beat 4)

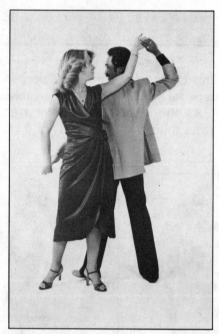

part B **step 1** (beat 1)

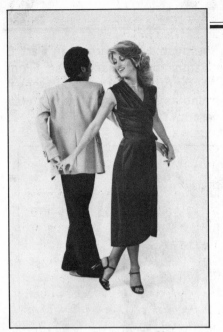

part B **step 2** (beat 2)

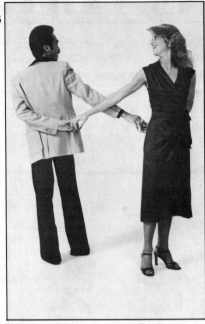

part B **step 3** (beat 3)

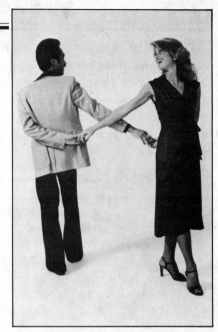

part B **step 4** (beat 4)

Part C;
SLIDING DOORS RIGHT

Since partners did, somehow or other, manage to slide to their left, they can bloody well slide back to the right. Thus, on beats 1-3 (steps 1-3) partners take 3 steps towards their right, as they pass *behind* each other's back. After sliding right, partners complete steps 4-7 (on beats 4-6) in the Left Parallel Position. 🕺

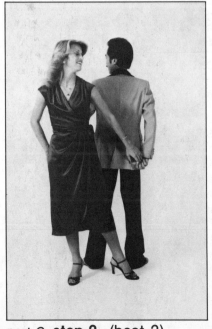

part C **step 2** (beat 2)

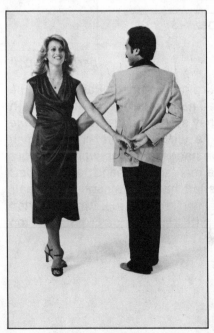

part C **step 3** (beat)

WOMAN'S AIRPLANE

The WOMAN'S AIRPLANE is a jet-age variation designed for those who enjoy flying high. Divided into 3 parts, each section of this variation contains the same basic 7 steps, completed in 6 syncopated beats of music, with all changes made on the first 3 beats. In Part A partners flip-flop their hands into the double hand cross. In Part B the woman zooms into her Airplane (Half Right Holding Underarm Turn). In Part C the woman makes a crash landing as she soars through a Half Left Holding Underarm Turn. 🕴

Part A:
HAND CROSS

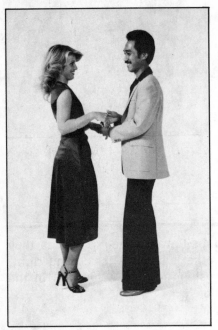

part A **step 3** (beat 3)

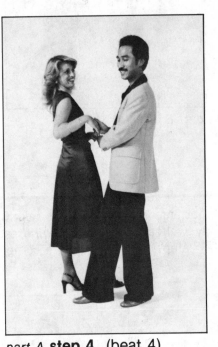

part A **step 4** (beat 4)

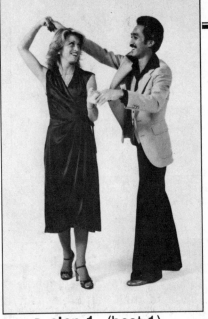

part B **step 1** (beat 1)

The Woman's Airplane begins in Part A with the double hand cross. Thus, as partners wing through their Basic Step, they switch hands into the *double hand cross*. In the double hand cross, which resembles a double handshake, the woman's right hand is held in the man's right hand, and her left hand is held in his left hand. Although either pair of clasped hands may rest on top, this variation will be performed with right hands crossed on top of the left hands. 🕴

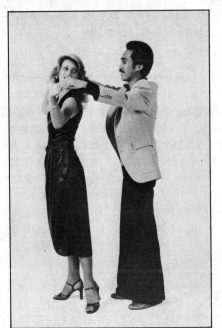

part B **step 2** (beat 2)

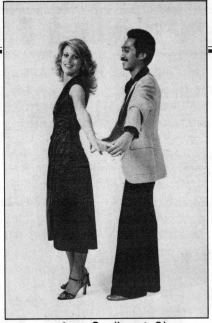

part B **step 3** (beat 3)

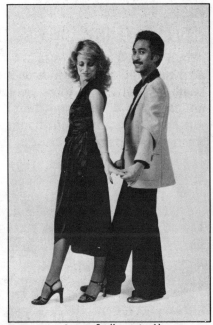

part B **step 4** (beat 4)

Part B:
WOMAN'S AIRPLANE

In Part B the man takes 3 steps in place on beats 1-3 (steps 1-3), while the woman makes her Airplane (Half Right Holding Underarm Turn) in 3 steps forward. As the woman turns, her right hand, uplifted in the man's right hand, rotates clockwise over her head. After the woman zooms 180 degrees clockwise, she stands directly in front of the man, with her back facing his stomach (remember the Shadow?) In addition, partners slightly flair their hands out to the side, as they complete steps 4-7 (on beats 4-6) in the Airplane Position. 🕺

Part C:
UNWIND

In Part C the man takes 3 steps in place on beats 1-3 (steps 1-3), while the woman unwinds by making a Half Left Holding Underarm Turn (180 degrees counter-clockwise) in 3 steps forward. After the woman unwinds, both partners switch hands back into the two-hand hold, then complete steps 4-7 (on beats 4-6) in the Holding Dance Position. 🕺

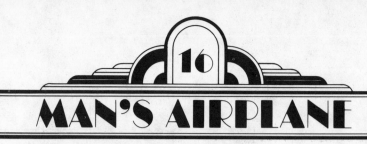

MAN'S AIRPLANE

The MAN'S AIRPLANE gives the man the chance to earn his wings. Divided into three parts, this variation begins in Part A with the Basic Step, as partners switch both pairs of hands into the *double hand cross*. In Part B the man soars through his Airplane (Half Right Holding Underarm Turn). In Part C the man glides home with a Half Left Holding Underarm Turn. 🕴

Part A: DOUBLE HAND CROSS

In Part A partners prepare for flight, as they zing through one sequence of their Basic Step. On beat 3 (step 3) partners switch hands into the *double hand cross,* then they complete steps 4-7 (on beats 4-6) with right hands crossed on top of their left hands. 🕴

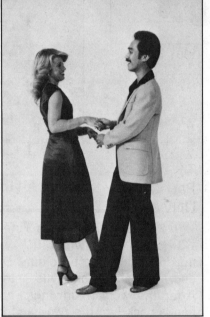

part A **step 4** (beat 4)

Part B: MAN'S AIRPLANE

In Part B the man lifts off into the wild blue yonder as he makes his Airplane (Half Right Holding Underarm Turn) in 3 steps forward on beats 1-3 (steps 1-3). As the man turns, his right hand rotates clockwise over his head. After the man completes his turn, he stands directly in front of the woman, with his back facing her stomach. With hands slightly flaired, partners complete steps 4-7 in the stratospheric Airplane Position. 🕴

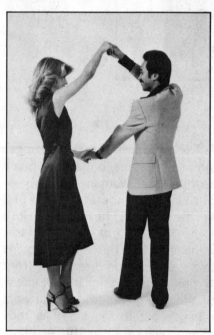

part B **step 1** (beat 1)

Part C:
UNWIND

Whenever the thrill of flight wanes, the man unwinds by making a Half Left Holding Underarm Turn (180 degrees counter-clockwise) in 3 steps forward on beats 1-3 (steps 1-3). As the man turns, his right hand rotates counter-clockwise over his head. After the man makes a smooth landing, both partners switch hands back into the two-hand hold, then complete steps 4-7 in the Holding Dance Position.

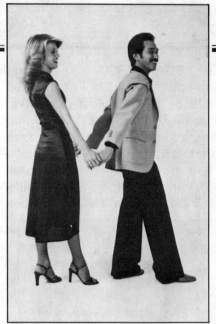

part B **step 4** (beat 4)

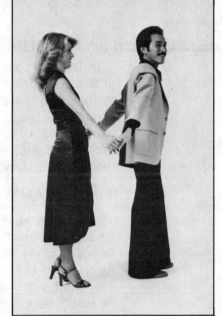

part B **step 3** (beat 3)

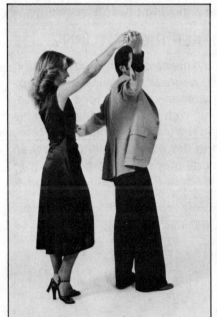

part B **step 2** (beat 2)

LATIN STREET HUSTLE

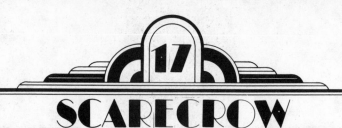

The SCARECROW is a twisting, turning, flip-flopping variation guaranteed to impress friends or foes. Divided into five sections, the Scarecrow begins in Part A with the Basic Step, as partners switch hands into the *double hand cross*. In Part B the man makes a Half Right Holding Underarm Turn, then scoots back next to the woman in the Right Side Parallel Position. In Part C partners switch into the Left Side Parallel Position, as they make dual holding underarm turns in opposite directions. In Part D partners switch back into the Right Side Parallel Position, as they zip through dual holding underarm turns in opposite directions. In Part E the man makes a Half Left Holding Underarm Turn, then partners conclude this variation in the Holding Dance Position.

Part A: DOUBLE HAND CROSS

In Part A, partners whip through one sequence of their Basic Step, while switching hands into the *double hand cross* on beat 3 (step 3). After stamping forward in the Right Parallel Position on beat 4 (step 4), partners conclude their triple step (on beats 5 & 6) with two steps back, rotating left, then one step forward, moving towards each other.

Part B: MAN'S HALF RIGHT TURN

In Part B the man makes a Half Right Holding Underarm Turn (180 degrees clockwise) in 3 steps forward, while the woman takes 3 steps in place. As the man turns, his right hand rotates clockwise over his head. After the man completes his turn, he scoots back next to the woman's right side, then both partners conclude steps 4-7 (on beats 4-6) in the Right Side Parallel Position.

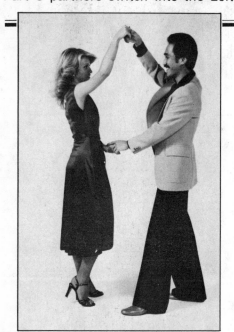

part B **step 1** (beat 1)

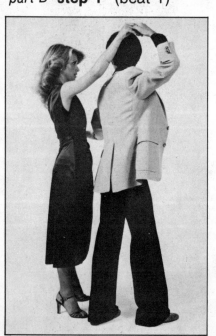

part B **step 2** (beat 2)

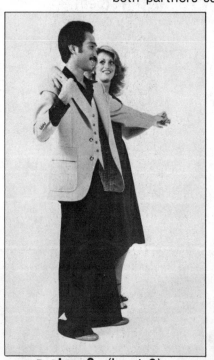

part B **step 3** (beat 3)

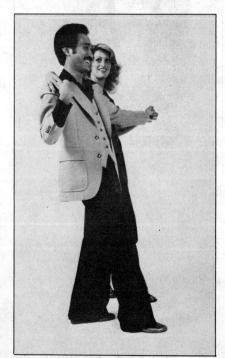

part B **step 4** (beat 4)

Part C:
SWITCH, WITH DUAL TURNS

In Part C partners switch places with each other by making dual holding underarm turns in opposite directions. On beat 1 (step 1) partners begin switching sides, as the man makes a Half Left Holding Underarm Turn (180 degrees counter-clockwise), and the woman makes a Half Right Holding Underarm Turn (180 degrees clockwise). As partners make their first set of dual turns, their clasped *right* hands rotate over their heads. On beat 2 (step 2) partners are halfway home, as their hands extend out to the sides and the man stands behind the woman. On beat 3 (step 3) partners complete their switch, as the man makes another Half Left Holding Underarm Turn (180 degrees counter-clockwise), and the woman makes another Half Right Holding Underarm Turn (180 degrees clockwise). While partners are making their second set of dual turns, their clasped *left* hands rotate over their heads. After completing their dual turns, partners conclude steps 4-7 (on beats 4-6) in the Left Side Parallel Position. 🕴

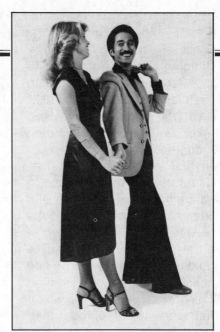

part C **step 4** (beat 4)

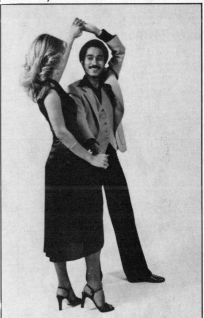

part C **step 3** (beat 3)

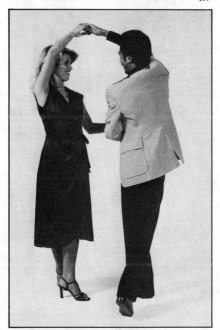

part C **step 1** (beat 1)

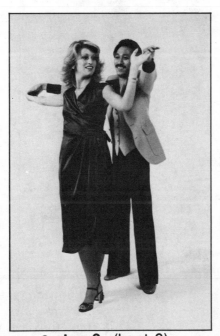

part C **step 2** (beat 2)

LATIN STREET HUSTLE

Part D:
SWITCH, WITH DUAL TURNS

In Part D partners once again switch places by making dual half holding turns in opposite directions. On beat 1 (step 1) partners begin switching sides, as the man makes a Half Right Holding Underarm Turn (180 degrees clockwise), and the woman makes a Half Left Holding Underarm Turn (180 degrees counter-clockwise). As partners make their first set of dual half turns, their clasped *left* hands rotate over their heads. On beat 2 (step 2) partners are halfway to the opposite side, as their hands extend out to the sides and the man stands behind the woman. On beat 3 (step 3) partners complete their switch, as the man makes another Half Right Holding Underarm Turn, and the woman makes another Half Left Holding Underarm Turn (180 degrees counter-clockwise). As partners make their second set of dual half turns, their clasped *right* hands rotate over their heads. After completing their dual turns, partners conclude steps 4-7 (on beats 4-6) in the Right Side Parallel Position.

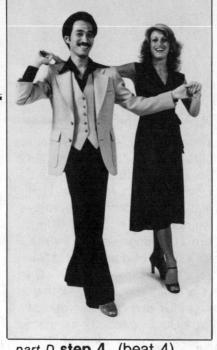

part D **step 4** (beat 4)

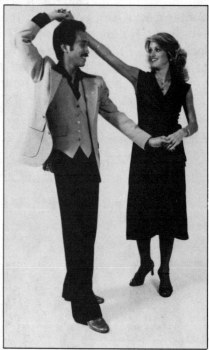

part D **step 3** (beat 3)

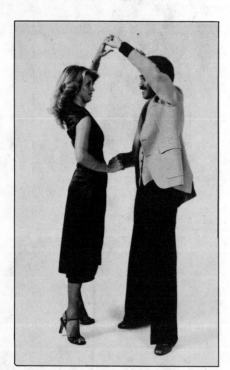

part D **step 1** (beat 1)

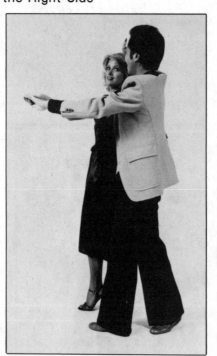

part D
step 2 (beat 2)

Part E:
MAN'S HALF LEFT TURN

To unwind, the man makes a Half Left Holding Underarm Turn (180 degrees counter-clockwise) in 3 steps forward, while the woman takes 3 steps in place. As the man turns, his right hand rotates counter-clockwise over his head. After the man unwinds, both partners conclude steps 4-7 (on beats 4-6) in the Holding Dance Position.

DISCO SLOW

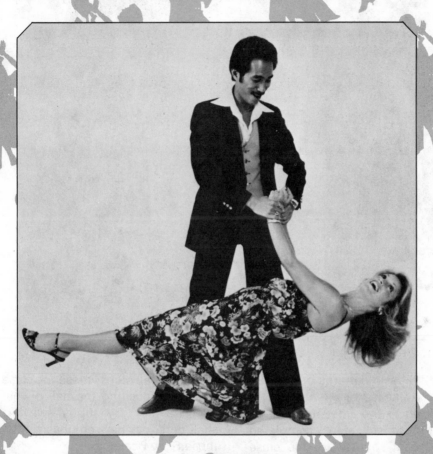

On those dreamy nights when you long to melt into your lover's arms, that's the perfect time to try some SLOW DISCO. Nothing, but nothing, could be more romantic than swaying to a heart throbbing disco song such as Donna Summer's *McArthur Park Suite.* In this chapter you learn how to do the lilting Trot, sexy Box, free-wheeling Pinwheel, and death-defying Slow Drop. Love to love you, baby!

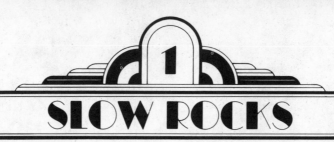
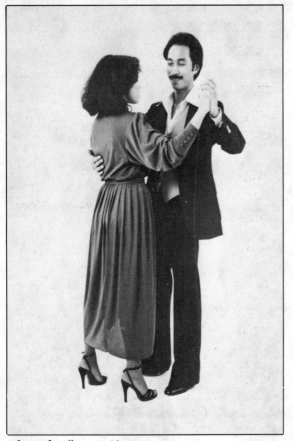

step 1 (beat 1)

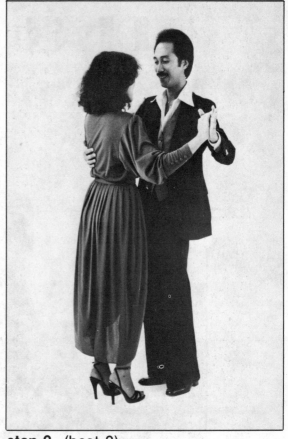

step 2 (beat 2)

SLOW ROCKS contain basic patterns of 4 steps, completed in 4 beats (1 measure) of music. The walk steps may be taken to the side, forward, or back. Alternated with these walk steps, completed on the odd-numbered beat counts, are toe close steps, taken on the even-numbered beat counts.

Similar to tap steps, these toe close steps are made by lightly touching the ball of the foot next to the opposite foot. By subtly swaying their hips and shoulders, partners emphasize the sensuousness of these Slow Rocks.

Man's Part:

Beat Steps

- (1) 1. Left foot side
- (2) 2. Right foot toe next to left foot
- (3) 3. Right foot side
- (4) 4. Left foot toe next to right foot

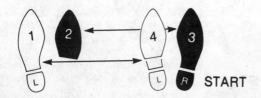

Woman's Part:

Beat Side

- (1) 1. Right foot side
- (2) 2. Left foot toe next to right foot
- (3) 3. Left foot side
- (4) 4. Right foot toe next to left foot

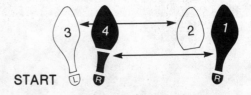

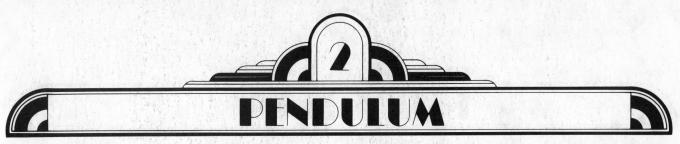

PENDULUM

Another basic pattern of 4 steps, completed in 4 beats (1 measure) of music, is the PENDULUM, which alternates forward and backward steps with toe close steps. Similar to the Slow Rocks, the Pendulum includes walk steps on the even-numbered beat counts, followed with toe close steps on the odd-numbered beat counts. On the toe close steps, no weight is placed on the ball of the foot that lightly touches next to the opposite foot. Unlike the previous variation, however, this variation contains walk steps which may be taken either diagonally forward or diagonally back. To emphasize the pendulum effect, tilt torso slightly back on the forward steps, then tilt torso slightly forward on the back steps, but straighten to an upright position on every toe close step.

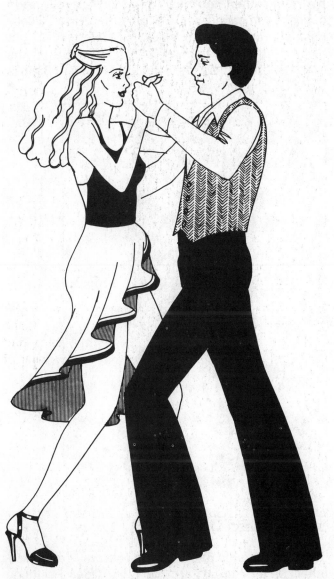

step 1 (beat 1)

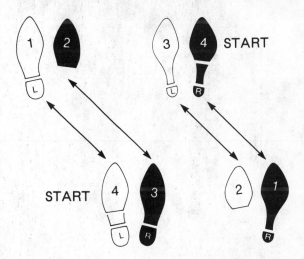

Man's Part:

Beat Steps
- (1) 1. Left foot diagonally forward
- (2) 2. Right foot toe next to left foot
- (3) 3. Right foot diagonally back
- (4) 4. Left foot toe next to right foot

Woman's Part:

Beat Steps
- (1) 1. Right foot diagonally back
- (2) 2. Left foot toe next to right foot
- (3) 3. Left foot diagonally forward
- (4) 4. Right foot toe next to left foot

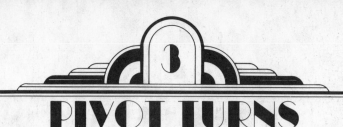

3
PIVOT TURNS

PIVOT TURNS dress up the plain Jane Slow Rocks by adding dual quarter turns to the walk steps. Similar to the previous two variations, walk steps, taken on the odd-numbered beat counts, are alternated with toe close steps, taken on the even-numbered beat counts. In this variation, however, dual quarter turns are made on the walk steps, as partners alternate pivoting away from, then turning towards each other.

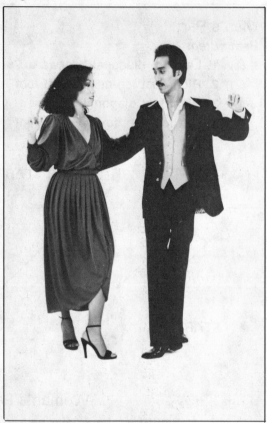

step 1 (beat 1)

On beat 1 (step 1) partners pivot away from each other as they break into the Conversation Position. Thus, the man steps back on his left foot, as he breaks away from the woman by making a ¼ *Left* Turn (90 degrees counter-clockwise). The woman, on the other hand, steps back on her right foot, as she breaks away from the man by making a ¼ *Right* Turn (90 degrees clockwise). As partners pivot away from each other and open to the Conversation Position, the man's left hand releases from the woman's right hand. On beat 2 (step 2) partners complete their toe close steps, while standing in the Conversation Position (Open Position, with woman's left side parallel to the

man's right side).

On beat 3 (step 3) partners return to the Closed Dance Position by pivoting towards each other. This time, however, the man steps forward on his right foot, as he turns towards the woman by making a ¼ *Right* Turn (90 degrees clockwise). Conversely, the woman steps forward on her left foot, as she turns towards the man by making a ¼ *Left* Turn (90 degrees counter-clockwise). After partners complete their dual quarter turns in opposite directions, they resume the Closed Dance Position, as the man clasps the woman's right hand in his left hand. While embraced in the Closed Position, partners complete their toe close steps on beat 4 (step 4).

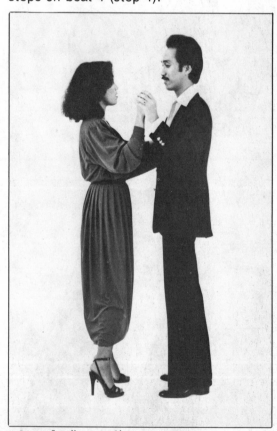

step 4 (beat 4)

On beat 5 (step 5) partners pivot away from each other, as they break into the Right Open Position. The man, therefore, steps back on his left foot, as he breaks away from the woman by making a ¼ *Right* Turn (90 degrees clockwise). Conversely, the woman steps back on her right foot, as she breaks away from the man by making a ¼ *Left* Turn (90 degrees counter-clockwise). As partners pivot away from each other and open to the Right Open Position, the man removes his right hand from the woman's waist, and the woman removes her left hand from the man's shoulder. On beat 6 (step 6) partners complete their toe close steps, while standing in the Right Open Position (Open Position, with woman's right side parallel to the man's left side).

On beat 7 (step 7) partners return to the Closed Dance Position by pivoting towards each other. This time, however, the man steps forward on his right foot, as he turns towards the woman by making a ¼ *Left* Turn (90 degrees counter-clockwise). Conversely, the woman steps forward on her left foot, as she turns towards the man by making a ¼ *Right* Turn (90 degrees clockwise). After partners complete their dual quarter turns in opposite directions, they resume the Closed Dance Position, as the man places his right hand on the woman's back, and the woman places her left hand on the man's shoulder. While embraced in the Closed Dance Position, partners complete their toe close steps on beat 8 (step 8). 🕴

Man's Part:
Beat Steps

- (1) 1. Left foot back, turning ¼ left
- (2) 2. Right foot toe next to left foot
- (3) 3. Right foot forward, turning ¼ right
- (4) 4. Left foot toe next to right foot
- (5) 5. Left foot back, turning ¼ right
- (6) 6. Right foot toe next to left foot
- (7) 7. Right foot forward, turning ¼ left
- (8) 8. Left foot toe next to right foot

Woman's Part:
Beat Steps

- (1) 1. Right foot back, turning ¼ right
- (2) 2. Left foot toe next to left foot
- (3) 3. Left foot forward, turning ¼ left
- (4) 4. Right foot toe next to left foot
- (5) 5. Right foot back, turning ¼ left
- (6) 6. Left foot toe next to right foot
- (7) 7. Left foot forward, turning ¼ right
- (8) 8. Right foot toe next to left foot

DISCO SLOW

DISCO FORWARD TROT

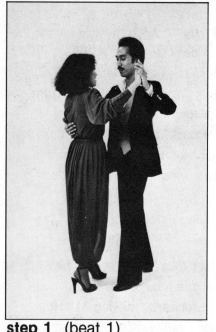

step 1 (beat 1)

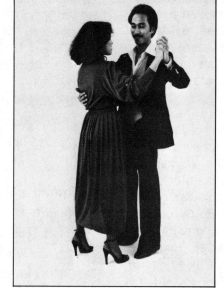

step 5 (beat 5)

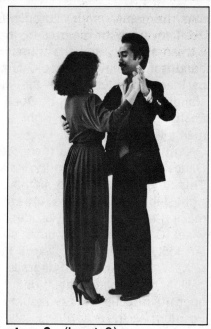

step 6 (beat 6)

Skippy Blair defines the trot as a "lilting movement of little running steps, stepping on every beat." Unlike the Slow Rocks, therefore, the DISCO FORWARD TROT is composed of 6 small, quick steps, completed in 6 beats (1-½ measures) of music, with weight placed directly on the foot on

each step. This variation begins on beats 1-4 (steps 1-4) with walk steps, as the man takes 4 walk steps forward, and the woman takes 4 walk steps back. This pattern concludes on beats 5-6 (steps 5-6) with a chassé, as both partners step side, then close side (draw feet together).

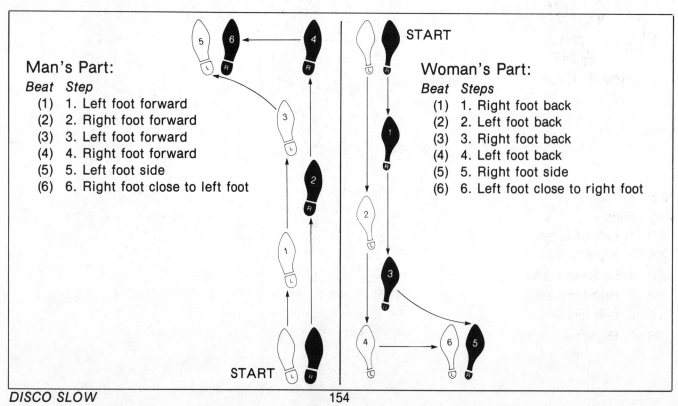

Man's Part:

Beat Step
- (1) 1. Left foot forward
- (2) 2. Right foot forward
- (3) 3. Left foot forward
- (4) 4. Right foot forward
- (5) 5. Left foot side
- (6) 6. Right foot close to left foot

Woman's Part:

Beat Steps
- (1) 1. Right foot back
- (2) 2. Left foot back
- (3) 3. Right foot back
- (4) 4. Left foot back
- (5) 5. Right foot side
- (6) 6. Left foot close to right foot

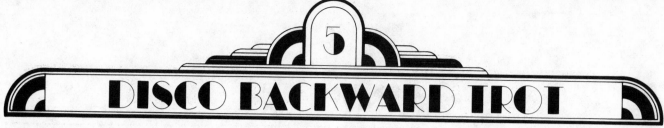

DISCO BACKWARD TROT

As the name implies, the DISCO BACKWARD TROT reverses the direction of the walk steps used in the previous variation, although the pattern still contains 6 small, lively steps, completed in 6 beats (1½ measures) of music. This variation begins with walk steps on beats 1-4 (steps 1-4), as the man takes 4 walk steps back, and the woman takes 4 walk steps forward. The pattern concludes on beats 5-6 (steps 5-6) with a chassé, as both partners step side, then close side (draw feet together).

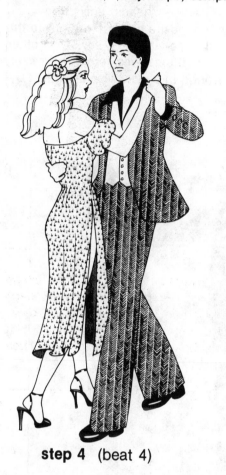

step 4 (beat 4)

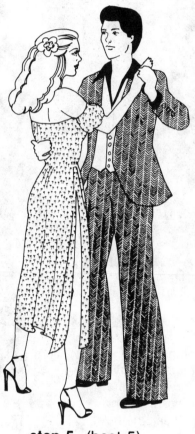

step 5 (beat 5)

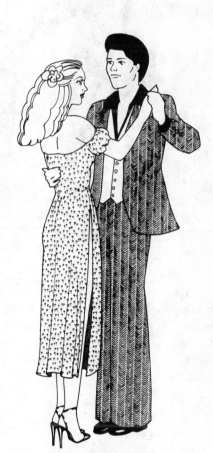

step 6 (beat 6)

Man's Part:
Beat Steps

(1) 1. Left foot back
(2) 2. Right foot back
(3) 3. Left foot back
(4) 4. Right foot back
(5) 5. Left foot side
(6) 6. Right foot close to left foot

Woman's Part:
Beat Steps

(1) 1. Right foot forward
(2) 2. Left foot forward
(3) 3. Right foot forward
(4) 4. Left foot forward
(5) 5. Right foot side
(6) 6. Left foot close to right foot

DISCO SLOW

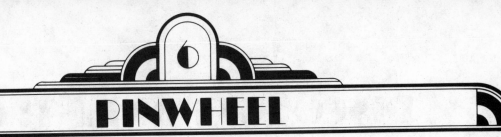

PINWHEEL

Although the PINWHEEL can be performed with almost any Salsa pattern, it looks particularly elegant in slow motion. Similar to most Salsa variations described in Chapter 5, the Pinwheel Right Parallel Position, with the woman's right side parallel to the man's right side. Many partners prefer to use the two-hand hold (both pairs of hands clasped), although others prefer the waist hold (one pair of hands encircling each other's waist, with opposite hands flung out to the side). Sensational free-wheelers, on the other hand, prefer to lock themselves into the Pretzel, before twirling around in a clockwise direction. 🕺

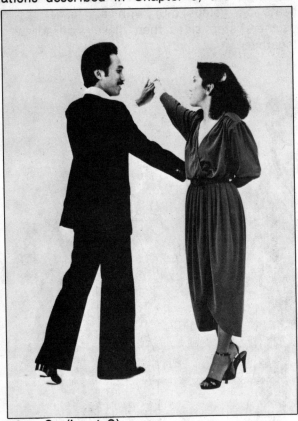

step 2 (beat 2)

contains a basic pattern of 4 steps, completed in 4 beats (1 measure) of music. In this variation, however, both the man and the woman walk in the same direction, as they rotate clockwise. More important, partners perform the Pinwheel in the

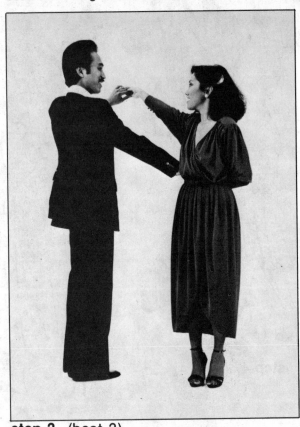

step 3 (beat 3)

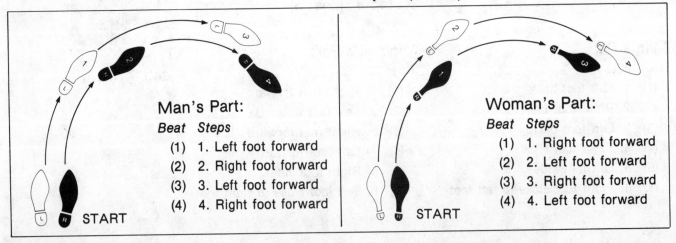

Man's Part:

Beat   Steps

(1) 1. Left foot forward

(2) 2. Right foot forward

(3) 3. Left foot forward

(4) 4. Right foot forward

Woman's Part:

Beat   Steps

(1) 1. Right foot forward

(2) 2. Left foot forward

(3) 3. Right foot forward

(4) 4. Left foot forward

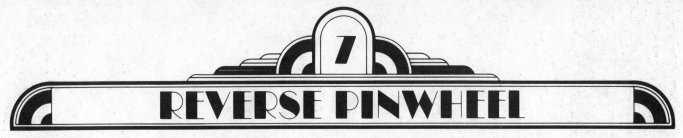

REVERSE PINWHEEL

As the name implies, the REVERSE PINWHEEL twirls in the opposite direction, as both the man and the woman rotate counter-clockwise. Similar to the Pinwheel, the Reverse Pinwheel contains a basic pattern of 4 steps, completed in 4 beats (1 measure) of music. Unlike the previous variation, however, the Reverse Pinwheel is performed in the Left Parallel Position, with the woman's left side parallel to the man's left side. Partners may choose, of course, their hand position, as they join hands in the two-hand hold, wrap their arms around each other's waist in the waist hold, or twist themselves into the Reverse Pretzel.

step 2 (beat 2)

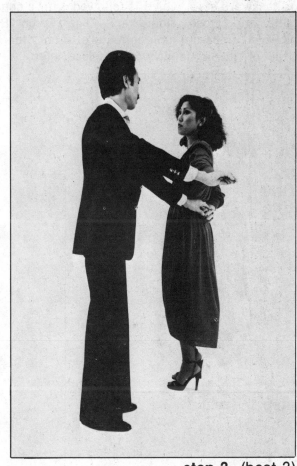

step 3 (beat 3)

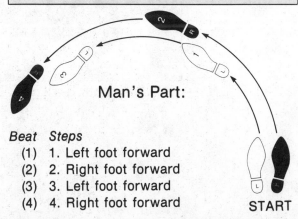

Man's Part:

Beat	Steps
(1)	1. Left foot forward
(2)	2. Right foot forward
(3)	3. Left foot forward
(4)	4. Right foot forward

START

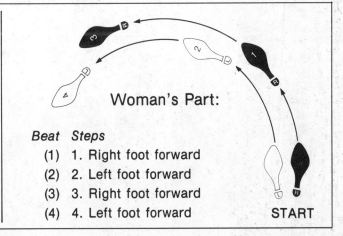

Woman's Part:

Beat	Steps
(1)	1. Right foot forward
(2)	2. Left foot forward
(3)	3. Right foot forward
(4)	4. Left foot forward

START

DISCO SLOW

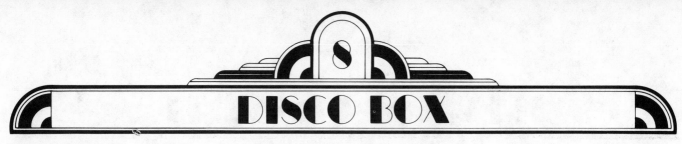

DISCO BOX

The DISCO BOX, sometimes called the BLACK WALTZ, combines the sensuous movements of the Slow Disco with the Basic Box Step. Similar to other box patterns, such as the Waltz Box or the Samba Caixo, the Disco Box starts with a forward or backward step, which is followed with a chassé (side and close side step). The Disco Box, however, adds one unique feature: a hold for one beat of music follows each close step. Thus, for the Disco Box the pattern contains 6 steps, completed in 8 beats (2 measures) of music.

For the first half of the pattern which contains steps 1-3 (completed on beats 1-4), the man steps forward on his left foot, as the woman steps back on her right foot, then both partners step side, close side (draw feet together), and hold the close position for one beat of music. The second half of the pattern, which contains steps 4-6 (completed on beats 4-8), partners reverse the direction of their steps; thus, the man steps forward on his right foot, as the woman steps back on her left foot, then both partners step side, close side (draw feet together), and hold the close position for the last beat count of music.

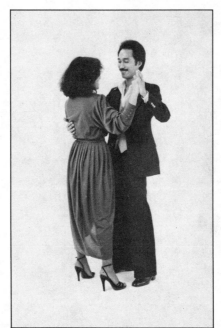

step 1 (beat 1)

step 2 (beat 2)

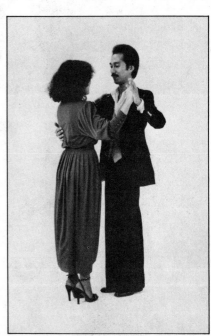

step 3 (beats 3-4)

Man's Part:

Beat *Steps*
- (1)   1. Left foot forward
- (2)   2. Right foot side
- (3-4) 3. Left foot close to right foot / hold
- (5)   4. Right foot back
- (6)   5. Left foot side
- (7-8) 6. Right foot close to left foot / hold

Woman's Part:

Beat *Steps*
- (1)   1. Right foot back
- (2)   3. Left foot side
- (3-4) 3. Right foot close to left foot / hold
- (5)   4. Left foot forward
- (6)   5. Right foot side
- (7-8) 6. Left foot close to right foot / hold

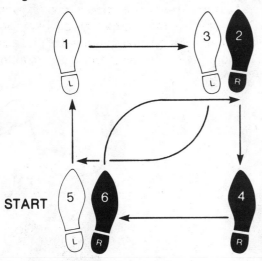

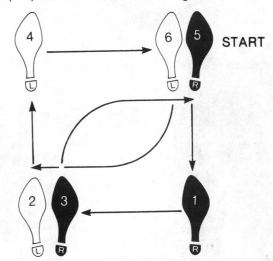

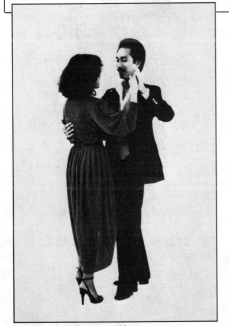

step 4 (beat 5)

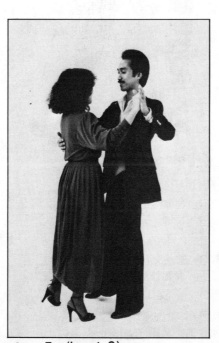

step 5 (beat 6)

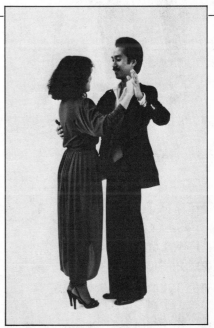

step 6 (beats 7-8)

DISCO SLOW

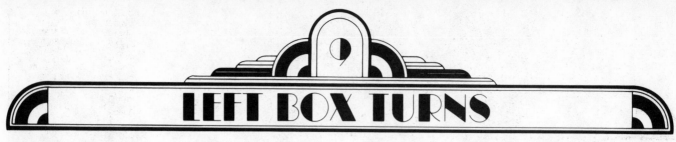

LEFT BOX TURNS

In the pattern for LEFT BOX TURNS, dual left turns are made on each step in the basic Box. Before partners take each step, therefore, they glance over their own left shoulders, then they simultaneously make dual *left turns* (counter-clockwise). Despite the addition of these left turns, however, the pattern still resembles a box configuration, in which each forward or backward step is followed with a chassé (side and close step), but concludes with a "hold" for one beat count of music.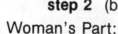

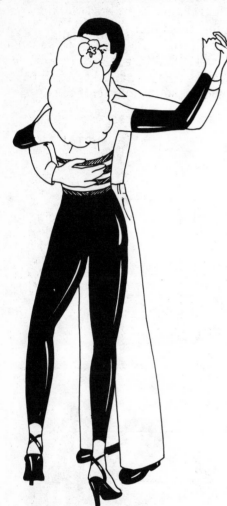

step 1 (beat 1)

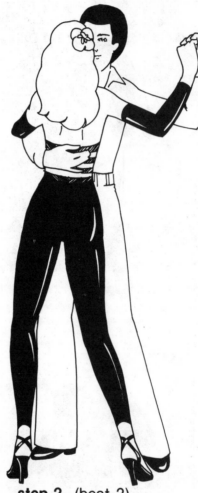

step 2 (beat 2)

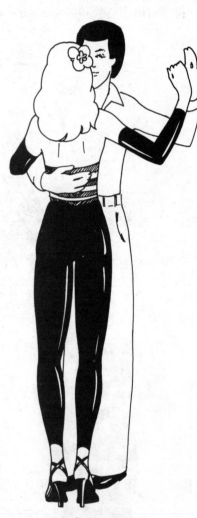

step 3 (beats 3-4)

Man's Part:
Beat Steps

(1)	1. Left foot forward
(2)	2. Right foot side
(3-4)	3. Left foot close to right foot / hold
(5)	4. Right foot back
(6)	5. Left foot side
(7-8)	6. Right foot close to left foot / hold

Woman's Part:
Beat Steps

(1)	1. Right foot back
(2)	2. Left foot side
(3-4)	3. Right foot close to left foot / hold
(5)	4. Left foot forward
(6)	5. Right foot side
(7-8)	6. Left foot close to right foot / hold

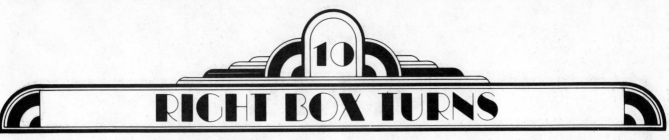
The pattern for RIGHT BOX TURNS differs from the previous pattern in two significant ways. Unlike the Left Box Turns, Right Box Turns incorporate dual right turns into the basic Box. Before taking each step, therefore, partners glance over their own right shoulders, then they both complete dual right turns (clockwise) on each step.

In addition to incorporating right turns, rather than left turns, this pattern also contains a unique combination of steps, which reverses the step sequence used for the Left Box. Although partners still trace a box configuration on the floor, the man starts by stepping back on his left foot, and the woman starts by stepping forward on her right foot. Although the direction changes, each forward or backward step is still followed with a chassé, as partners step side, then close side (draw feet together). On the last beat count of each measure of music, partners "hold" the close position.

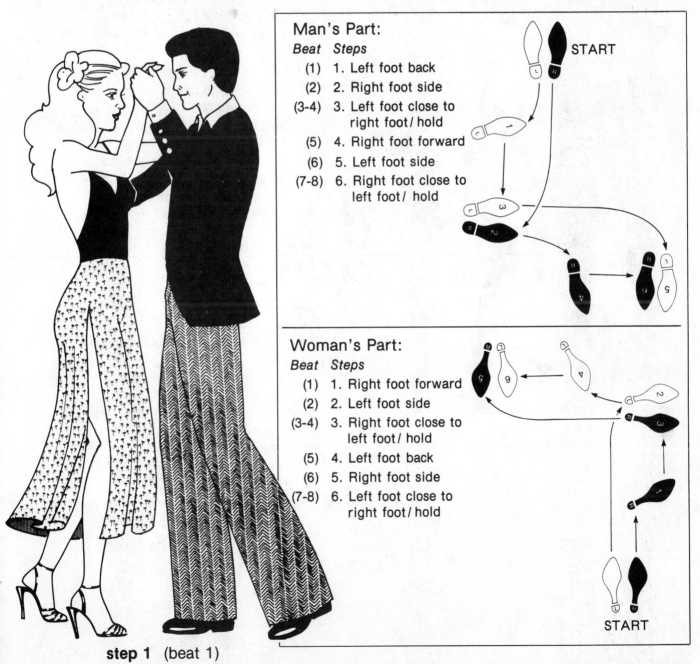

Man's Part:

Beat *Steps*

(1)	1. Left foot back
(2)	2. Right foot side
(3-4)	3. Left foot close to right foot / hold
(5)	4. Right foot forward
(6)	5. Left foot side
(7-8)	6. Right foot close to left foot / hold

Woman's Part:

Beat *Steps*

(1)	1. Right foot forward
(2)	2. Left foot side
(3-4)	3. Right foot close to left foot / hold
(5)	4. Left foot back
(6)	5. Right foot side
(7-8)	6. Left foot close to right foot / hold

step 1 (beat 1)

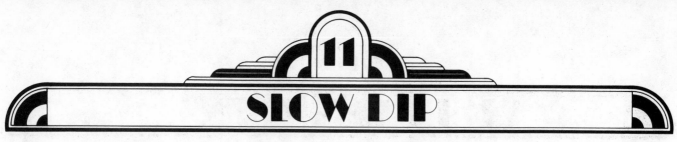
In the elegant and exquisitely sexy SLOW DIP, the man dips the woman back, until the woman's upper torso is perpendicular to the floor. This variation begins on beats 1-4 (steps 1-4) with side steps alternated with toe close steps, performed in the Closed Dance Position. On beats 5-7 (steps 5-7) the man holds the woman in the Dip by bracing her back with his right hand, without releasing her left hand from his right hand. To make her dip, the woman balances her weight on her right foot, lifts her left foot off the floor, and drops her head back. This variation concludes on beat 8 (step 8), as the man pulls the woman up out of her neck-stretching Dip.

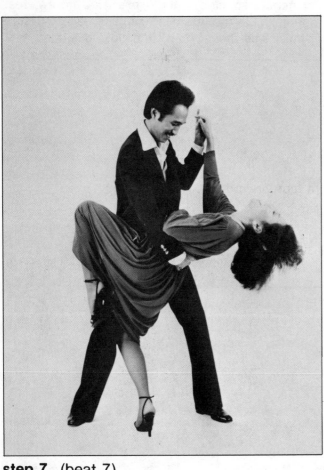

step 7 (beat 7)

Man's Part:

Beat Steps

(1) 1. Left foot side

(2) 2. Right foot toe next to left foot

(3) 3. Right foot side

(4) 4. Left toe next to right foot

(5) 5. Left foot side, bend left knee and dip woman back

(6) 6. Left foot holds his weight, as he balances the woman in Dip

(7) 7. Left foot holds his weight, as he balances the woman in the Dip

(8) 8. Right foot step in place, as he lifts woman out of the Dip

Woman's Part:

Beat Steps

(1) 1. Right foot side

(2) 2. Left foot toe next to right foot

(3) 3. Left foot side

(4) 4. Right foot toe next to left foot

(5) 5. Right foot side, pivoting ¼ left, as woman leans torso back

(6) 6. Right foot holds her weight, as woman lifts left foot off the floor and bends her left knee, while in the Dip

(7) 7. Right foot holds her weight as woman remains in the Dip

(8) 8. Left foot step in place, as the woman straightens torso, and lifts out of Dip

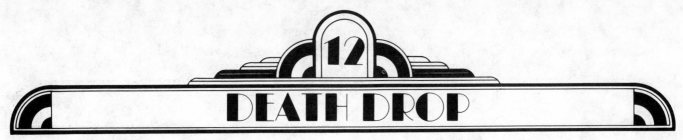

DEATH DROP

Performing a DEATH DROP in slow motion promises to be a rather terrifying, but unforgettable experience. Slowly, ever so slowly, the woman descends to the floor, as she balances all of her weight on her right foot. Of course, it's up to the Herculean man to grab both of the woman's wrists, then fling her down and hold her a few inches off the floor. Although any one of a number of step sequences can be used with the Death Drop, one popular pattern begins with side steps alternated with toe close steps on beats 1-4 (steps 1-4), completed in the Closed Dance Position. This variation concludes with the Death Drop on beats 5-8 (steps 5-8).

Man's Part:
Beat Steps

- (1) 1. Left foot side
- (2) 2. Right foot toe next to left foot
- (3) 3. Right foot side
- (4) 4. Left foot toe next to right foot
- (5) 5. Left foot side, as he grabs the woman's wrists, then flings her into the Death Drop
- (6) 6. Left foot holds his weight, as he lowers the woman further down into the Drop
- (7) 7. Left foot holds his weight as he balances the woman in the Death Drop
- (8) 8. Right foot step in place, as he lifts the woman up out of the Drop

Woman's Part:
Beat Steps

- (1) 1. Right foot side
- (2) 2. Left foot toe next to right foot
- (3) 3. Left foot side
- (4) 4. Right foot toe next to left foot
- (5) 5. Right foot side, pivoting ¼ left, as woman drops down with her right knee bent
- (6) 6. Right foot holds her weight, as she lifts her left foot off the floor, then drops further down
- (7) 7. Right foot holds her weight, while she remains in the Death Drop.
- (8) 8. Left foot step in place, as woman straightens up out of the Drop.

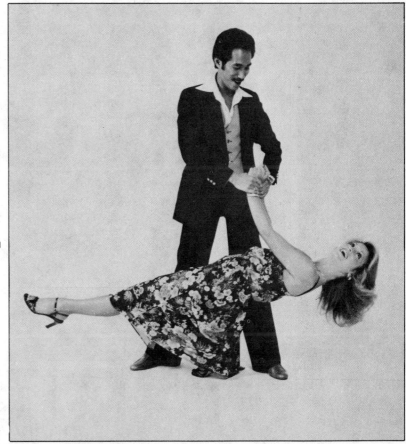

step 7 (beat 7)

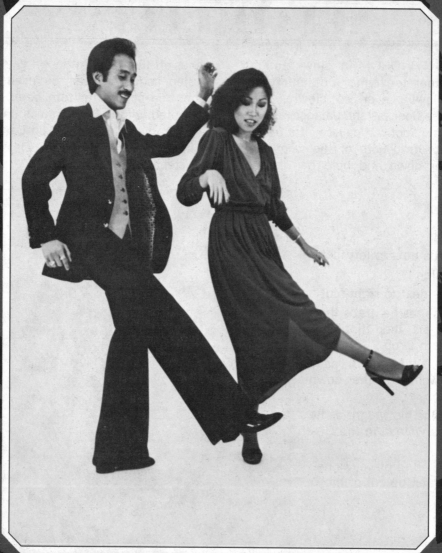

PART III

FREE-STYLE DISCO

CHAPTER 8

DISCO BODY DANCES

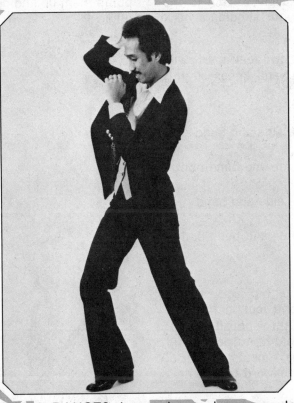

BODY DANCES have always been popular, because they are easy to perform as well as self-expressive. The earliest body dances were pantomime or mimetic dances. In the 1900s, body dances in the form of "animal dances" were performed to ragtime music. In the late 1950s and early 1960s, the country went crazy over body dances such as the Twist, Jerk, Hitchhike, and Mashed Potato. Today, disco dances, such as the Freak, the Bump, and the Rock are back in style like never before.

Sensual hip movement is the single most important ingredient that separates hot from lukewarm disco body dancers. Whether you sway, swish, flip, or shake your hips, you should move them as often and as emphatically as you possibly can. Once you've conquered the basic hip movements, you will be ready to stun everyone with your versatile, but rhythmically controlled, disco style!

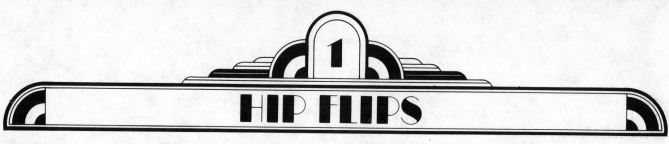

HIP FLIPS

The saucy flipping of the hips from side to side adds zip to your disco style. With feet spread about two feet apart and knees slightly bent, flip your hips from side to side and bounce your knees up and down on each beat of music. To flip effectively, lift your hip up and push it out to the side. For added zing, shake your shoulders back and forth, as you fling your hips from side to side. While doing these hip flips, move your hands frequently and expressively: for example, you might want to prop one or both hands on your hips, fling them up into the air (Travolta style), pump them up and down, or roll them around each other.

STANCE:

Start with feet spread about two feet apart, with weight balanced on both feet, and knees slightly bent.

Beat   Movement

(1)   1. Flip right hip out to the side and bend both knees down-up.

(2)   2. Flip left hip out to the side and bend both knees down-up.

(3)   3. Flip right hip out to the side and bend both knees down-up.

(4)   4. Flip left hip out to the side and bend both knees down-up.

ALTERNATE PATTERN

To add additional zest to your hip flips, spread feet diagonally apart (place one foot in front of, but slightly to the side of, the opposite foot). Continue to flip hips on each beat of music, but tilt your torso slightly forward for 4 beats of music, then lean your torso slightly backward for the next 4 beats.

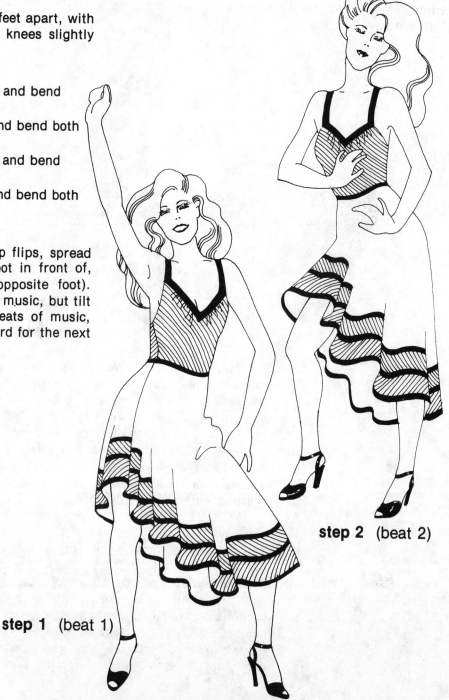

step 2 (beat 2)

step 1 (beat 1)

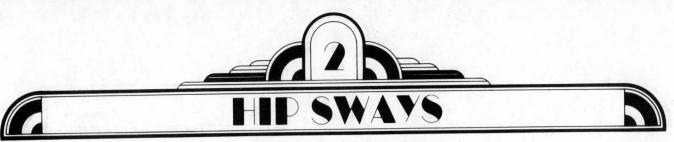

HIP SWAYS

Unlike the bouncy hip flips, the HIP SWAYS are smooth, sensuous and fluid. A gentle rocking motion is added, as you slowly shift your weight from one foot to the other. While rocking, sway your hips from side to side, letting your body drift with the rhythm of the music. To heighten the illusion of a flowing motion, swing both arms straight and across your chest, moving them either with or in opposition to the direction in which your hips are swaying.

Beat **Movement**

(1) 1. Rock weight to right foot and tilt left hip out to the side.

(2) 2. Rock weight to left foot and tilt right hip out to the side.

(3) 3. Rock weight to right foot and tilt left hip out to the side

(4) 4. Rock weight to left foot and tilt right hip out to the side

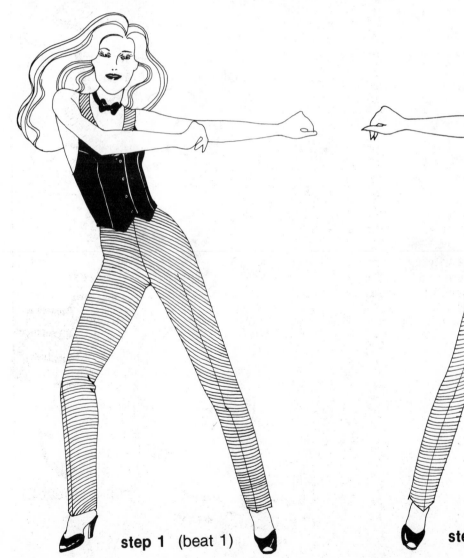

step 1 (beat 1)

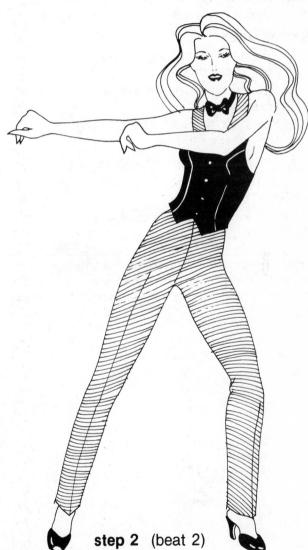

step 2 (beat 2)

STANCE:
Start with feet spread about two feet apart, with weight balanced on both feet, and knees slightly bent.

DISCO BODY DANCES

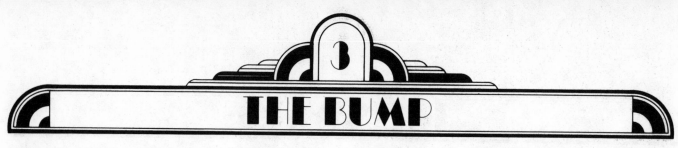

THE BUMP

For almost ten years now, disco dancers have spent many a night bumping to the disco beat. Similar to other body dances, such as the Freak, the BUMP comes in many sizes, shapes, and figures. Arms, shoulders, back, and rump, as well as hips, can be used to bump. Thus, the Bump, which can be done either solo or with a partner, becomes as individual as you are.

The basic Single Bump pattern substitutes a

STANCE:

Start with feet spread about two feet apart, with weight balanced equally on both feet.

bump for a step on every even-numbered beat count: step, bump, step, bump. To add a dash of flash to your bumping technique, a more complicated Triple Bump pattern begins with a diagonally forward step, followed by three quick bumps in succession. For full bumping power, keep knees relaxed, as you flip your hips and swing your arms freely.

Beat Movement
(1) 1. Right foot step diagonally forward
(2) 2. Bump left hip out, with weight on right foot
(3) 3. Left foot step diagonally forward
(4) 4. Bump right hip out, with weight on left foot

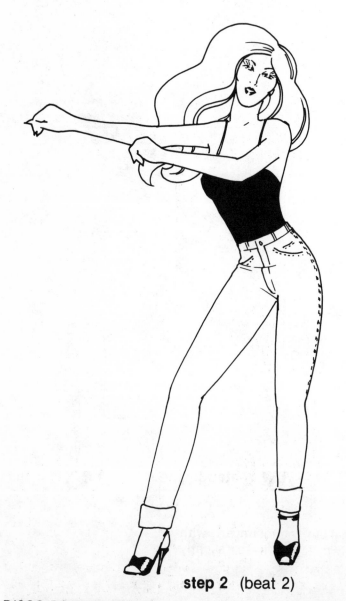

step 2 (beat 2)

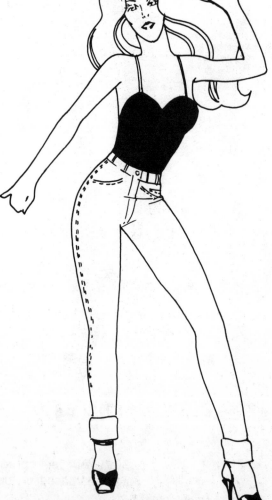

step 4 (beat 4)

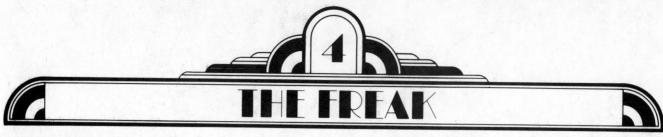

THE FREAK

The FREAK, a wild and crazy dance, started a disco trend quickly picked up by other funky body dances such as the *Spank,* the *Snake* and the *Feel.* Although both the dance and the song have freaked out the entire country, there's no right or wrong way to do the Freak correctly. Of course, the rhythm is obvious, which makes it easy to get the body moving in tune with the tempo. (Even DJs in roller skating rinks report that "le Freak" is one song often requested, due to its unbeatable beat.)

On the West Coast, a favorite Freak movement is the hand rotation in which the hands circle around the head. In another Freak technique done with feet spread about shoulder width apart, the dancer bobs up and down, while lifting and lowering his shoulders. A third technique, popular on the East Coast, turns the Freak into an up-dated, up-tempo Charleston in which the feet swivel back and forth, as the body jiggles to the rhythm. Whichever style you choose, remember to keep your knees relaxed, as you bounce up and down, 'cause the Freak is chic!

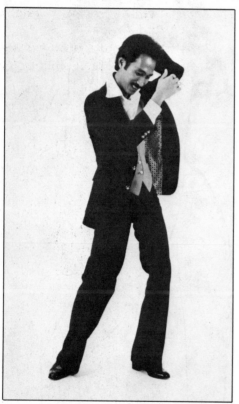

step 1 (beat 1)

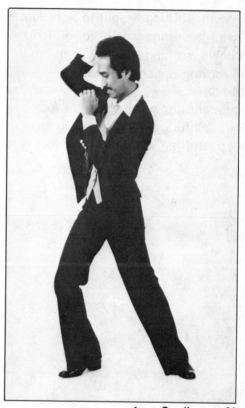

step 3 (beat 2)

STANCE:

Start with feet spread a comfortable distance apart, with weight balanced on both feet, and knees flexed.

Beat Movement

(1) 1. Swivel towards left, bend left knee, dip left shoulder, and rotate hands around your head.

(&) 2. Straighten up.

(2) 3. Swivel towards right, bend right knee, dip right shoulder, and rotate hands around your head.

(&) 4. Straighten up.

ALTERNATE PATTERN:

Hands may be extended down, with arms kept close to the body, and feet spread shoulder width apart. Maintain the same basic syncopated rhythm, but bounce up and down, shifting weight from one foot to the other, while flexing the knees, and lifting up from the shoulders.

DISCO BODY DANCES

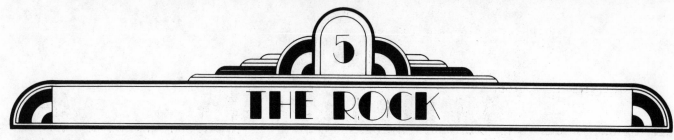
The ROCK, another sensuous free-style dance that can be transformed into a line or partner dance, combines hip flips with a rocking motion. Most of the hip-swaying motion is created by a smooth shifting of weight from one foot to the other. As you slowly descend to the floor, then rock yourself back up, knees should remain bent, with weight evenly distributed on both feet. If the Rock is performed with a partner, no hands are held, although the partners may rock into different positions, such as back to back, or into the Cradle Wrap.

STANCE:

Start with feet spread about two feet apart, with weight balanced on both feet, and knees relaxed.

Beat   Movement

(1)   1. Begin rocking down, shifting weight to left foot

(2)   2. Rock down, shifting weight to right foot

(3)   3. Rock down, shifting weight to left foot

(4)   4. Rock down, shifting weight to right foot

(5)   5. Begin rocking up, shifting weight to left foot

(6)   6. Rock up, shifting weight to right foot

(7)   7. Rock up, shifting weight to left foot

(8)   8. Rock up, shifting weight to right foot

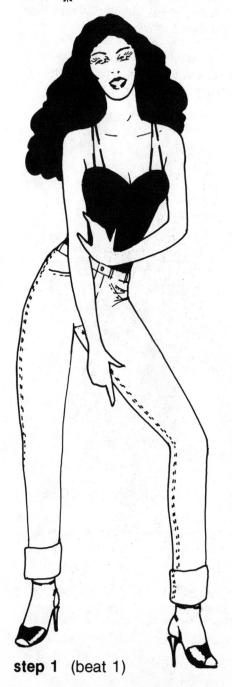

step 1   (beat 1)

DOLPHIN ROLLS

Although John Travolta may not be a Sea World porpoise, he sure knows how to dolphin roll his body. These DOLPHIN ROLLS, which combine hip shakes with body shimmies, are done with feet spread diagonally apart. On each beat of music, shake your hips and shimmy your shoulders, as you roll back and forth, shifting your weight from the backward to the forward foot.

STANCE:

Start with feet spread diagonally apart, with left foot forward and weight on left foot.

For a change of pace, place the right foot forward, then repeat the DOLPHIN ROLLS, rocking back and forth, as you shake your hips and shimmy your shoulders.

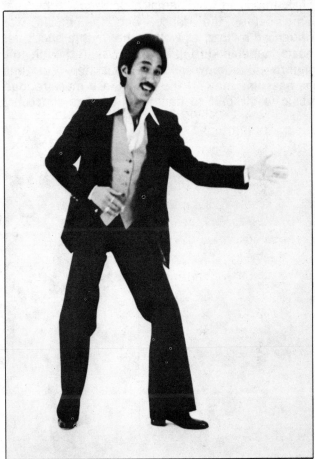

step 2 (beat 2)

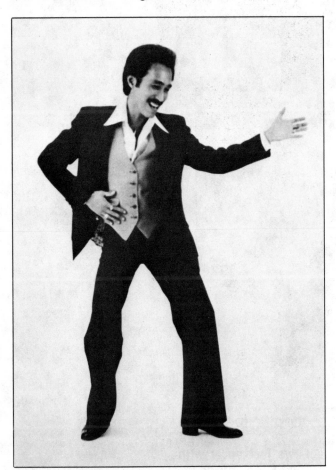

step 1 (beat 1)

Beat Movement

(1) 1. Roll weight backward onto right foot.
(2) 2. Roll weight forward onto left foot.
(3) 3. Roll weight backward onto right foot.
(4) 4. Roll weight forward onto left foot.

7 RIDE-A-BIKE

The RIDE-A-BIKE is a solo dance which first became popular during the early 1970s. Still a favorite among free-form enthusiasts, the Ride-a-Bike was originally performed to *reggae,* blues music imported from Jamaica. In *reggae,* the beat came before the dance, and the music was influenced by jazz, as well as the rhythm and blues music popular during the 1950s. Although the rhythm guitar plays all four beats, the drum and the bass line play off the beat. Since most *reggae* music is difficult to dance to, dancers concocted their own, rather simplified patterns, such as the Ride-A-Bike.

The Ride-a-Bike, which is performed with feet spread about two feet apart and knees flexed, pantomimes the actions of a cyclist. To mimic a bike rider, the dancer crouches down, bends his knees, and pretends to grab onto the handlebars. On each beat of music, the dancer pulls the handlebars from side to side, as he shifts his weight from one foot to the other. 🕺

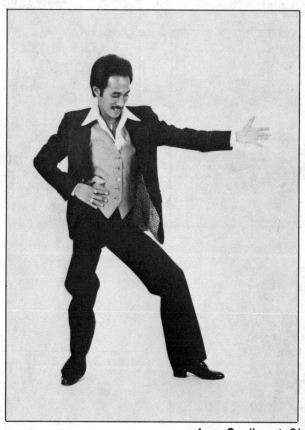

step 3 (beat 3)

STANCE:
Start with feet spread about two feet apart with weight balanced on both feet, and knees flexed.

Beat *Movement*
- (1) 1. Crouch down on knees, and pretend to hold handlebars of a bike.
- (2) 2. Turn bike right, throwing right shoulder and hip up.
- (3) 3. Turn bike left, swiveling left shoulder and hip up.
- (4) 4. Turn bike right, throwing right shoulder and hip up.

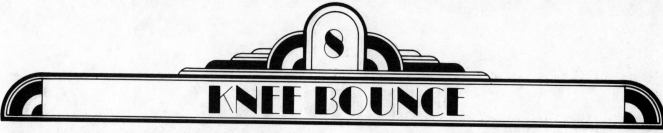

KNEE BOUNCE

Knees, as well as hips and thighs, get a terrific workout with the KNEE BOUNCE. Designed to keep you bouncing to the beat, this body dance is excellent for free-style dancing, but it can also be turned into a fantastic exercise that will tone and firm weak muscles. For all you ski buffs, this dance is especially effective for getting legs into shape to take the toughest mogul on the mountain. To add style to the Knee Bounce, shimmy your shoulders back and forth, as you bounce up and down.

STANCE:

Start with feet together in the parallel (close) position, with weight balanced on your left foot.

Beat   Movement

(1)   1. Right foot diagonally forward, bend right knee, tilt left hip up, reach right hand down.

(&)   2. Bounce both knees down, with weight on both feet.

(2)   3. Left foot close to right foot and flex both knees.

(&)   4. Bounce both knees down, with weight on both feet.

(3)   5. Left foot diagonally forward, bend left knee, tilt right hip up, reach left hand down.

(&)   6. Bounce both knees down, with weight on both feet.

(4)   7. Right foot close to left foot and flex both knees.

(&)   8. Bounce both knees down, with weight on both feet.

step 1 (beat 1)

173   *DISCO BODY DANCES*

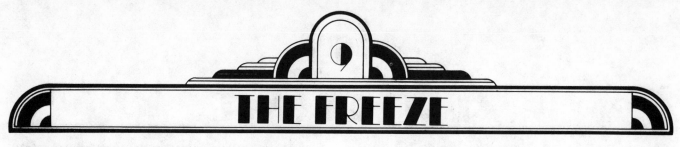

THE FREEZE

The FREEZE is a free-style body dance popular in some regions of the country, including Dallas, Texas, according to dance instructor Diane Johnson. The Freeze is made up of four distinct parts, with each part completed in 4 beats (1 measure) of music: Walk Steps; Hip Movements; Freeze; ¼ Line Turn. As the last part indicates, the Freeze can be done as a line dance, as well as a free-style dance.

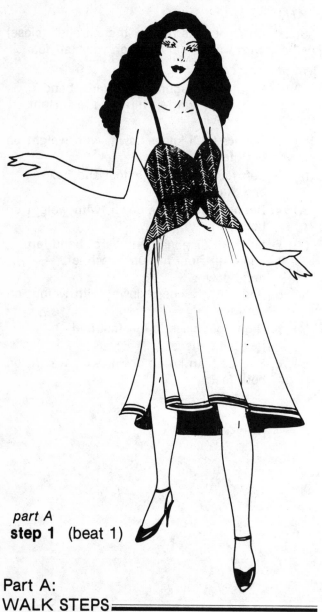

part A
step 1 (beat 1)

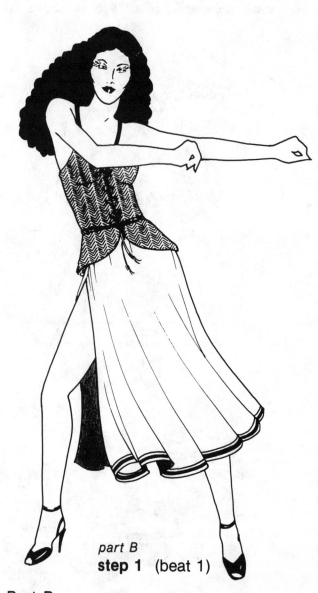

part B
step 1 (beat 1)

Part A:
WALK STEPS

Part A is composed of four walk steps, completed in four beats of music. Although these walk steps may be taken in any direction that you choose, begin walking with your right foot. While taking your walk steps, swing your arms freely back and forth and thrust your chest in and out.

Part B:
HIP MOVEMENTS

In Part B, you will flip, shake, or sway your hips in any direction you choose, as long as the 4 hip movements are completed in 4 beats of music. Of course, plenty of dynamic arm movement and knee bounce should accent the hip movements.

Part C:
FREEZE

In Part C you will strike one pose and freeze in that position for 4 beats of music. For added effect, the arms and body can be held in an unusual or angular position, using the locking technique of the L.A. Lock.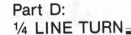

Part D:
¼ LINE TURN

The last sequence of steps in the Freeze begins with 3 tap steps (tap forward, tap back, tap side) and ends with a ¼ line turn. As most line hoofers know, the line turn enables the dancers to make one sweeping ¼ left turn (90 degrees counter-clockwise) to face the next wall. To make this ¼ turn, swing your right foot to the left, while pivoting around on your left foot. After completing your line turn, repeat the entire Freeze pattern, beginning with the walk steps in Part A.

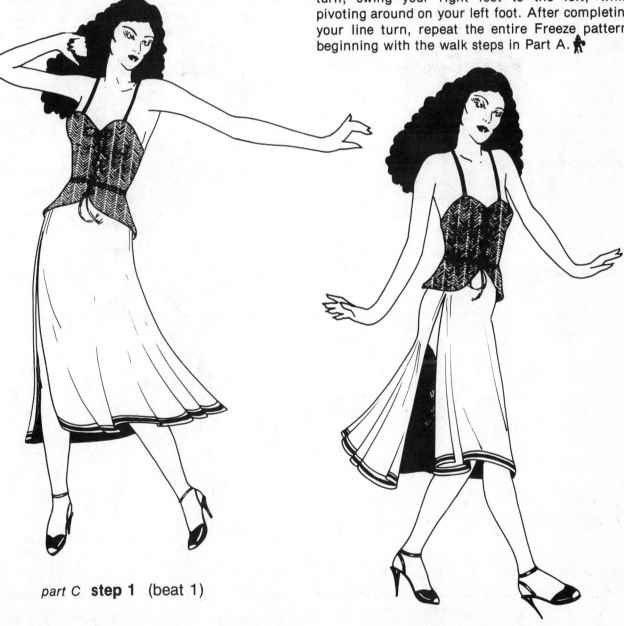

part C **step 1** (beat 1)

part D **step 4** (beat 4)

DISCO BODY DANCES

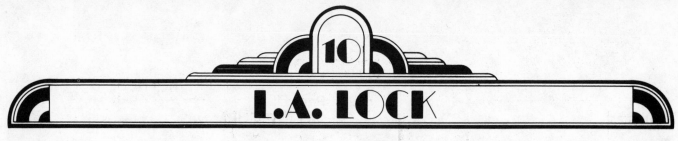

L.A. LOCK

The Lockers, perhaps the hottest group of free-style dancers in the world, have created their own unique dancing style, which is currently sweeping the country. Just a few of the free-form dances that the Lockers have made famous include the *Robot, Slow Motion, Skeeter Rabbit, Stop and Go, Samba Splits,* and the *Scoobie Doo.* The L. A. LOCK, which fits into the disco category of funky, adopts the Lockers' dance technique in which the joints of the body are locked into position.

Unlike most body dances which can be broken down to fit into a basic beat versus body movement, the L.A. Lock does not conform to any strict pattern. In general, the dancer locks into one unusual position for one or two beats of music. This locked pose is then followed with a series of quick, sharp movements. Double takes, in which the dancer turns his head and takes several quick glances in succession, are called fast locks. Many lock routines include splits, jumps and other gymnastic stunts.

STANCE

Start with feet spread about a foot apart, with weight balanced equally on both feet.

Beat   Movement
- (1)   1. Strike an unusual or angular pose and lock joints into position.
- (2)   2. Hold position, with joints locked.
- (3)   3. Take a fast double take.
- (&)   4. Take a fast double take.
- (4)   5. Take a fast double take.

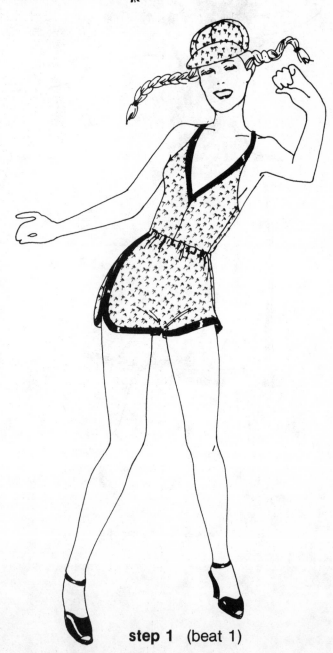

step 1 (beat 1)

CHAPTER 9

FREE-STYLE COMBINATION DANCES

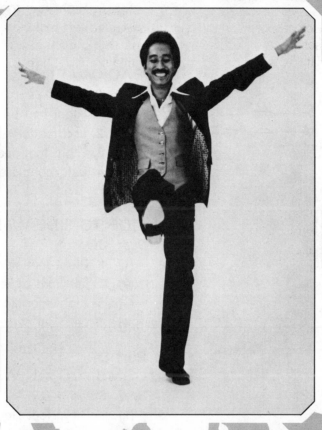

This chapter explores a variety of FREE-STYLE or FREE-FORM disco dances. To most of you, some patterns may appear extremely simple. For example, the Disco Strut combines a series of walking steps, and the Disco Tap Out yokes together various tap steps. Nevertheless, these step combinations are frequently used in both free-style and line dances.

In addition, these combination dances give you ample opportunity to practice your pivots, spins, kicks, and swivels. Moreover, you'll have the chance to coordinate steps with sexy body movements such as hip thrusts, shoulder shakes, and body shimmies. After you master the patterns described in this secton, you'll never have to worry about sticking out like a sore thumb on the dance floor. Instead, you'll be able to ''do your own thing'' with undeniable class!

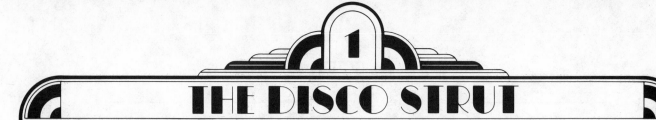

THE DISCO STRUT

Strut is the only word that adequately describes how to walk in true disco style. Swing your arms, dip your shoulders, thrust your chest in and out, and bounce your knees to the disco rhythm. Think of the way Travolta could strut and sway as he swung those buckets of paint in *Saturday Night Fever.*

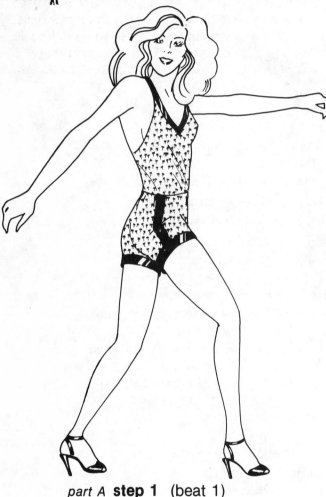

part A **step 1** (beat 1)

BODY MOVEMENTS
The body weight shifts naturally as the feet move. On each walking step forward, backward or to the side, bend the knee that steps. On all tap close steps, bend the opposite knee. While stepping to the side, tilt opposite hip out. While stepping forward, tilt body slightly backward. While stepping backward, tilt body slightly forward.

Part A:
FORWARD WALK
Beat Steps
- (1) 1. Right foot forward
- (2) 2. Left foot close to right foot
- (3) 3. Right foot forward
- (4) 4. Left foot close to right foot

Part B:
BACKWARD WALK
Beat Steps
- (1) 1. Right foot back
- (2) 2. Left foot close to right foot
- (3) 3. Right foot back
- (4) 4. Left foot close to right foot

Part C:
SIDE TO SIDE WALK
Beat Steps
- (1) 1. Right foot side
- (2) 2. Left foot close to right foot
- (3) 3. Right foot side
- (4) 4. Left foot close to right foot

Part D:
COMBINATION WALK WITH TAP STEPS
Beat Steps
- (1) 1. Right foot side
- (2) 2. Left foot close to right foot
- (3) 3. Right foot side
- (4) 4. Left foot tap next to right foot
- (5) 5. Left foot back
- (6) 6. Right foot close to left foot
- (7) 7. Left foot back
- (8) 8. Right foot tap next to left foot
- (9) 9. Right foot forward
- (10) 10. Left foot close to right foot
- (11) 11. Right foot forward
- (12) 12. Left foot tap next to right foot
- (13) 13. Left foot side
- (14) 14. Right foot close to right
- (15) 15. Left foot side
- (16) 16. Right foot tap next to left foot

TAXI DRIVER

The TAXI DRIVER, a relatively easy free-style dance, became popular after Travolta's hip thrusting performance in *Saturday Night Fever*. The first 8 beats (8 steps) contain simple walking steps which demand a strutting style, as you swing your shoulders back and forth, and thrust your chest in and out. The last 4 beats of music emphasize hip flips, as your hips thrust from side to side, while your arms fling up, then reach down. 🤷

BODY MOVEMENTS

As you take your 8 walking steps, *strut:* i.e., stick your chest in and out, wiggle your rear from side to side, and bend those knees. On the hip thrusts, alternate throwing out your hips, while tilting or leaning in the opposite direction. Pretend that you are trying to hail a taxi in the middle of a blizzard.

Beat   Steps

- (1)   1. Left foot forward
- (2)   2. Right foot forward
- (3)   3. Left foot forward
- (4)   4. Right foot forward
- (5)   5. Left foot back
- (6)   6. Right foot back
- (7)   7. Left foot back
- (8)   8. Right foot back
- (9)   9. Left hip out (bend right knee, lift right hand up)
- (10) 10. Right hip out (bend left knee, bring right hand down)
- (11) 11. Left hip out (bend right knee, lift right hand up)
- (12) 12. Right hip out (bend left knee, bring right hand down)

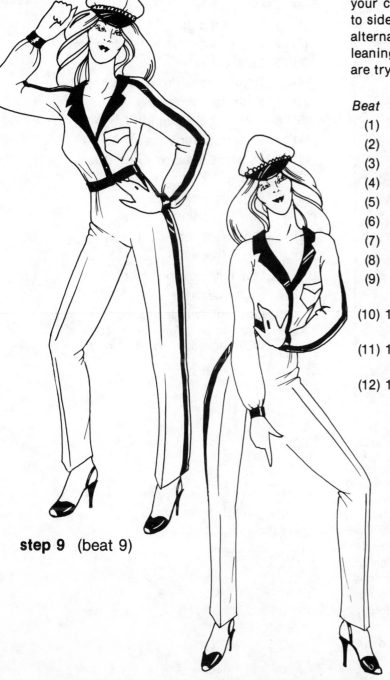

step 9 (beat 9)

step 10 (beat 10)

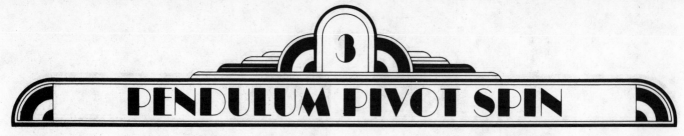

PENDULUM PIVOT SPIN

The PENDULUM PIVOT SPIN combines double chassés with forward and backward walk steps and includes tap close steps on every fourth beat of music. On the last step of this 16 beat pattern, a Pivot Spin is substituted for the tap step. To make a Pivot Spin, balance your weight on your right foot, as you swing your left foot around the right foot, and complete a Full Right Turn by spinning 360 degrees clockwise. (If you prefer, however, a Lift may replace the Pivot Spin, as you lift your left leg off the floor and bend it at the knee, crossing it in front of your right leg.)

Beat Steps

- (1) 1. Left foot side
- (2) 2. Right foot close to left foot
- (3) 3. Left foot side
- (4) 4. Right foot tap next to left foot
- (5) 5. Right foot forward
- (6) 6. Left foot close to left foot
- (7) 7. Right foot forward
- (8) 8. Left foot tap next to right foot
- (9) 9. Left foot back
- (10) 10. Right foot close to left foot
- (11) 11. Left foot back
- (12) 12. Right foot tap next to left foot
- (13) 13. Right foot side
- (14) 14. Left foot close to right foot
- (15) 15. Right foot side
- (16) 16. Left foot swings around right foot, pivoting in a Full Right Turn (360 degrees clockwise) on the right foot

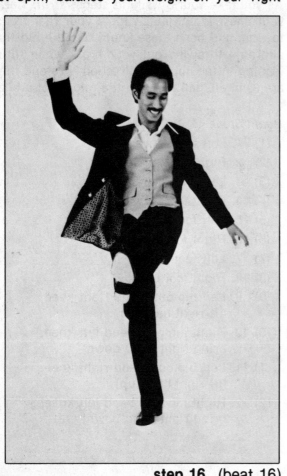

step 16   (beat 16)

ARM MOVEMENTS
Swing arms freely, flinging them up and down.

BODY MOVEMENTS
On the odd-numbered beat counts, tilt your body in the direction that is opposite to the direction of the step: on the side steps, flip hip out to the opposite side; on the forward steps, lean torso slightly back; on the back steps, lean torso slightly forward. On the even-numbered beat counts, straighten hips and align your body, as you draw your feet together.

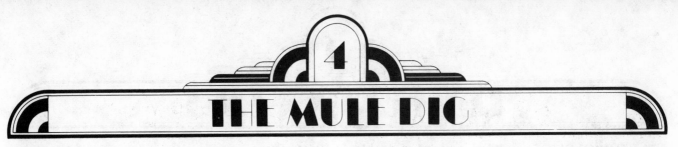

The MULE DIG is a simple dance pattern, done in place (in one position), in which the toe of one foot digs into the ground. Similar to the tap step, a stub or dig step is done while balancing the weight on the opposite foot. The leg that supports the body while you stub forward should be bent slightly. In Part A, a simple digging or stubbing pattern is described. In Part B, syncopated beats are added as you stub then kick forward. These two parts may be repeated sequentially or separately as many times as you choose. Moreover, to do this dance effectively, you should pretend that you are a stubborn mule who balks at moving forward.

Part A:
MULE DIG

Beat Steps

(1) 1. Left foot dig forward (stub left toes against floor, bend left knee, as weight shifts to right foot)

(2) 2. Right foot dig forward (stub right toes against floor, bend right knee, as weight shifts to left foot)

(3) 3. Left foot dig forward (stub left toes against floor, bend left knee, as weight shifts to right foot)

(4) 4. Right foot dig forward (stub right toes against floor, bend right knee, as weight shifts to left foot)

Part B:
DIG-KICK STEP

Beat Steps

(1) 1. Left foot dig forward (short, stubbing step with weight on right foot, as left knee bends slightly)

(&) 2. Left foot kick forward (small, short kick forward, with weight on right foot, straighten left leg)

(2) 3. Left foot close back (swing left foot back, next to right foot, placing weight on left foot)

(3) 4. Right foot dig forward (short, stubbing step with weight on left foot, as right knee bends slightly)

(&) 5. Right foot kick forward (small, short kick forward, with weight on left foot, straighten right leg)

(4) 6. Right foot close back (swing right foot back, next to left foot, placing weight on right foot)

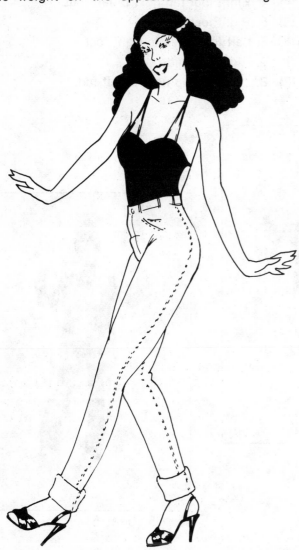

part B **step 2** (beat ''and'')

ARM MOVEMENTS
Swing arms back and forth with a free and vibrant motion, as if walking through a cornflower field at dawn.

BODY MOVEMENTS
Bend knee slightly on the stub or dig step; straighten one knee and bend opposite knee, as you shift your weight.

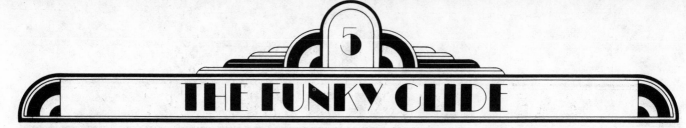

THE FUNKY GLIDE

The FUNKY GLIDE combines a series of double chassés, incorporating a tap close step on every fourth beat of music. On the chassé, each side step is followed with a close step in which feet are drawn together. In essence, the Funky Glide is an up-dated version of the *Chuckie,* a disco free-style dance that alternated single chassés, popular during the early 1970s. 🕺

Beat	Steps
(1)	1. Left foot side
(2)	2. Right foot close to left foot
(3)	3. Left foot side
(4)	4. Right foot tap next to left foot
(5)	5. Right foot side
(6)	6. Left foot close to right foot
(7)	7. Right foot side
(8)	8. Left foot tap next to left foot

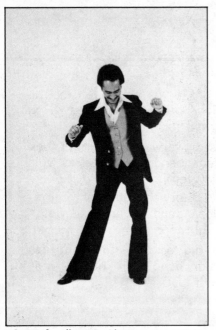

step 1 (beat 1)

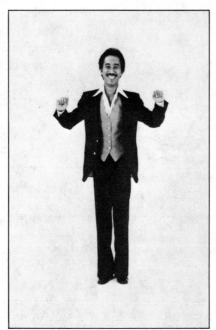

step 2 (beat 2)

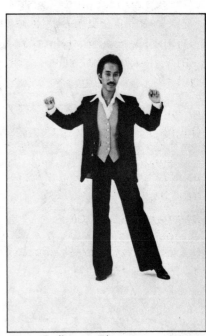

step 5 (beat 5)

ARM MOVEMENTS
Swing arms from side to side, as you slip slide away.

BODY MOVEMENTS
As you step side on the odd-numbered beats, stick your hip out, tilt your torso, and bend one knee. As you draw feet together (close) on the even-numbered beats, straighten hips, align the body, and flex knees.

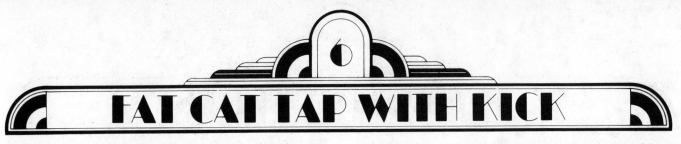

FAT CAT TAP WITH KICK

Two short, snappy kicks are finagled into this syncopated pattern. To make your kick, swing your foot forward, lifting it off the ground. After you have kicked your foot forward, immediately swing it back into place and put your weight on it. Since the entire kick and swing (close back) takes only one beat of music, you'd better hot foot it and kick fast. Mastery of this kick step will make it easy for you to incorporate kicks into other dance patterns.

Beat	Steps
(1)	1. Right foot tap side
(2)	2. Right foot step side
(3)	3. Left foot tap next to right foot
(&)	4. Left foot kick forward (short kick)
(4)	5. Left foot swing (close) back
(5)	6. Right foot step in place
(6)	7. Left foot tap side
(7)	8. Left foot step side
(8)	9. Right foot tap next to left foot
(&)	10. Right foot kick forward (short kick)
(9)	11. Right foot swing (close) back
(10)	12. Left foot step in place

BODY MOVEMENTS
On the tap steps, tilt hip up, but bend the opposite knee. On side steps, bend the knee that steps, and straighten body. On the short kick steps, straighten the leg, flex the opposite knee, and slightly tilt head and shoulders back.

ARM MOVEMENTS
On the side steps, swing arms back and forth. On the kick steps, swing arms up and out to the side.

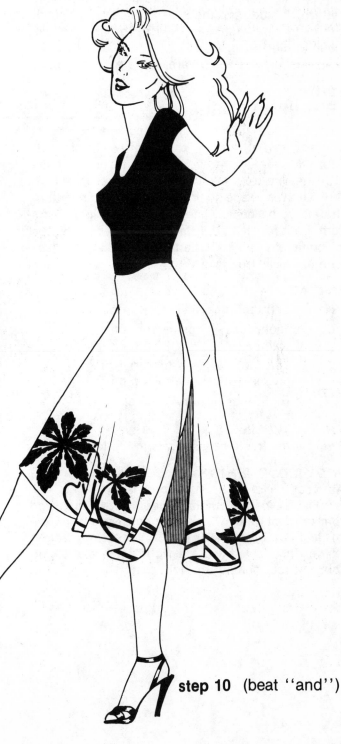

step 10 (beat ''and'')

FREE-STYLE DANCES

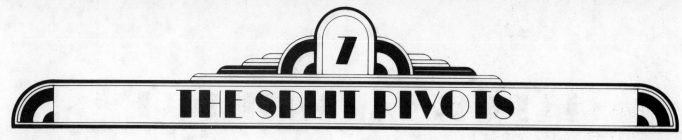

THE SPLIT PIVOTS

The SPLIT PIVOTS nudge their way into many free-style variations, including some line dances such as the *Midnight Fever Line Dance*. Similar to Pivot Spins, these Split Pivots (Dual Half Pivot Turns) also form complete turns in a circular pattern. In addition, the Split Pivots may be made either to the right (clockwise) or to the left (counter-clockwise).

Nevertheless, there are several differences between these two types of pivot turns. First of all, most Pivot Spins are made in one beat of music, but Split Pivots take 4 beats to complete. Secondly, Pivot Spins are made with one foot planted on the floor, while the opposite foot swings around. In a Split Pivot, the feet switch right smack in the middle. Therefore, Split Pivots are composed of two Half Turns, each made in the same direction, but with alternate feet.

Part A:
LEFT PIVOT TURNS

Left Pivot Turns, completed in 4 beats (1 measure) of music, combine two Half Left Turns. Moreover, the first Half Left Turn is made with the left foot pivoting, while the second Half Left Turn is made with the right foot pivoting. Therefore, on beat 3 (step 3), your weight shifts from the left foot to the right foot, as you continue to complete a Full Left Turn (360 degrees counter-clockwise).

Beat   Steps

  (1)   1. Left foot diagonally forward

  (2)   2. Right foot swings in front of left foot, pivoting in a ½ Left Turn on left foot

  (3)   3. Left foot swings behind right foot, pivoting in a ½ Left Turn on right foot

  (4)   4. Right foot close to left foot

ARM MOVEMENTS
Swing arms freely as you pivot to the left.

BODY MOVEMENTS
As your Pivot Left Turn begins on beats 1-2 (steps 1-2), bend your left knee slightly, pivot on your left foot, and swing your right foot around the left foot. On beats 3-4 (steps 3-4) shift your weight to the right foot, bend the right knee, and swing your left foot behind the right foot.

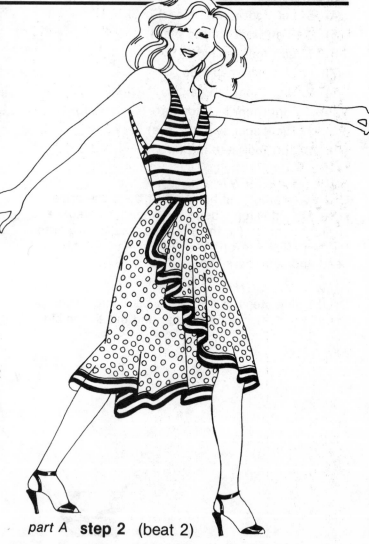

part A **step 2** (beat 2)

Part B:
RIGHT PIVOT TURNS

Right Pivot Turns, completed in 4 beats (1 measure) of music, combine two Half Right Turns. Moreover, the first Half Right Turn is made with the right foot pivoting, while the second Half Right Turn is made with the left foot pivoting. Therefore, on beat 3 (step 3) your weight shifts from the right foot to the left foot, as you continue to complete a Full Right Turn (360 degrees clockwise).

ARM MOVEMENTS:
Swing arms freely as you pivot to the right.

Beat   Steps
(1)   1. Right foot diagonally forward
(2)   2. Left foot swings in front of right foot, pivoting in a ½ Right Turn on right foot
(3)   3. Right foot swings behind left foot, pivoting in a ½ Right Turn on left foot
(4)   4. Left foot close to right foot

BODY MOVEMENTS
As your Pivot Right Turn begins on beats 1-2 (steps 1-2), bend your right knee slightly, pivot right on your right foot, and swing your left foot around your right foot. On beats 3-4 (steps 3-4), shift your weight to your left foot, bend the left knee slightly, and swing your right foot behind the left foot.

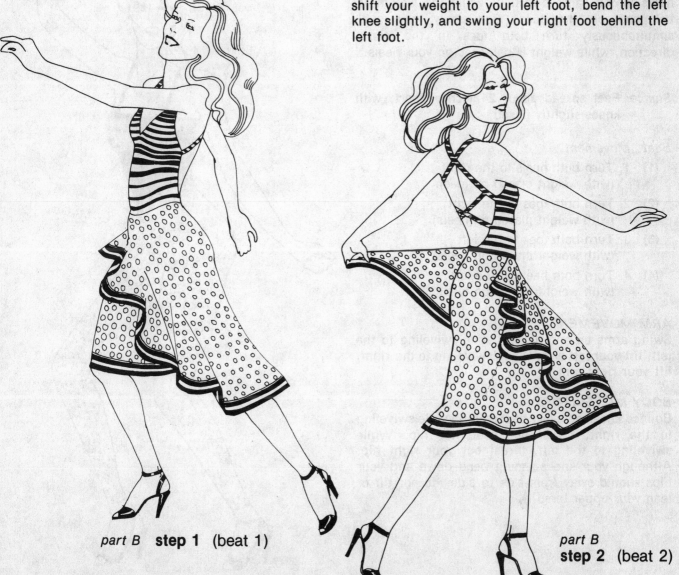

part B **step 1** (beat 1)

part B
step 2 (beat 2)

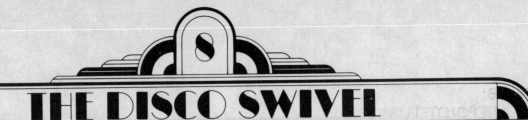

THE DISCO SWIVEL

The DISCO SWIVEL is a free-style dance that combines two different types of foot swivels. Part A uses side-to-side swivels in which both heels or both toes simultaneously swivel in the same direction. Part B is composed of in-and-out swivels in which "roach toes" are alternated with "pigeon toes." In the "roach toe," heels are pointed towards each other, and toes are turned out. In the "pigeon toe," heels are turned out, and toes are pointed towards each other. 🕺

Part A:
SIDE-TO-SIDE SWIVELS

In Part A your feet will be spread about 24 inches (shoulder width) apart, as you swivel from side to side. Instead of turning heels towards or away from each other, however, you will turn both heels in the same direction, while the weight is balanced on the toes. Conversely, you will simultaneously turn both toes in the same direction, while weight is balanced on your heels.

Stance: Feet spread about 24 inches apart, with knees slightly flexed.

Beat   Movement
  (1) 1. Turn both heels to the right
        (with weight placed on toes).
  (2) 2. Turn both toes to the right
        (with weight placed on heels)
  (3) 3. Turn both toes to the left
        (with weight placed on heels).
  (4) 4. Turn both heels to the left
        (with weight placed on toes).

ARM MOVEMENTS
Swing arms up and down. While swiveling to the left, lift your left arm. While swiveling to the right, lift your right arm.

BODY MOVEMENTS
Bounce knees on every beat count. While swiveling to the right, thrust out your left hip. While swiveling to the left, thrust out your right hip. Although your knees should bend down and your hips should sway from side to side, do not tilt or lean your upper torso. 🕺

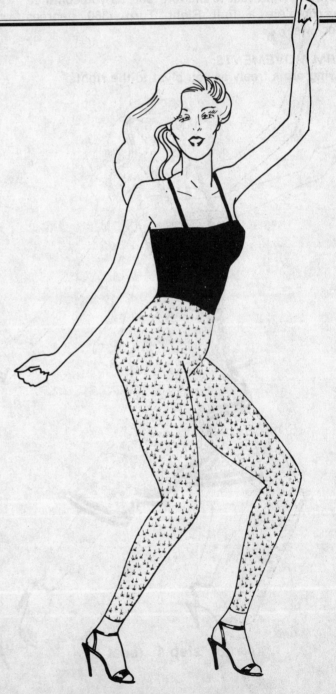

part A **step 1** (beat 1)

Part B:
IN AND OUT SWIVELS

Part B contains some odd but amusing foot movements in which both heels or both toes swivel towards each other, then split apart. Whenever both heels are pointing towards each other, with both toes pointing in opposite directions, the position is called the *roach toe.* Conversely, whenever both heels are pointing in opposite directions, with both toes pointing towards each other, the position is called the *pigeon toe.* This section combines both the roach toe and the pigeon toe positions, varying the stance as the heels and toes alternate swiveling in and out.

In addition, as you move towards the right (on odd numbered beats), your weight should shift to your right heel and left toe. As you move towards the left (on even numbered beats), your weight should shift to the left heel and right toe. Moreover, this entire sequence is done with feet planted about 24 inches apart (approximately shoulder width apart).

Stance: Feet spread about 24 inches apart, with knees slightly flexed.

Beat   Movement

(1)   1. Swivel Out (roach toe): Point both heels towards each other, with toes turned out (with weight on right heel and left toe)

(2)   2. Swivel In (pigeon toe): Turn both heels out, with toes turned in (with weight on left heel and right toe)

(3)   3. Swivel Out (roach toe): Point both heels towards each other, with toes turned out (with weight on right heel and left toe)

(4)   4. Swivel In (pigeon toe): Turn both heels out, with toes turned in (with weight on left heel and right toe)

BODY MOVEMENTS
As heels swivel towards each other, with toes spread apart, lean torso backward, and thrust the left hip out. As heels spread apart, with toes pointing towards each other, scrunch torso forward and thrust the right hip out.

ARM MOVEMENTS
When your heels are pointing towards each other and toes are spread apart (on odd numbered beats), push both elbows back. When your heels are spread apart, with toes pointing towards each other (on even numbered beats), lift elbows out to the sides.

part A **step 2** (beat 2)

187

JAZZ SQUARE WALK

The JAZZ SQUARE WALK is a popular dance pattern that can be performed as either a free-style dance or as a touch dance. If jazzed up to become a partner dance, as a Salsa variation, the basic pattern is not altered, which means that the man's part is exactly the same as the woman's part!

As a free-style dance, the Jazz Square Walk makes any dancer look like a pro. This illusion is created perhaps by the pattern which contains pass (cross) steps, back steps, side steps and tap steps. Of course, all of these steps are easy to do, but they still look classy to onlookers.

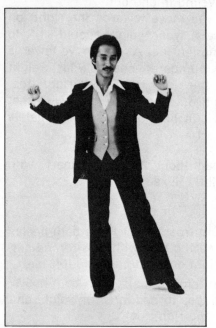

step 4 (beat 4)

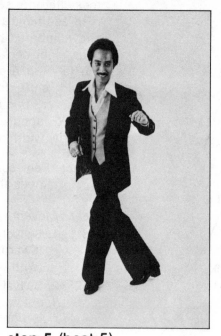

step 5 (beat 5)

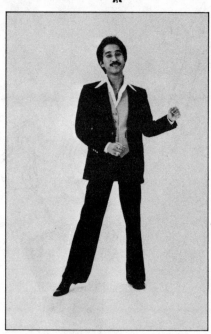

step 8 (beat 8)

Beat Step

(1) 1. Right foot pass forward
     (cross in front of left foot)

(2) 2. Left foot pass forward
     (cross in front of right foot)

(3) 3. Right foot back

(4) 4. Left foot tap side

(5) 5. Left foot pass forward
     (cross in front of right foot)

(6) 6. Right foot pass forward
     (cross in front of left foot)

(7) 7. Left foot back

(8) 8. Right foot tap side

FREE-STYLE DANCES

CHAPTER 10

LINE DANCES

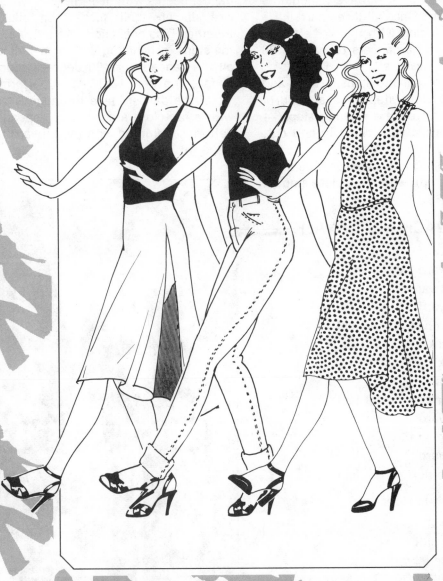

From pre-historic times, dancers have joined together to perform LINE DANCES. During the 1930s, at the height of theatrical dancing in motion pictures and musical comedies, Busby Berkeley choreographed spectacular production numbers. Some of the best movie musicals, which contain stunning dance numbers, include *An American in Paris* (1951), *Singin' in the Rain* (1952), *Seven Brides for Seven Brothers* (1954), and *West Side Story* (1957). The popular movie *Saturday Night Fever* indicates that line dancing is back in style on the disco floor.

Although any number of people — from two to fifty — can perform in a line dance, there are a few standard rules that apply to most line dances. First of all, dancers stand and face the same direction. Secondly, every dancer in the line performs the exact same sequence of steps. Thirdly, each line dance concludes with a ¼ Left Line Turn. To make their ¼ turn, all the dancers in the line kick their right foot forward, while pivoting 90 degrees counter-clockwise on their left foot. Once the dancers have completed their turn, they should be facing the next wall, as they repeat the entire line dance from beginning to end.

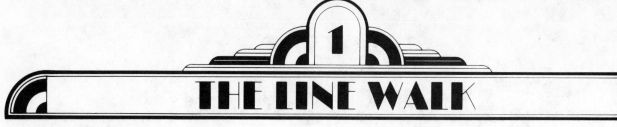

THE LINE WALK

The LINE WALK, a 38 step line dance completed in 38 beats of music, can be divided into three distinct parts. Each part, however, should be performed consecutively. Once all three parts have been performed, concluding with the ¼ Left Line Turn and 4 steps back, the dancers repeat the 38 steps, while facing the next wall.

Part A is composed of walking steps forward and backward, with a tap close step on every fourth beat. Remember to strut on the walking steps — bounce your knees, thrust your chest in and out, and swing those shoulders!

Part B is made up of double chassés (side step, followed with a close step), with a tap close step on every fourth beat.

Part C, the most radical part of this basic line dance, begins with heel clicks in which the dancers rise up on their toes, then click their heels together. The heel clicks are followed with tap and toe steps, concluding with a ¼ Left Line Turn, as all the dancers turn 90 degrees counter-clockwise to face the next wall. After performing the Line Turn, the dancers take three steps back, followed with a tap close step, before repeating the entire pattern, beginning with the forward and backward walk. 🕺

Part A:
FORWARD AND BACKWARD WALK

Beat Steps
- (1) 1. Left foot forward
- (2) 2. Right foot forward
- (3) 3. Left foot forward
- (4) 4. Right foot tap next to left foot
- (5) 5. Right foot back
- (6) 6. Left foot back
- (7) 7. Right foot back
- (8) 8. Left foot tap next to right foot
- (9) 9. Left foot forward
- (10) 10. Right foot forward
- (11) 11. Left foot forward
- (12) 12. Right foot tap next to left foot

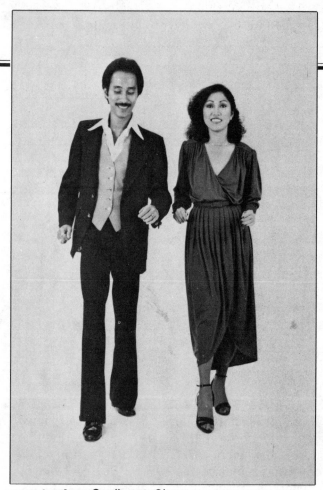

part A **step 2** (beat 2)

Part B:
SIDE-TO-SIDE WALK

Beat Steps

(1) 1. Right foot side
(2) 2. Left foot close to right foot
(3) 3. Right foot side
(4) 4. Left foot tap next to right foot
(5) 5. Left foot side
(6) 6. Right foot close to left foot
(7) 7. Left foot side
(8) 8. Right foot tap next to left foot
(9) 9. Right foot side
(10) 10. Left foot tap next to right foot
(11) 11. Left foot side
(12) 12. Right foot tap next to left foot

Part C:
HEEL CLICKS, TAP STEPS, AND ¼ LINE TURN

Beat Steps

(1) 1. Click heels (lift up on toes and click heels together)
(2) 2. Click heels (lift up on toes and click heels together)
(3) 3. Right foot tap forward
(4) 4. Right foot tap forward
(5) 5. Right foot tap back
(6) 6. Right foot tap back
(7) 7. Right foot toe forward
(8) 8. Right foot toe back
(9) 9. Right foot toe side
(10) 10. Right foot kick forward, pivoting ¼ left on left foot
(11) 11. Right foot back
(12) 12. Left foot back
(13) 13. Right foot back
(14) 14. Left foot tap next to right foot

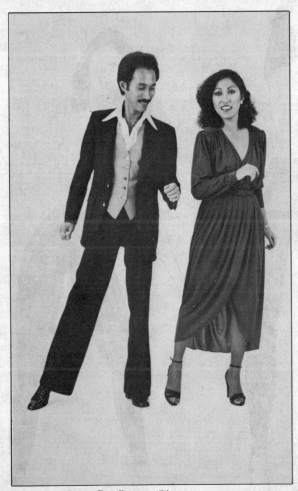

part B **step 5** (beat 5)

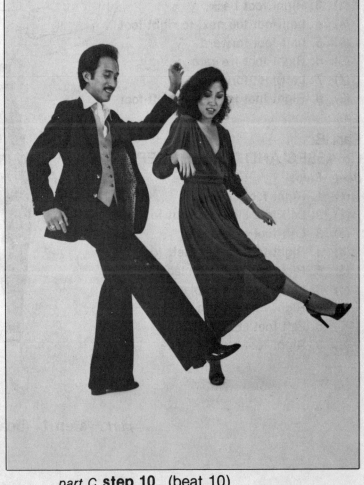

part C **step 10** (beat 10)

LINE DANCES

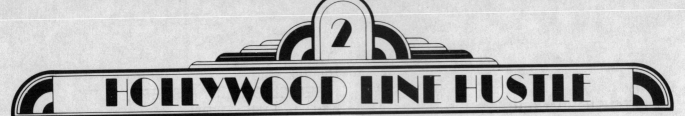

HOLLYWOOD LINE HUSTLE

The HOLLYWOOD LINE HUSTLE, sometimes called the L.A. LINE DANCE, is suspiciously similar to the Line Walk previously described. Nevertheless, there are a few minor differences that do make this line dance a particular favorite in some areas of the country. One difference is that, unlike the Line Walk, the Hollywood or L.A. Line Hustle contains 33 steps completed in 32 beats of music. In addition, for emphasis, we have divided this line dance into 4 sections, each containing a total of 8 beats (2 measures) of music.

Part A begins with a backward walk, ending on beat 4 with a toe (close) back, then a sequence of forward walk steps, ending on beat 8 with a toe (close) forward. To make your toe step, remember to point your toe, without placing any weight on the ball of the foot.

Part B begins with double chassés, but concludes with 6 steps in place. Moreover, the last three steps in place form a *triple step*, since these 3 steps (steps 7-9) are completed in 2 syncopated beats of music (beats 7 and 8).

Part C contains Left Pivot Turns, followed with walk and toe steps. This line dance concludes in Part D with a series of toe steps, ending with a ¼ Left Line Turn, as dancers turn 90 degrees counter-clockwise, before repeating the entire pattern, while facing the next wall.

Part A:
LINE WALK

Beat   Steps

- (1)   1. Right foot back
- (2)   2. Left foot back
- (3)   3. Right foot back
- (4)   4. Left foot toe next to right foot
- (5)   5. Left foot forward
- (6)   6. Right foot forward
- (7)   7. Left foot forward
- (8)   8. Right foot toe next to left foot

Part B:
CHASSES AND TRIPLE STEPS

Beat   Steps

- (1)   1. Right foot side
- (2)   2. Left foot close to right foot
- (3)   3. Left foot side
- (4)   4. Right foot close to left foot
- (5)   5. Right foot step in place
- (6)   6. Left foot step in place
- (7)   7. Right foot step in place
- (&)   8. Left foot step in place
- (8)   9. Right foot step in place

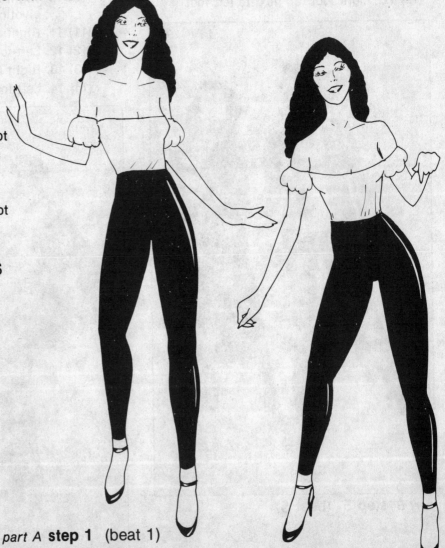

part A **step 1**   (beat 1)

part B **step 3**   (beat 3)

Part C:
LEFT PIVOT TURNS

Beat Steps

(1) 1. Left foot diagonally forward

(2) 2. Right foot swings in front of left foot, pivoting in a ½ Left Turn on left foot

(3) 3. Left foot swings behind right foot, pivoting in a ½ Left Turn on right foot

(4) 4. Right foot close to left foot

(5) 5. Left foot step in place

(6) 6. Right foot step in place

(7) 7. Left foot toe side

(8) 8. Left foot toe next to right foot

Part D:
TOE STEPS, WITH ¼ LEFT TURN

Beat Steps

(1) 1. Left foot toe side

(2) 2. Left foot toe next to right foot

(3) 3. Left foot forward

(4) 4. Right foot step in place

(5) 5. Left foot back

(6) 6. Right foot toe next to left foot

(7) 7. Right foot toe side

(8) 8. Right foot kick forward, pivoting ¼ left on left foot

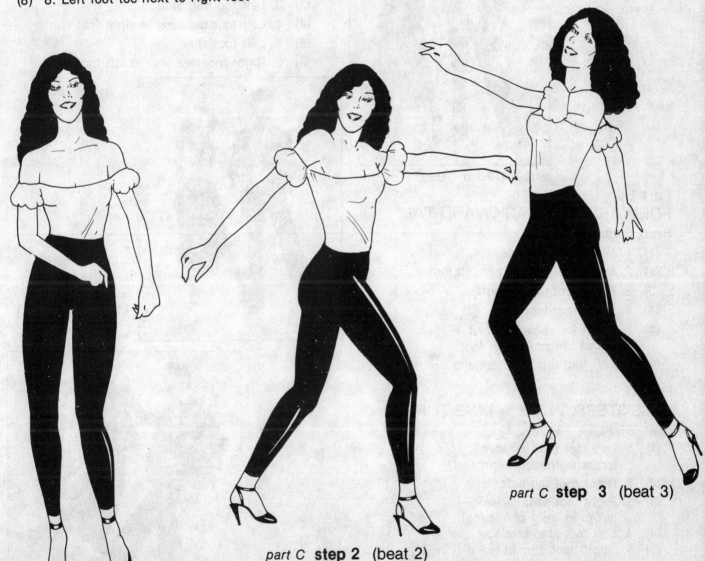

part C **step 3** (beat 3)

part C **step 2** (beat 2)

part B **step 4** (beat 4)

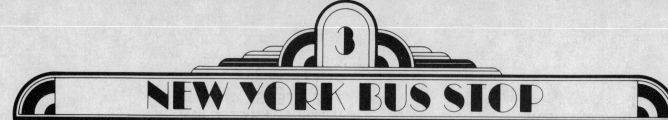

NEW YORK BUS STOP

The label, NEW YORK BUS STOP, has been glued onto a wide variety of step patterns. For example, one version contains walk steps followed by hip thrusts. Another version sticks a few kicks in. The version described here, however, contains a basic 18 beat (18 step) pattern. Part A includes a series of double side tap steps. Part B contains forward and backward tap steps. Part C mixes pass steps with tap steps and concludes with a ¼ Left Line Turn.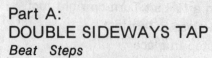

Part A:
DOUBLE SIDEWAYS TAP

Beat Steps
- (1) 1. Left foot tap side
- (2) 2. Left foot tap next to right foot
- (3) 3. Left foot tap side
- (4) 4. Left foot tap next to right foot
- (5) 5. Left foot side
- (6) 6. Right foot tap next to left foot

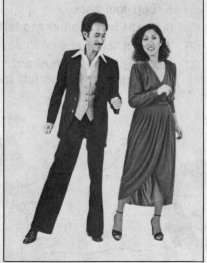

part A **step 5** (beat 5)

Part B:
FORWARD AND BACKWARD TAP

Beat Steps
- (1) 1. Right foot tap side
- (2) 2. Right foot tap next to left foot
- (3) 3. Right foot tap forward
- (4) 4. Right foot tap back
- (5) 5. Right foot pass forward
       (cross in front of left foot)
- (6) 6. Left foot tap to left side

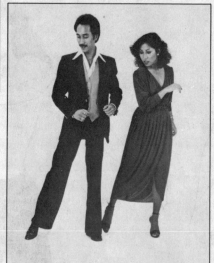

part B
step 1 (beat 1)

Part C:
PASS STEPS, WITH ¼ LINE TURN

Beat Steps
- (1) 1. Left foot pass forward
       (cross in front of right foot)
- (2) 2. Right foot tap side
- (3) 3. Right foot pass forward
       (cross in front of left foot)
- (4) 4. Left foot step in place
- (5) 5. Right foot step in place
- (4) 4. Left foot step in place
- (5) 5. Right foot tap side
- (6) 6. Right foot kick forward,
       pivoting ¼ left on left foot

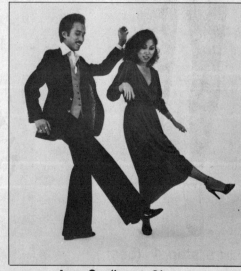

part C **step 6** (beat 6)

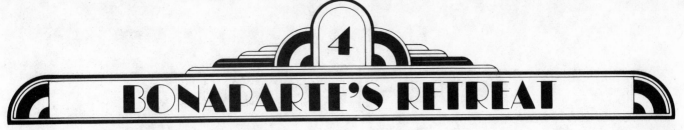

BONAPARTE'S RETREAT

Although BONAPARTE'S RETREAT is sometimes called the HOT CHOCOLATE LINE DANCE, we feel that the former name is more appropriate, because first the dancers mobilize, as they move in a line down the side, then they "retreat" backward and perform a "holding" action, before wheeling to the left and "defending" in another direction. This entire line dance of 16 steps, completed in 16 beats of music, neatly divides into two parts:

Part A (mobilization of forces) with pass and toes steps; and, Part B (retreat, hold, defend) with walk and rock steps, ending with a ¼ Left Line Turn. Throughout this line dance, your arms, with elbows bent, should swing from side to side, as your hips sway in the opposite direction. Ready—Aim—Fire! ♣

Part A:
PASS AND TOE FORWARD STEPS

Beat *Steps*
- (1) 1. Right foot side
- (2) 2. Left foot pass forward (cross in front of right foot)
- (3) 3. Right foot side
- (4) 4. Left foot toe forward
- (5) 5. Left foot side
- (6) 6. Right foot pass forward (cross in front of left foot)
- (7) 7. Left foot side
- (8) 8. Right foot toe forward

Part B:
WALK STEPS, WITH ¼ LINE TURN

Beat *Steps*
- (1) 1. Right foot back
- (2) 2. Left foot back
- (3) 3. Right foot back
- (4) 4. Left foot toe forward
- (5) 5. Left foot step in place (lean forward)
- (6) 6. Right foot step in place (lean back)
- (7) 7. Left foot step in place (lean forward)
- (8) 8. Right foot kick forward, piovting ¼ left on left foot

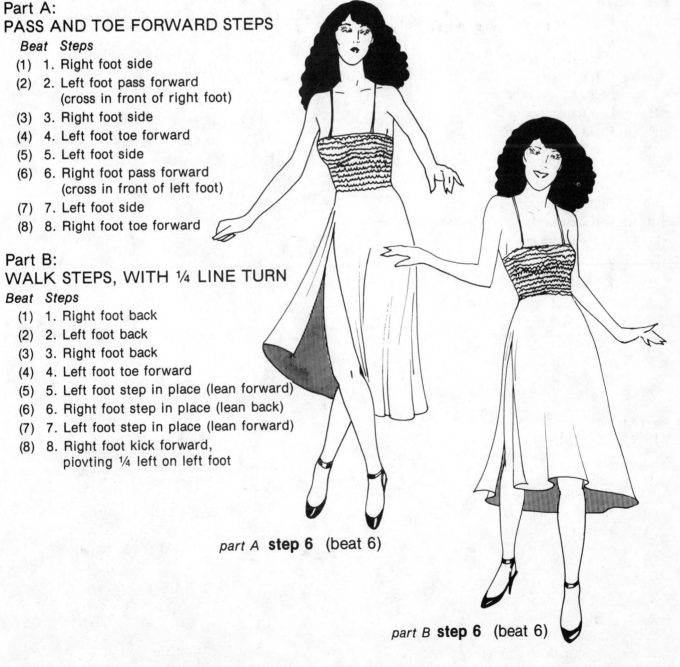

part A **step 6** (beat 6)

part B **step 6** (beat 6)

195

CALIFORNIA BUS STOP

The CALIFORNIA BUS STOP, often called the CALIFORNIA HUSTLE, is a foot stomping 36 beat count (36 step) line dance. Part A begins with the backward and forward walk. On every 4th beat, however, stamp your foot (keeping weight on the opposite foot) and clap your hands. Part B, the Side to Side Walk, includes a series of pass back (cross behind) steps and another series of foot stamps with hand claps. Part C, which returns to a semi-normal sequence, begins with in and out foot swivels, followed with a series of tap steps that end with a ¼ Left Line Turn. 🎞

Part A:
BACKWARD AND FORWARD WALK

Beat Steps

(1) 1. Right foot back

(2) 2. Left foot back

(3) 3. Right foot back

(4) 4. Left foot slap (close) back, and clap hands

(5) 5. Left foot forward

(6) 6. Right foot forward

(7) 7. Left foot forward

(8) 8. Right foot slap (close) forward, and clap hands

(9) 9. Right foot back

(10) 10. Left foot back

(11) 11. Right foot back

(12) 12. Left foot slap (close) back, and clap hands

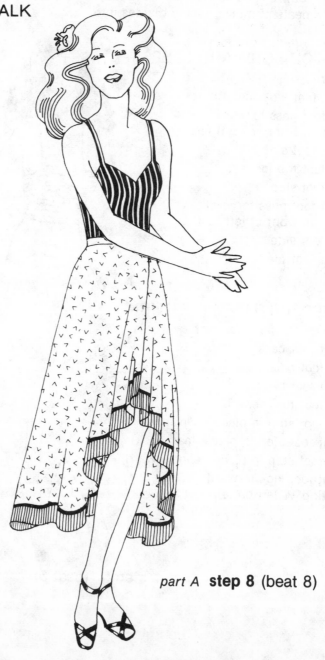

part A **step 8** (beat 8)

Part B:
SIDE TO SIDE WALK

Beat Steps
- (1) 1. Left foot side
- (2) 2. Right foot pass back
  (cross behind left foot)
- (3) 3. Left foot side
- (4) 4. Right foot slap (close) next to
  left foot, and clap hands
- (5) 5. Right foot side
- (6) 6. Left foot pass back
  (cross behind right foot)
- (7) 7. Right foot side
- (8) 8. Left foot slap (close) next to
  right foot, and clap hands
- (9) 9. Left foot side
- (10) 10. Right foot slap (close) next to
  left foot, and clap hands
- (11) 11. Right foot side
- (12) 12. Left foot slap (close) next to
  right foot, and clap hands

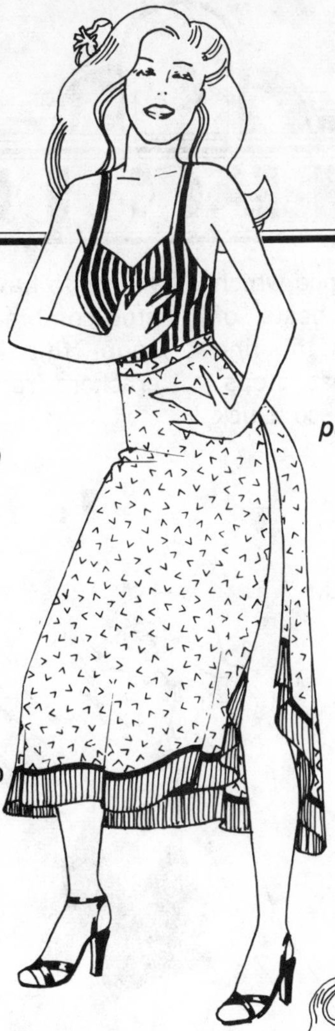

part B **step 1** (beat 1)

Part C:
SWIVEL AND TOE-TAP STEP

Beat Steps
- (1) 1. Swivel heels apart, then together
- (2) 2. Swivel heels apart, then together
- (3) 3. Right foot tap forward
- (4) 4. Right foot tap forward
- (5) 5. Right foot tap back
- (6) 6. Right foot tap back
- (7) 7. Right foot tap forward
- (8) 8. Right foot tap back
- (9) 9. Right foot tap forward
- (10) 10. Right foot tap back
- (11) 11. Right foot tap side
- (12) 12. Right foot kick forward,
  pivoting ¼ left on left foot

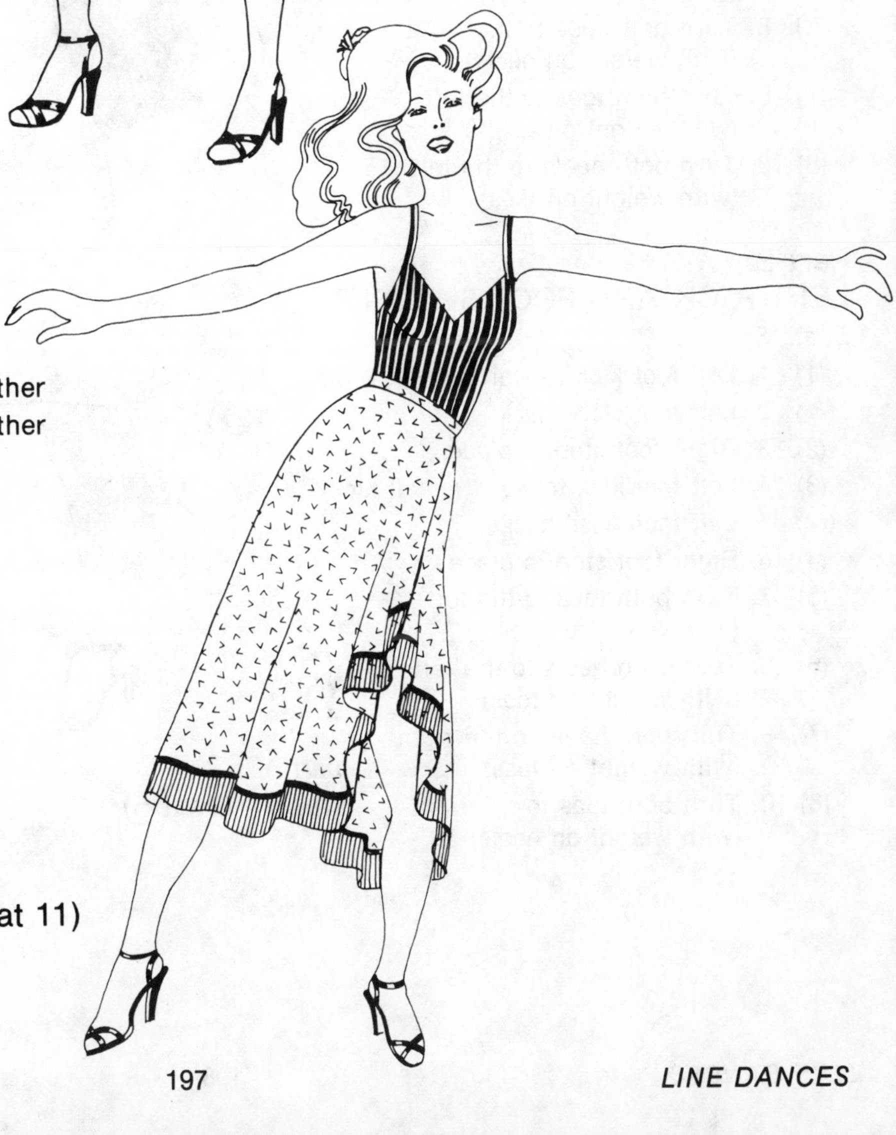

part C **step 11** (beat 11)

LINE DANCES

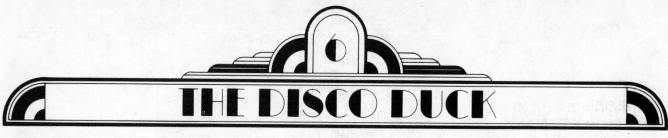

THE DISCO DUCK

The DISCO DUCK is a whacky line dance which contains 40 steps, completed in 32 beats of syncopated music. Divided into four parts, this line dance contains kicks, foot swivels, pass steps, chassés, and toe steps. In fact, the Disco Duck seems to have roped together almost every type of step combination. So, while it might not be duck soup, this line dance will surely separate the crackers from the quackers.

Part A:
RIGHT KICK AND FOOT SWIVELS
Beat *Steps*

- (1) 1. Right foot kick forward (small kick)
- (&) 2. Right foot close back
- (2) 3. Left foot step in place
- (3) 4. Right foot kick forward (small kick)
- (&) 5. Right foot close back
- (4) 6. Left foot step in place
- (5) 7. Turn both heels to the right (with weight on toes)
- (6) 8. Turn both toes to the right (with weight on heels)
- (7) 9. Turn both toes to the left (with weight on heels)
- (8) 10. Turn both heels to the left (with weight on toes)

Part B:
LEFT KICK AND FOOT SWIVELS
Beat *Steps*

- (1) 1. Left foot kick forward (small kick)
- (&) 2. Left foot close back
- (2) 3, Right foot step in place
- (3) 4. Left foot kick forward (small kick)
- (&) 5. Left foot close back
- (4) 6. Right foot step in place
- (5) 7. Turn both toes to the left (with weight on heels)
- (6) 8. Turn both heels to the left (with weight on toes)
- (7) 9. Turn both heels to the right (with weight on toes)
- (8) 10. Turn both toes to the right (with weight on heels)

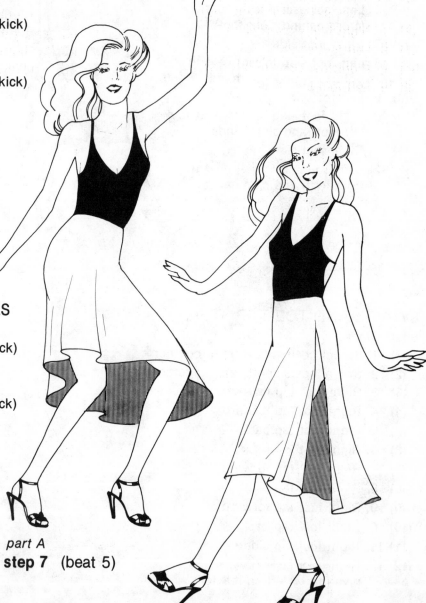

part A
step 7 (beat 5)

part B **step 1** (beat 1)

Part C:
PASS FORWARD
WITH SIDE STEPS

Beat **Steps**

(1) 1. Right foot pass forward
(cross in front of left foot)

(2) 2. Left foot step in place

(3) 3. Right foot side

(&) 4. Left foot close to right foot

(4) 5. Right foot side

(5) 6. Left foot pass forward
(cross in front of right foot)

(6) 7. Right foot step in place

(7) 8. Left foot side

(&) 9. Right foot close to left foot

(8) 10. Left foot step side

Part D:
RIGHT KICK, TOE STEPS,
AND ¼ LINE TURN

Beat **Steps**

(1) 1. Right foot kick forward (small kick)

(&) 2. Right foot close back

(2) 3. Left foot step in place

(3) 4. Right foot kick forward (small kick)

(&) 5. Right foot close back

(4) 6. Left foot step in place

(5) 7. Right foot toe forward

(6) 8. Right foot toe back

(7) 9. Right foot toe side

(8) 10. Right foot kick forward,
pivoting ¼ left on left foot

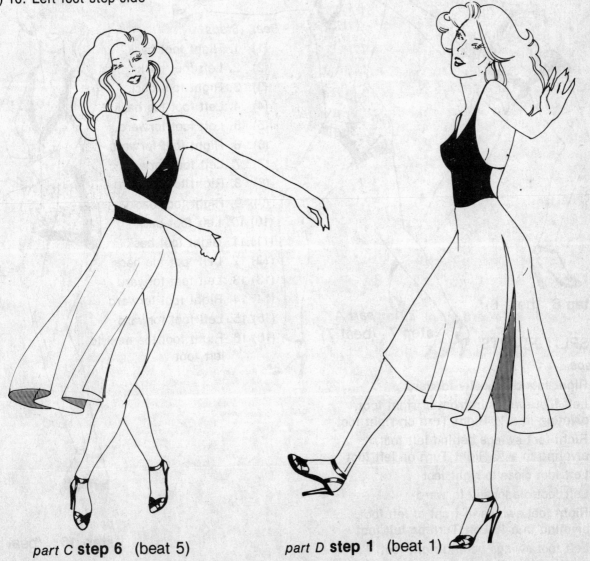

part C **step 6** (beat 5)   *part D* **step 1** (beat 1)

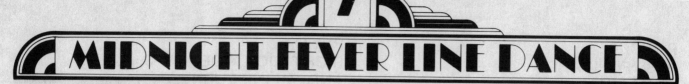

MIDNIGHT FEVER LINE DANCE

The MIDNIGHT FEVER LINE DANCE is, without a doubt, the most exciting line dance of all. Although not difficult to do, this dance does require some stamina, because it contains a whopping total of 52 steps that must be completed in 46 beats of music. But length alone does not a fever make, quoth the raven. Indeed, this dance is so crammed with pivots, kicks, taps, shooting arms, hip flips, and heel clicks that it becomes virtually impossible to resist. But be forewarned—once ignited, the midnight fever cannot be quenched. ✦

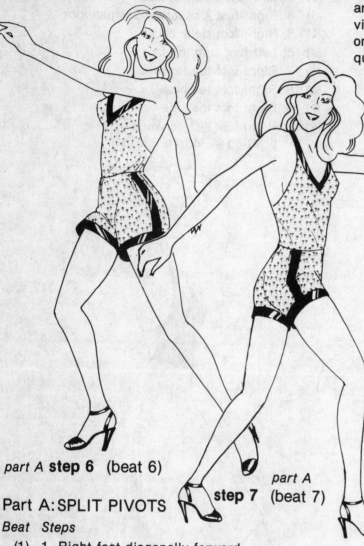

part A **step 6** (beat 6)

part A
step 7 (beat 7)

Part A: SPLIT PIVOTS

Beat Steps

(1) 1. Right foot diagonally forward

(2) 2. Left foot swings in front of right foot, pivoting in a ½ Right Turn on right foot

(3) 3. Right foot swings behind left foot, pivoting in a ½ Right Turn on left foot

(4) 4. Left foot close to right foot

(5) 5. Left foot diagonally forward

(6) 6. Right foot swings in front of left foot, pivoting in a ½ Left Turn on left foot

(7) 7. Left foot swings behind right foot, pivoting in a ½ Left Turn on right foot

(8) 8. Right foot close to left foot

Part B:
BACKWARD AND FORWARD WALK, WITH TOE STEPS

Beat Steps

(1) 1. Right foot back

(2) 2. Left foot back

(3) 3. Right foot back

(4) 4. Left foot toe back

(5) 5. Left foot forward

(6) 6. Right foot forward

(7) 7. Left foot forward

(8) 8. Right toe forward

(9) 9. Right foot back

(10) 10. Left foot back

(11) 11. Right foot back

(12) 12. Left foot toe back

(13) 13. Left foot forward

(14) 14. Right foot forward

(15) 15. Left foot forward

(16) 16. Right foot toe next to left foot

part B
step 16 (beat 16)

Part C:
KICK AND SHOOTING ARM MOVEMENT

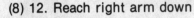

Beat Steps

(1) 1. Right foot kick forward
(&) 2. Right foot close back
(2) 3. Left foot step in place
(3) 4. Right foot kick forward
(&) 5. Right foot close back
(4) 6. Left foot step in place
(5) 7. Lift right arm up
(&) 8. Bend right arm at waist
(6) 9. Reach right arm down
(7) 10. Lift right arm up
(&) 11. Bend right arm at waist

(8) 12. Reach right arm down
(9) 13. Lift right arm up
(&) 14. Bend right arm at waist
(10) 15. Reach right arm down
(11) 16. Lift right arm up
(&) 17. Bend right arm at waist
(12) 18. Reach right arm down

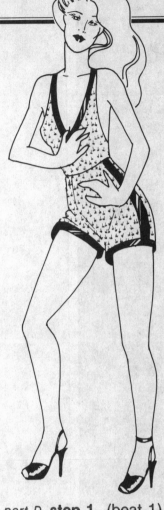

part D **step 1** (beat 1)

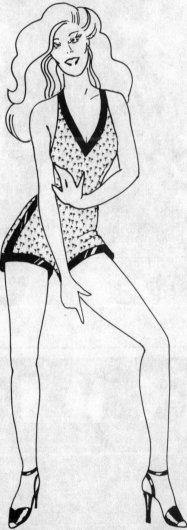

part C **step 9** (beat 6)

Part D:
ARM ROLLS, HEEL CLICKS, AND ¼ LINE TURN

Beat Steps

(1) 1. Left hip tilt up, roll arms
(2) 2. Right hip tilt up, roll arms
(3) 3. Left hip tilt up, roll arms
(4) 4. Right hip tilt up, roll arms
(5) 5. Click heels together, flap arms
(6) 6. Click heels together, flap arms
(7) 7. Right foot tap forward
(8) 8. Right foot tap back
(9) 9. Right foot kick forward,
    pivoting ¼ left on left foot
(10) 10. Right foot extended forward,
    ready to repeat pattern

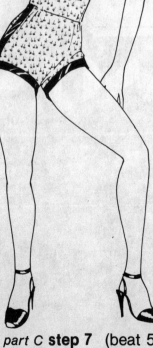

part C **step 7** (beat 5)

LINE DANCES

PART IV

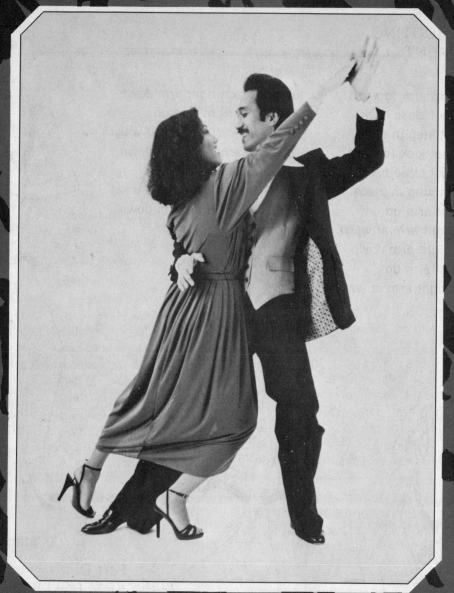

BALLROOM DANCES

CHAPTER 11

WALTZ

Despite some ambiguity concerning names and dates, the WALTZ, according to most dance historians, did develop from earlier folk and peasant dances. Moreover, the roots of this refined and elegant dance are implanted firmly in the not-so-refined round dances popular in Germany, specifically Bavaria, from the 15th to the 18th centuries. These popular round dances, also tagged "wooing dances," included such frenzied versions as the *Landler, Weller, Spinner,* and *Waltzer,* among others.

In addition to the Bavarian folk dances, however, another potential predecessor to the modern Waltz, cited by many prominent historians, is a rollicking round dance called *La Volta.* Invented in Northern Italy and popular in Italian courts during the 16th century, *La Volta,* which means "turning dance," was considered risque in its day.

Introduced to Austrian courts as early as the 17th century, the Waltz was originally considered vulgar by those who were accustomed to the dignity and control of the minuet. Nevertheless, by the late 18th or early 19th century, the rough edges had been honed down sufficiently to make this dance acceptable to the majority. In addition, the forward and backward leaps had been modified into smoother, smaller, and more graceful looking steps. A gliding motion was also introduced which eliminated any jumps, leaps, or kicks. At approximately the same time, the Waltz acquired its characteristic step pattern, which incorporates a side step on the second beat, with a closing step on the third beat, although the forward and backward steps still emphasized the strongly accented first beat.

BASIC WALTZ RHYTHM AND MOTION

Basic step patterns in Waltz are composed of 6 steps, completed in 6 beats (2 measures) of music. The first beat count of each measure of music corresponds to a forward or backward step. Moreover, each forward step is taken *between* the feet of one's partner. The last two beat counts of each measure of music correspond to either a chassé (side step, followed with a close step) or a balance step ("hold" for two counts).

The basic movement for the Waltz is the rise and fall. According to dance expert Skippy Blair, the movement is "down on count one—2/3 of the way up on count two— and all the way up on count three." On each forward step, taken on the first beat count, touch the floor with the heel first, then roll forward onto the ball of the foot. Conversely, on each step back, taken on the first beat count, touch the floor with the toe first, then roll back onto the ball of the foot. On the last two beat counts, however, rise up on the toes. (In dance jargon, the word "toes" refers to the *ball* of the foot. Thus, to rise up on your toes, press the ball of the foot onto the floor.)

For an elegant Waltz style, keep your back straight, chin up, and lean slightly back with both shoulders. In addition, you should use the Contrabody Movement with all Waltz patterns. Thus, as you step forward with your left foot, pull your left shoulder back and hold it back for the next two beats of music. Conversely, as you step forward with your right foot, pull your right shoulder back and hold it back for the next two beat counts.

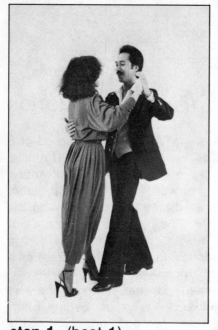

step 1 (beat 1)

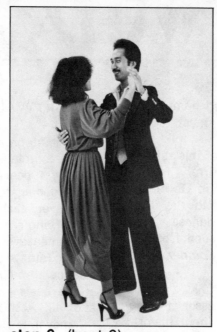

step 2 (beat 2)

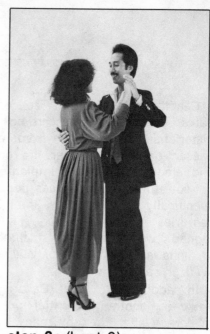

step 3 (beat 3)

The basic step pattern in Waltz is the LEFT BOX STEP. Composed of 6 steps, completed in 6 beats (2 measures) of music, the Left Box Step forms a box or square configuration on the floor. Moreover, the Left Box Step consists of two parts or halves which can be viewed as mirror images of each other: "Forward Waltz Step" and "Backward Waltz Step."

The first half of the pattern, the "Forward Waltz Step," includes steps 1-3 (completed on beats 1-3). On the first beat count, the man steps forward with the heel of his left foot touching the floor, as the woman steps back with the toe of her right foot touching the floor. On the next two beat counts, both the man and the woman slowly rise up on their toes as they step side and close side (draw feet together).

The second half of the pattern, the "Backward Waltz Step," which mirrors the first part, contains steps 4-6 (completed on beats 4-6). On the fourth beat count, the man steps back with the toe of his right foot touching the floor, as the woman steps forward with the heel of her left foot touching the floor. On the last two beat counts, both the man and the woman slowly rise up on their toes, as they step side and close side (draw feet together).

While waltzing through their Left Box Step, partners should emphasize the Contrabody Movement. Thus, as the man steps forward on his left foot, he pulls his left shoulder diagonally back and holds it back for the next two beat counts. As the woman steps back on her right foot, she pushes her right shoulder forward and holds it forward for the next two beat counts.

The Left Box Step is, of course, the pattern which forms the basis for most other partner dances. The Waltz, however, is a progressive dance in which partners glide across the floor, while turning in the Line of Direction (counter-clockwise). The next two variations, Left Box Turns and Right Box Turns, describe the ways in which turns can add flair and fluidity to the basic Left Box Step.

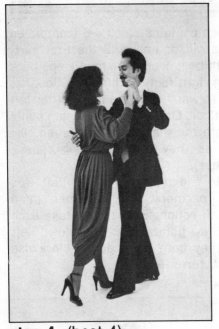 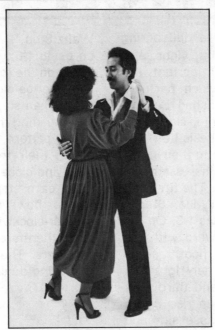 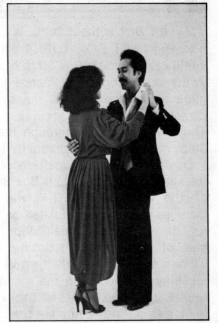

step 4 (beat 4)   **step 5** (beat 5)   **step 6** (beat 6)

Man's Part:

Beat   Steps

  (1) 1. Left foot forward
  (2) 2. Right foot side
  (3) 3. Left foot close to right foot
  (4) 4. Right foot back
  (5) 5. Left foot side
  (6) 6. Right foot close to left foot

Woman's Part:

Beat   Steps

  (1) 1. Right foot back
  (2) 2. Left foot side
  (3) 3. Right foot close to left foot
  (4) 4. Left foot forward
  (5) 5. Right foot side
  (6) 6. Left foot close to right foot

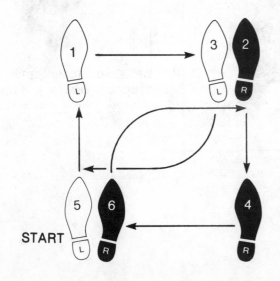 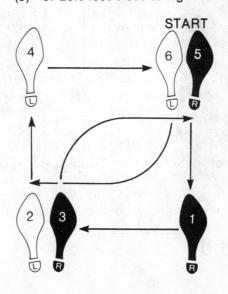

WALTZ

A Left Box without turns is only a dull boring box. But LEFT BOX TURNS add vim, vigor, and vitality to the basic Box Step. Most important, the Waltz is a progressive dance in which partners glide across the floor in the established Line of Direction which is, of course, counter-clockwise. Thus, while waltzing through their basic Left Box Step, partners should gradually turn to their left.

Of course, the step pattern remains essentially the same as the basic Left Box Step. The first half of the pattern, the "Forward Waltz Step," includes steps 1-3, completed on beats 1-3. On the first beat count, the man steps forward with the heel of his left foot touching the floor, as the woman steps back with the toe of her right foot touching the floor. On the second and third beat counts, both the man and the woman rise up on their toes as they complete their chassé (side and close steps).

The second half of the pattern, the "Backward Waltz Step," which contains steps 4-6 (completed on beats 4-6), is a mirror image of the first part. Thus, on the fourth beat count, the man steps back with the toe of his right foot touching the floor, as the woman steps forward with the heel of her left foot touching the floor. On the last two beat counts of the pattern, both the man and the woman rise up on their toes as they complete their chassé (side and close steps).

On each step in the pattern for the Left Box Turns, however, partners turn together in a counter-clockwise direction. Before they take each step, therefore, they glance over their own left shoulders. Then they both turn counter-clockwise by making dual *left* turns.

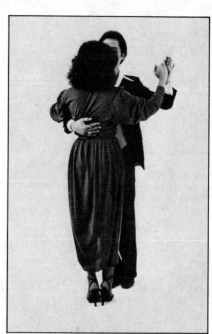

step 3 (beat 3)

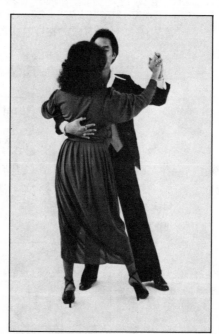

step 2 (beat 2)

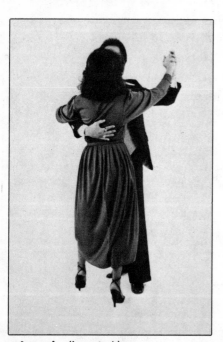

step 1 (beat 1)

Man's Part:

Beat   Steps

(1)   1. Left foot forward
(2)   2. Right foot side
(3)   3. Left foot close to right foot
(4)   4. Right foot back
(5)   5. Left foot side
(6)   6. Right foot close to left foot

The man turns gradually to his left

Woman's Part:

Beat   Steps

(1)   1. Right foot back
(2)   2. Left foot side
(3)   3. Right foot close to left foot
(4)   4. Left foot forward
(5)   5. Right foot side
(6)   6. Left foot close to right foot

The woman turns gradually to her left

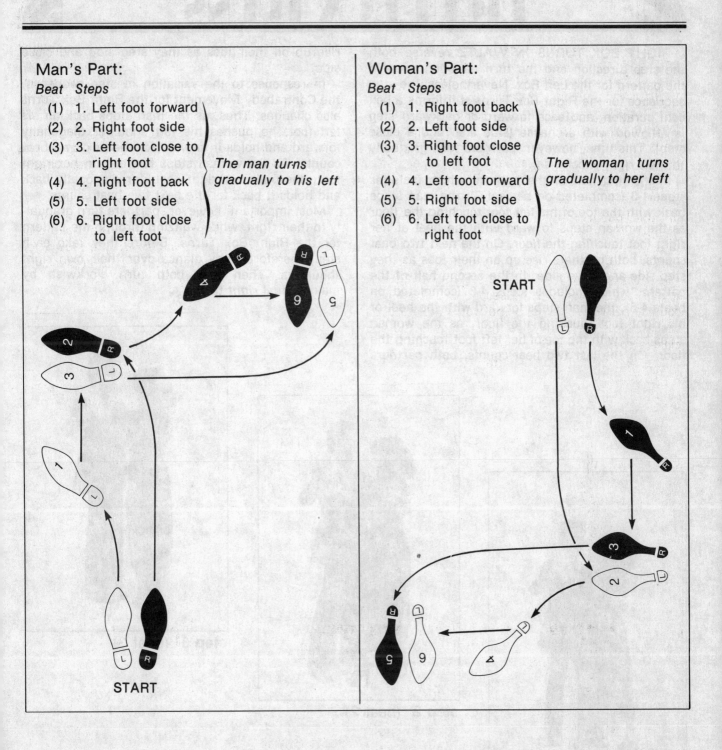

START

START

START

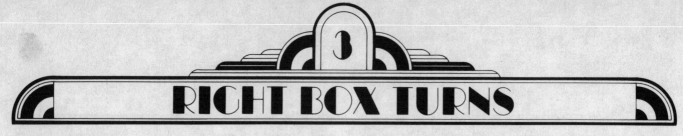

RIGHT BOX TURNS

RIGHT BOX TURNS IN WALTZ reverse both the step direction and the turn direction used in the pattern for the Left Box. Nevertheless, the step sequence for the Right Box Turns still forms a box configuration, and each forward or backward step is followed with a chassé (side step and a close step). This time, however, partners turn gradually to their right (clockwise).

In the first half of the pattern, which includes steps 1-3 (completed on beats 1-3), the man steps back with the toe of his left foot touching the floor as the woman steps forward with the heel of her right foot touching the floor. On the next two beat counts, both partners rise up on their toes as they step side and close side. In the second half of the pattern, which includes steps 4-6 (completed on beats 4-6), the man steps forward with the heel of his right foot touching the floor, as the woman steps back with the toe of her left foot touching the floor. On the last two beat counts, both partners

rise up on their toes as they step side and close side.

In response to the variation in step sequence, the Contrabody Movement for the Right Box Turns also changes. Thus, as the man steps back on his left foot, he pushes his left shoulder diagonally forward and holds it forward for the next two beat counts. As the woman steps forward on her right foot, she pulls her right shoulder diagonally back and holds it back for the next two beat counts.

Most important, however, partners turn gradually to their right, while waltzing through the pattern for the Right Box Turns. Before they take each step, therefore, they glance over their own right shoulders. Then they both turn clockwise by making dual *right* turns.

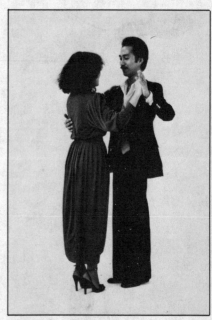

step 3   (beat 3)

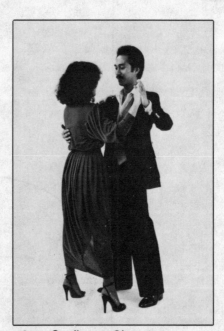

step 2   (beat 2)

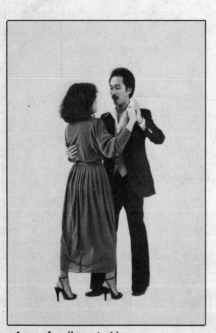

step 1   (beat 1)

Man's Part:

Beat   Steps

(1) 1. Left foot back
(2) 2. Right foot side
(3) 3. Left foot close to right foot
(4) 4. Right foot forward
(5) 5. Left foot side
(6) 6. Right foot close to left foot

The man turns gradually to his right (clockwise).

Woman's Part:

Beat   Steps

(1) 1. Right foot forward
(2) 2. Left foot side
(3) 3. Right foot close to left foot
(4) 4. Left foot back
(5) 5. Right foot side
(6) 6. Left foot close to right foot

The woman turns gradually to her right (clockwise).

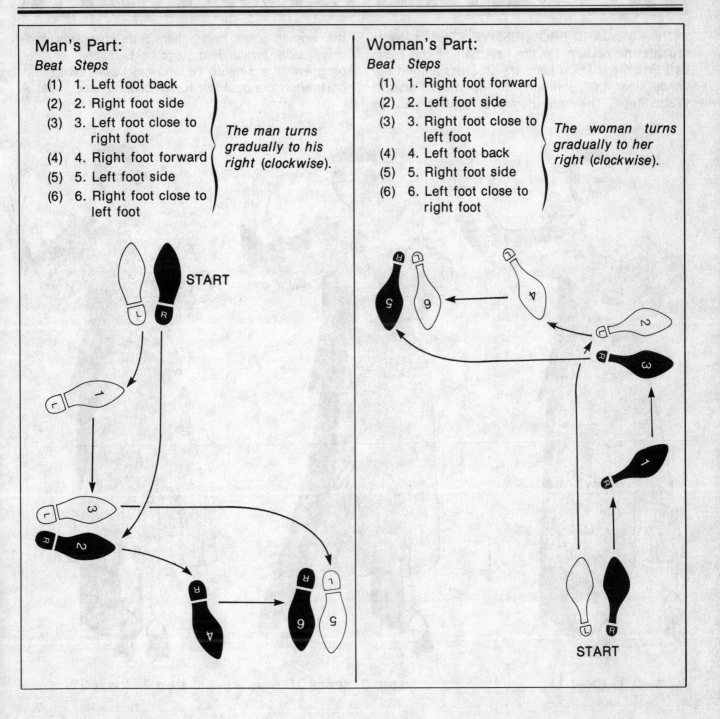

FORWARD PROGRESSIVE STEP

The FORWARD PROGRESSIVE STEP in Waltz repeats the pattern for the first half of the basic Left Box Step. Thus, partners progress around the dance floor by continuing to do the "Forward Waltz Step." The man, therefore, steps forward as the woman steps back, then both step side and close side (draw feet together). Moreover, to progress in a smooth counter-clockwise direction, partners make dual *left* turns (counter-clockwise).

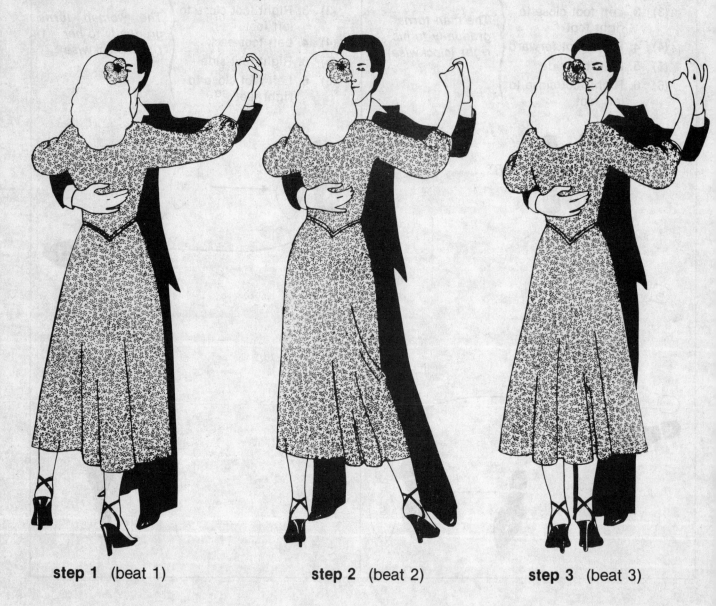

step 1 (beat 1)   **step 2** (beat 2)   **step 3** (beat 3)

Man's Part:

Beat Steps

(1) 1. Left foot forward

(2) 2. Right foot side

(3) 3. Left foot close to right foot

(4) 4. Right foot forward

(5) 5. Left foot side

(6) 6. Right foot close to left foot

Woman's Part:

Beat Steps

(1) 1. Right foot back

(2) 2. Left foot side

(3) 3. Right foot close to left foot

(4) 4. Left foot back

(5) 5. Right foot side

(6) 6. Left foot close to right foot

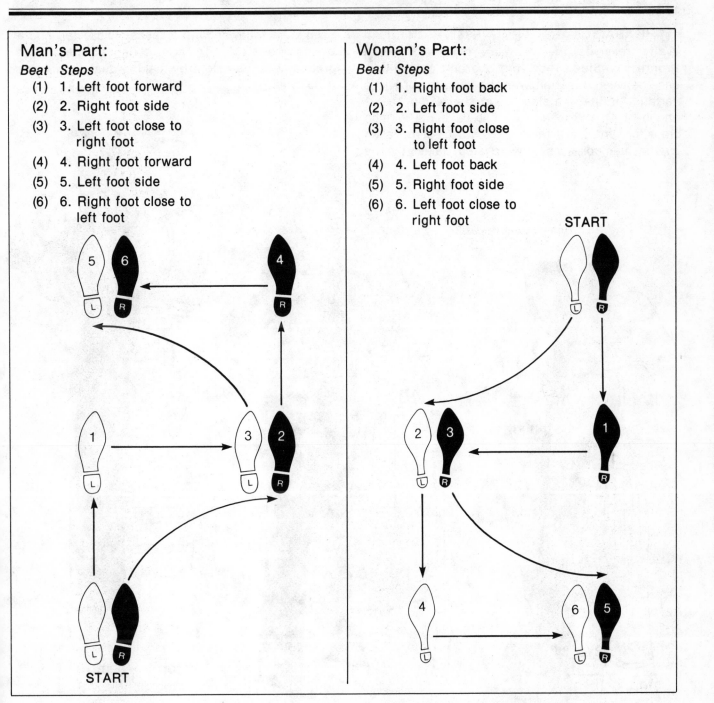

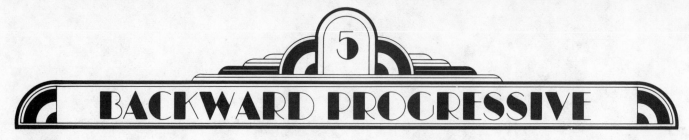

5
BACKWARD PROGRESSIVE

THE BACKWARD PROGRESSIVE STEP in Waltz reverses the direction of the Forward Progressive Step. Thus, the one and only difference between this Waltz variation and the previous variation is that, on step 1 and step 4 (on beat 1 and beat 4), the man steps back and the woman steps forward. Nevertheless, each back step, taken by the man, or each forward step, taken by the woman, is followed with a chassé (side step and a close side step). To add style, partners turn gradually to their right by making dual *right* turns (clockwise). ♣

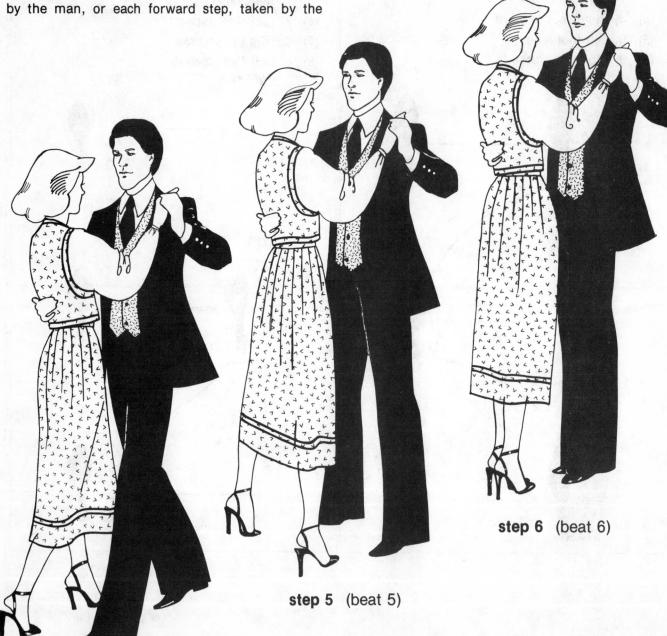

step 4   (beat 4)

step 5   (beat 5)

step 6   (beat 6)

Man's Part:

Beat   Steps

(1)   1. Left foot back

(2)   2. Right foot side

(3)   3. Left foot close
           to right foot

(4)   4. Right foot back

(5)   5. Left foot side

(6)   6. Right foot close
           to left foot

Woman's Part:

Beat   Steps

(1)   1. Right foot forward

(2)   2. Left foot side

(3)   3. Right foot close to
           left foot

(4)   4. Left foot forward

(5)   5. Right foot side

(6)   6. Left foot close to
           right foot

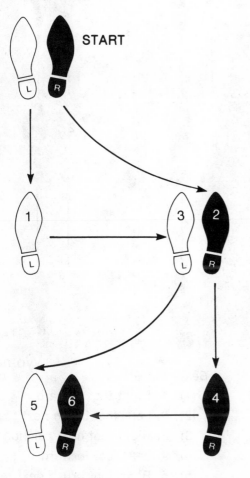

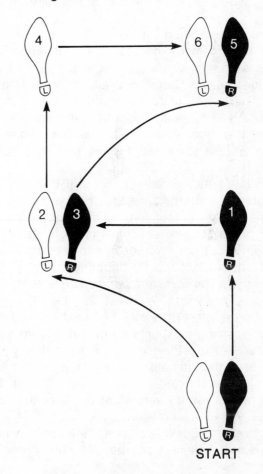

HESITATION WALTZ PATTERNS

In the early 1900s in North America, there developed a simple pattern of step-together-step, with a syncopated "hesitation" on the second and third beats. On this hesitation, dancers used the flat part of their foot, rather than their toes, to make a dipping movement. This dance, called the *Boston* or the *Hesitation Waltz*, eventually developed into the *Boston Dip* in which the man would lean directly over the woman. By 1914, however, this form of Hesitation Waltz gave way to the One-Step, which was probably just as well, since expert dancers, disgusted with the simplicity of the pattern, had nicknamed this dance the Ignoramus Waltz.

Although the Boston Dip is no longer one of the world's most famous dances, the Hesitation or Balance Steps in Waltz are still popular. The Hesitation Balance Steps in Waltz may be taken forward, backward, or to either side. What makes the Hesitation unique is that, after partners take a step on the first beat count, weight remains balanced on the same foot for the next two beat counts.

To visualize the movement that will be used in *all* Hesitation patterns, pretend that you have a huge blister on one foot (made, no doubt, by ten straight hours of disco dancing the night before). To alleviate your pain, you decide to take one step forward on beat 1 (step 1), hobbling towards the kitchen where you *think* the bandaids are kept. As you near the kitchen, on beat 2 (step 2), you gingerly draw (close) the sore foot next to the foot that is supporting all your weight. But, just as you draw your feet together, you remember that your brother used the bandaids two weeks ago after he nicked his chin shaving. Thus, on beat 3 (step 3) you hesitate as you try to remember where the box might be. As you hesitate, your feet remain in the same parallel (close) position, although your weight is still balanced on the foot that doesn't hurt.

Although this graphic description exaggerates the movement, the fundamentals remain the same. On the first step taken forward, backward, or sideways, weight will remain on this foot for the next 2 beats. In the diagrams that illustrate "Hesitation" patterns, a balance or weightless step is marked with a jagged footprint. 🐾

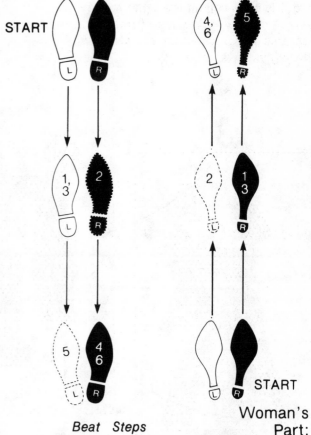

Man's Part:

Beat	Steps
(1)	1. Left foot back
(2)	2. Right foot brush next to left
(3)	3. Left foot hold position
(4)	4. Right foot back
(5)	5. Left foot brush next to right
(6)	6. Right foot hold position

Woman's Part:

Beat	Steps
(1)	1. Right foot forward
(2)	2. Left foot brush next to right
(3)	3. Right foot hold position
(4)	4. Left foot forward
(5)	5. Right foot brush next to left
(6)	6. Left foot hold position

FORWARD HESITATION

In the BALANCE FORWARD HESITATION the man steps forward, as the woman steps back. In addition, each forward or backward step is followed with a brush close step in which one foot drifts towards and lightly touches against the opposite foot, although *no* weight is placed on the foot that brushes. After drawing feet together in the parallel (close) position, partners "hold" the position for one beat of music. Most important, weight is balanced on the same foot for every three beats (1 measure) of music. (Notice that in the step diagrams the "weightless" steps are indicated with jagged footprints.)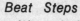

	Beat	Steps
Man's Part:	(1)	1. Left foot forward
	(2)	2. Right foot brush next to left
	(3)	3. Left foot hold position
	(4)	4. Right foot forward
	(5)	5. Left foot brush next to right
	(6)	6. Right foot hold position

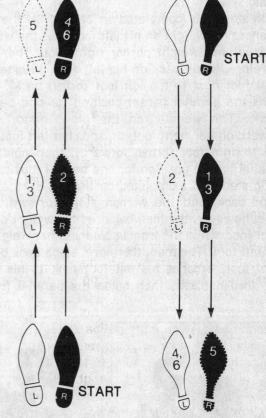

	Beat	Steps
Woman's Part:	(1)	1. Right foot back
	(2)	2. Left foot brush next to right
	(3)	3. Right foot hold position
	(4)	4. Left foot back
	(5)	5. Right foot brush next to left
	(6)	6. Left foot hold position

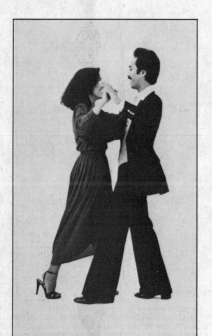

step 1 (beat 1)

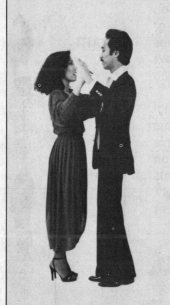

step 2 (beat 2)

BACKWARD HESITATION

In the BALANCE BACKWARD HESITATION the man steps back, and the woman steps forward. Each forward or backward step is followed with a brush close step in which one foot drifts towards, and lightly touches against, the opposite foot. After drawing feet together into the parallel (close) position, partners "hold" the position for one beat of music. Most important, weight is balanced on the same foot for every three beats (1 measure) of music.

On steps 1-3 (completed on beats 1-3), the man balances his weight on his left foot, but the woman balances her weight on her right foot. The man, therefore, steps back on his left foot, brushes his right foot next to his left foot (brush back), then holds the parallel (close) position for one beat of music. The woman, on the other hand, steps forward on her right foot, brushes her left foot next to her right foot (brush forward), then holds the parallel (close) position for one beat of music.

On steps 4-6 (completed on beats 4-6), the man steps back, and the woman steps forward. This time, however, the man balances his weight on his right foot, while the woman balances her weight on her left foot. The man, therefore, steps back on his right foot, brushes his left foot next to his right foot (brush back), then holds the parallel (close) position for one beat of music. The woman, on the contrary, steps forward on her left foot, brushes her right foot next to her left foot (close forward), then holds the parallel (close) position for one beat of music.

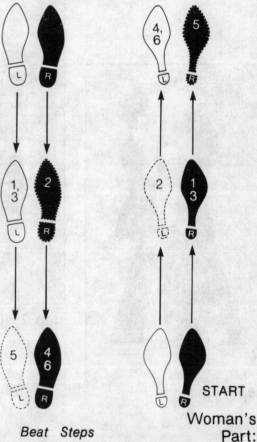

Man's Part:

Beat	Steps
(1)	1. Left foot back
(2)	2. Right foot brush next to left
(3)	3. Left foot hold position
(4)	4. Right foot back
(5)	5. Left foot brush next to right
(6)	6. Right foot hold position

Woman's Part:

Beat	Steps
(1)	1. Right foot forward
(2)	2. Left foot brush next to right
(3)	3. Right foot hold position
(4)	4. Left foot forward
(5)	5. Right foot brush next to left
(6)	6. Left foot hold position

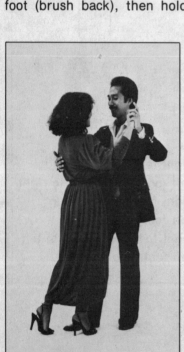

step 1 (beat 1)

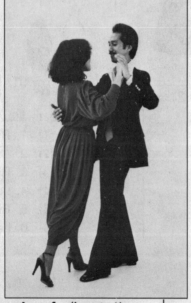

step 4 (beat 4)

BALANCE SIDE HESITATION

In the BALANCE SIDE HESITATION partners move from side to side, instead of forward or backward. Nonetheless, the basic movement (step, brush close, hold) remains the same. In the first half of the pattern, the "Left Side Hesitation," the man keeps his weight balanced on his left foot, and the woman keeps her weight balanced on her right foot. On steps 1-3 (beats 1-3), the man steps to his left side with his left foot, then brushes his right foot next to his left foot, and holds the position for one beat of music. Conversely, the woman steps to her right side with her right foot, then brushes her left foot next to her right foot, and holds the position for one beat of music.

In the second half of the pattern, the "Right Side Hesitation," the man and woman switch parts, as the man balances his weight on his right foot, and the woman balances her weight on her left foot. On beats 4-6 (steps 4-6), the man steps to his right side with his right foot, then brushes his left foot next to his right foot, and holds the position for the last beat of music. The woman, on the other hand, steps to her left side with her left foot, then brushes her right foot next to her left foot, and holds the position for the last beat of music.

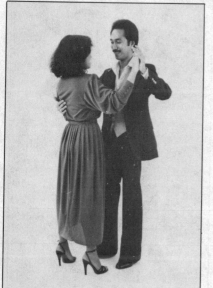

step 1 (beat 1)

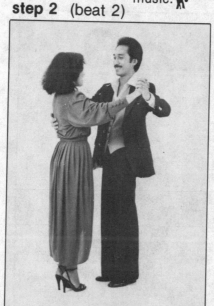

step 2 (beat 2)

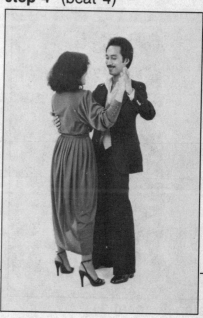

step 4 (beat 4)

Man's Part:
Beat Steps

(1) 1. Left foot side
(2) 2. Right foot brush next to left foot
(3) 3. Left foot hold position
(4) 4. Right foot side
(5) 5. Left foot brush next to right foot
(6) 6. Right foot hold position

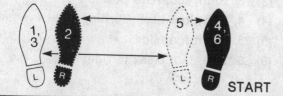

Woman's Part:
Beat Steps

(1) 1. Right foot side
(2) 2. Left foot brush next to right foot
(3) 3. Right foot hold position
(4) 4. Left foot side
(5) 5. Right foot brush next to left foot
(6) 6. Left foot hold position

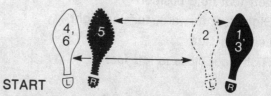

HESITATION RIGHT TURNS

The FORWARD HESITATION WITH RIGHT TURNS combines the first half of the pattern for the Forward Hesitation with the last half of the pattern for the Right Box Turns. This pattern begins on steps 1-3 (beats 1-3) with the Forward Hesitation. Throughout the first half of the pattern, the man keeps his weight balanced on his left foot, and the woman keeps her weight balanced on her right foot. Thus, the man steps forward on his left foot, brushes his right foot next to his left foot (brush forward), then holds the (close) position for one beat of music. The woman, on the other hand, steps back on her right foot, brushes her left foot next to her right foot (brush back), then holds the (close) position for one beat of music.

This pattern concludes on steps 4-6 (completed on beats 4-6) with the last half of the Right Box. The man, therefore, steps forward on his right foot, steps side on his left foot, then closes his right foot to his left foot. The woman, on the contrary, steps back on her left foot, steps side on her right foot, then closes her left foot to her right foot. Throughout the last half of the pattern, partners progress in a clockwise direction by making dual *right* turns (clockwise).

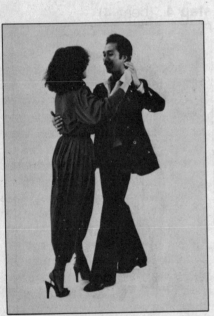

step 1 (beat 1)

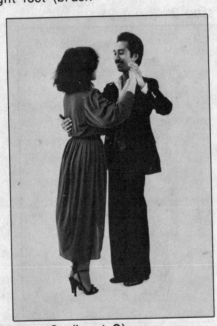

step 2 (beat 2)

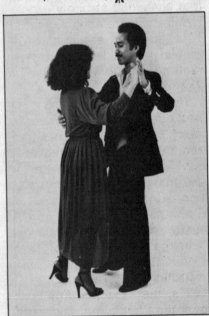

step 5 (beat 5)

Man's Part:

Beat *Steps*

(1) 1. Left foot forward

(2) 2. Right foot brush next to left foot

(3) 3. Left foot hold position

(4) 4. Right foot forward, turning right

(5) 5. Left foot side

(6) 6. Right foot close to left foot

Woman's Part:

Beat *Steps*

(1) 1. Right foot back

(2) 2. Left foot brush next to right foot

(3) 3. Right foot hold position

(4) 4. Left foot back, turning right

(5) 5. Right foot side

(6) 6. Left foot close to right foot

CHAPTER 12

FOX TROT

By the end of the 19th century, a wide variety of court and peasant dances had evolved, including the Mazurka, the Turkey Trot, the Schottische, the Polka, the Galop, and the Bunny Hug, as well as the One-Step and the Two-Step. All of these bouncy and febrile dances corresponded to music that contained strongly accented beats and lively, tempestuous tempos. Sometime between 1913 and 1914, however, music hall comedian and performer, Harry Fox, danced a series of fast walk steps to ragtime music during a performance in the Ziegfeld Follies.

Harry's ragtime walk was an instant smash, leading to the development of the FOX TROT which combined elements from both the One-Step and the Two-Step. Moreover, the popularity of the Fox Trot increased phenomenally after Vernon and Irene Castle standardized the steps, and dance teachers began to feature it as a ballroom dance. Consequently, before World War I broke out in 1914, the Fox Trot was the hottest craze in America since the Boston Dip.

Variations of the Fox Trot gradually evolved, reflecting the temper of the age. During the early 1920s, the "Flapper Age," everybody went crazy over the Charleston. Soon after, during the 1930s, syncopated music was added, which resulted in some swinging Swing variations, such as the Lindy Swing, commemorating Lindbergh's historic trans-Atlantic flight. Even today, many of the current disco touch dances, such as the Continental Hustle and Disco Trot are modified forms of the basic Fox Trot. More important, all of these patterns, both past and present, contain different accents of music, written in 4/4 time.

Moreover, different basic Fox Trot patterns have evolved, fluctuating with changes in cultural tastes, social preferences, types of music, and actual location of the dance. Just a few of the current Fox Trot forms that vary in terms of location include Nite Club, Discotheque, Country Club, and Ballroom patterns. Nevertheless, basic Fox Trot in any era, according to dance expert Skippy Blair, "refers to the current medium tempo, closed position dancing, danced to 4/4 time."

BASIC RHYTHM AND PATTERN

The modern ballroom version of the FOX TROT is smoother, slower, and more graceful looking than the form popular during the early 1900s. According to English dance master, Victor Silvester, the original Fox Trot used a series of brisk, almost frenetic steps, in which 4 slow walking steps were followed by 8 quick running steps. Compared with this older version, the modern day Fox Trot appears to be quite tame.

Indeed, the ballroom version of the Fox Trot currently in vogue contains a basic step pattern of 2 walks steps, alternated with 2 brush close steps for the first 4 beats, and concludes with a chassé (side step/ close step) on the last 2 beats of music. Similar to a tap or toe step, the brush step is made without placing any weight on the foot that brushes against or lightly touches the opposite foot. On the walk and chassé steps, however, weight is placed directly on the foot that steps.

In terms of rhythm, the Fox Trot may be counted in two ways. One way, usually preferred by most dance instructors, is to focus attention on the timing, formed by a combination of two slow beats followed by two quick beats: slow / slow / quick / quick. The two slow counts correspond to the two groups of walk and brush close steps, while the two quick counts correspond to the chassé (side step / close step).

Another equally easy method of keeping count emphasizes the beats which correspond to each step. Of course, the basic Fox Trot pattern contains a total of 6 steps, completed in 6 beats (1-½ measures) of music. Each step in the pattern, therefore, may be counted out individually. ♣

FORWARD PROGRESSIVE

In the BASIC FORWARD PROGRESSIVE FOX TROT, partners progress smoothly around the floor in a counter-clockwise direction. Similar to most Fox Trot patterns, the Basic Forward Progressive Step contains 4 steps, completed in 6 beats (1-½ measures of music). The basic rhythm and timing begins with two slow counts, followed with two quick counts: slow (beats 1-2)/ slow (beats 3-4)/ quick (beat 5)/ quick (beat 6).

On the two slow counts, the man takes two steps forward, as the woman takes two steps backward. Each of these two walk steps forward or backward must be followed through with a brush (close) step, taken in the same direction. Do *not* put any weight on the brush (close) step, as you slowly let one foot drift, until it is lightly touching next to the opposite foot. The Basic Forward Progressive Step concludes with a chassé in which partners take one step side (quick), followed with a close side step (quick). Unlike the brush step, the close step is made with weight placed on the foot that steps.

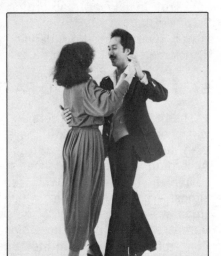

step 1 (beats 1-2)

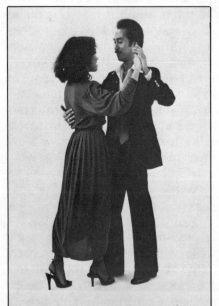

step 2 (beats 3-4)

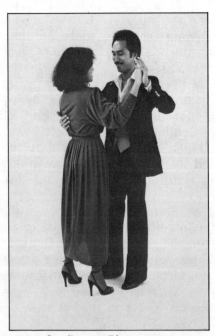

step 3 (beat 5)

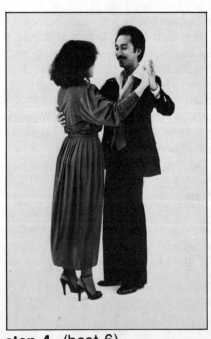

step 4 (beat 6)

Man's Part:

Time	Beat	Steps
Slow	(1-2)	1. Left foot forward / (R-brush forward)
Slow	(3-4)	2. Right foot forward/ (L-brush forward)
Quick	(5)	3. Left foot side
Quick	(6)	4. Right foot close to left foot

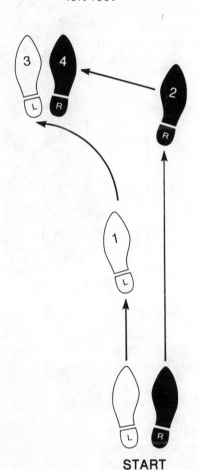

Woman's Part:

Time	Beat	Steps
Slow	(1-2)	1. Right foot back/ (L-brush back)
Slow	(3-4)	2. Left foot back/ (R-brush back)
Quick	(5)	3. Right foot side
Quick	(6)	4. Left foot close to right foot

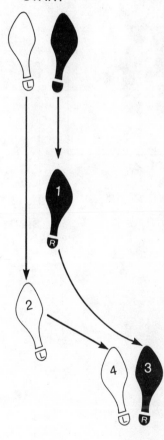

FOX TROT

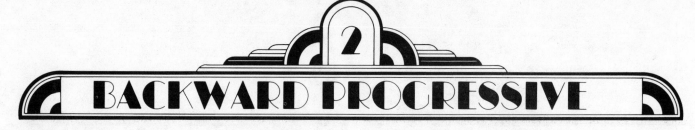

BACKWARD PROGRESSIVE

As the name implies, the BACKWARD PROGRESSIVE FOX TROT reverses the step direction used in the Basic Forward Progressive Step. This time, therefore, the man takes two steps backward, beginning with his left foot back, while the woman takes two steps forward, beginning with her right foot forward. Despite the change in step sequence for the Backward Progressive Step, both the timing and rhythm remain the same: slow (beats 1-2)/ slow (beats 3-4)/ quick (beat 5)/ quick (beat 6).

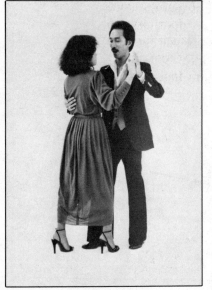

step 1 (beats 1-2)

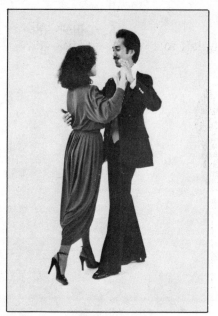

step 2 (beats 3-4)

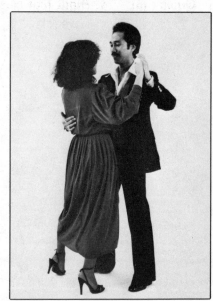

step 3 (beat 5)

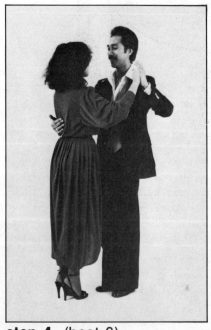

step 4 (beat 6)

Man's Part:

Time	Beat	Steps
Slow	(1-2)	1. Left foot back/ (R-brush back)
Slow	(3-4)	2. Right foot back/ (L-brush back)
Quick	(5)	3. Left foot side
Quick	(6)	4. Right foot close to left foot

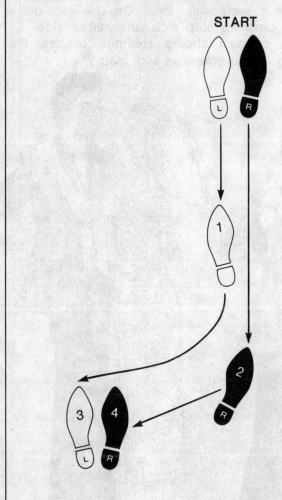

Woman's Part:

Time	Beat	Steps
Slow	(1-2)	1. Right foot forward/ (L-brush forward)
Slow	(3-4)	2. Left foot forward/ (R-brush forward)
Quick	(5)	3. Right foot side
Quick	(6)	4. Left foot close to right foot

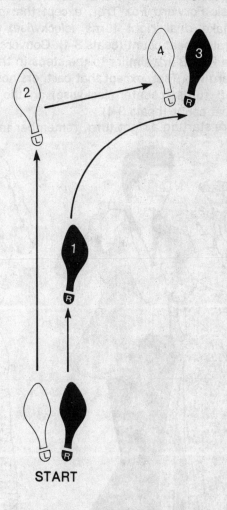

SENIOR FOX TROT

The SENIOR or COMBINATION WALK IN FOX TROT combines the Forward and Backward Step, but adds dual turns to the second slow beat count. Although the entire pattern contains a total of 8 steps, completed in 12 beats (3 measures) of music, it can be divided into two parts, with each part retaining the basic Fox Trot rhythm and timing: slow (beats 1-2)/ slow (beats 3-4)/ quick (beat 5)/ quick (beat 6).

The steps in Part A are similar to the steps in the Basic Forward Fox Trot, except that partners now make dual right turns (clockwise) on the second slow beat count (beats 3-4). Conversely, the steps in Part B are similar to the steps in the Basic Backward Fox Trot, except that partners now make dual left turns (counter-clockwise) on the second slow beat count (beats 3-4).

Before starting a right turn, remember to glance over your right shoulder. Conversely, to make a left turn, glance over your left shoulder. Your feet will indubitably follow the direction in which you are staring.

Despite the addition of these dual right and left turns, however, the SENIOR FOX TROT does resemble an amalgamation of the Basic Forward and Backward Steps. On the two slow counts, partners take two walk steps forward or backward, and then brush (close) one foot next to the opposite foot, after each walk step. On the two quick counts, partners step side, then close side. Of course, partners should continue to use the Contrabody Movement on each step.

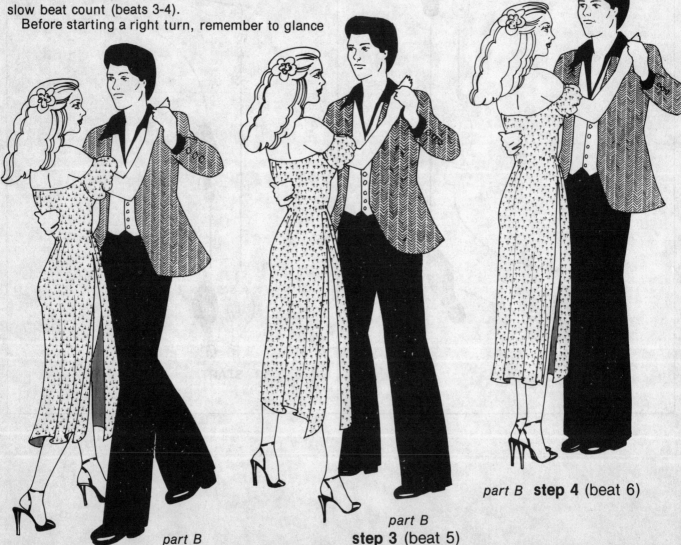

part B **step 4** (beat 6)

part B **step 3** (beat 5)

part B **step 2** (beats 3-4)

Part A:
SENIOR FOX TROT (BASIC FORWARD FOX TROT WITH RIGHT TURNS)

Man's Part:

Time	Beat	Steps
Slow	(1-2)	1. Left foot forward/ (R-brush forward)
Slow	(3-4)	2. Right foot forward, turning right/ (L-brush forward)
Quick	(5)	3. Left foot side
Quick	(6)	4. Right foot close to left foot

Woman's Part:

Time	Beat	Steps
Slow	(1-2)	1. Right foot back/ (L-brush back)
Slow	(3-4)	2. Left foot back, turning right/ (R-brush back)
Quick	(5)	3. Right foot side
Quick	(6)	4. Left foot close to right foot

Part B: SENIOR FOX TROT: BASIC BACKWARD STEP, WITH ONE-QUARTER LEFT TURN

Man's Part:

Time	Beat	Steps
Slow	(1-2)	1. Left foot back/ (R-brush back)
Slow	(3-4)	2. Right foot back, turning left/ (L-brush back)
Quick	(5)	3. Left foot side
Quick	(6)	4. Right foot close to left foot

Woman's Part:

Time	Beat	Steps
Slow	(1-2)	1. Right foot forward/ (L-brush forward)
Slow	(3-4)	2. Left foot forward, turning left/ (R-brush forward)
Quick	(5)	3. Right foot side
Quick	(6)	4. Left foot close to right foot

FOX TROT

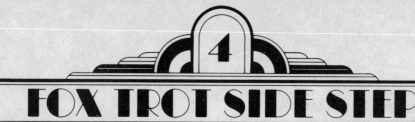
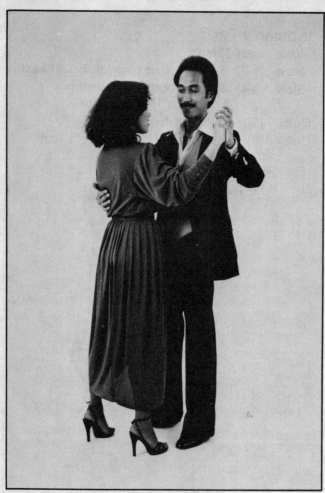

step 1 (beats 1-2)

In the FOX TROT SIDE STEP, partners continue to move in a sideways direction, as the man moves towards his left side, and the woman moves towards her right side. On the first slow count (beats 1-2), the man steps to his left side with his left foot, as the woman steps to her right side with her right foot. On the second slow count (beats 3-4), partners continue to move in the same sideways direction, as the man leads the woman into the Promenade Dance Position. On the second step sideways, therefore, partners move into the Promenade Position by crossing or passing one foot in front of the opposite foot (pass forward step): the man crosses his right foot in front of his left foot, as the woman crosses her left foot in front of her right foot. Notice that on the pass forward step, taken on the second slow count,

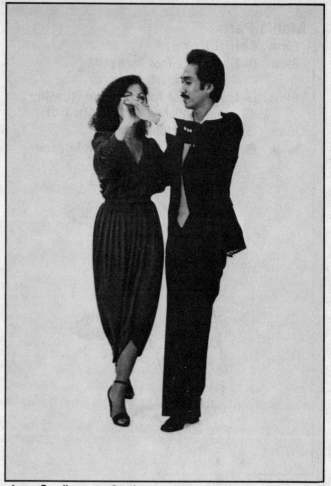

step 2 (beats 3-4)

partners break slightly away from each other, without releasing hands. Since *no* brush step follows either the side step or the pass forward step, partners must pause or "hold" position for one beat of music, after each step taken on the slow count.

The Fox Trot Side Step concludes with a chassé (side step, followed with a close side step). On the first quick count (beat 5), the man leads the woman back into the Social (Closed) Dance Position. As partners return to the Closed Position, the man steps towards his left side with his left foot, and the woman steps towards her right side with her right foot. On the last quick count (beat 6), the man closes his right foot to his left foot, as the woman closes her left foot to her right foot. 🎎

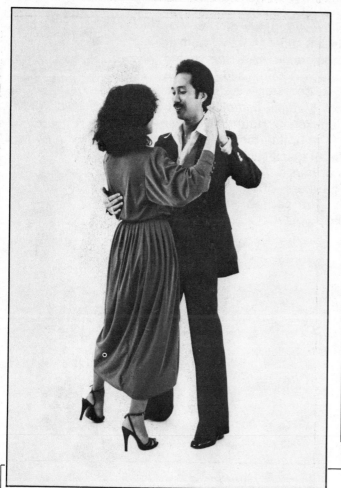

step 3 (beat 5)

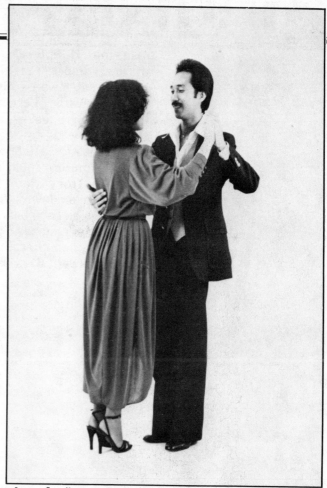

step 4 (beat 6)

Man's Part:

Time	Beat	Steps
Slow	(1-2)	1. Left foot side/ Hold
Slow	(3-4)	2. Right foot pass forward (cross in front of L-foot)/ Hold
Quick	(5)	3. Left foot side
Quick	(6)	4. Right foot close to left foot

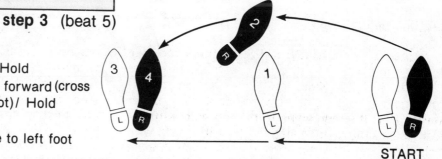

Woman's Part:

Time	Beat	Steps
Slow	(1-2)	1. Right foot side/ Hold
Slow	(3-4)	2. Left foot pass forward (cross in front of R-foot)/ Hold
Quick	(5)	3. Right foot side
Quick	(6)	4. Left foot close to right foot

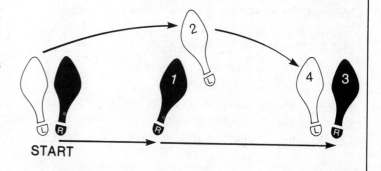

FOX TROT

TRIPLE CHASSES IN FOX TROT

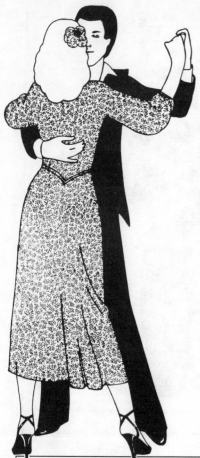

In the TRIPLE CHASSÉS, partners take all of their steps in a sideways direction, as the man moves towards his left side and the woman moves towards her right side. As the name implies, each chassé—which is composed of a side step, followed by a close step—is repeated three times for a total of 6 steps, completed in 6 beats of music. Thus, unlike the timing for most other Fox Trot patterns, the timing for this pattern can be broken down into all quick counts, with one step taken on each beat of music. After completing their triple chassés, partners often finish one sequence of another Fox Trot pattern, such as the Basic Backward Step.

Man's Part:

Time	Beat	Steps
Quick	(1)	1. Left foot side
Quick	(2)	2. Right foot close to left
Quick	(3)	3. Left foot side
Quick	(4)	4. Right foot close to left
Quick	(5)	5. Left foot side
Quick	(6)	6. Right foot close to left

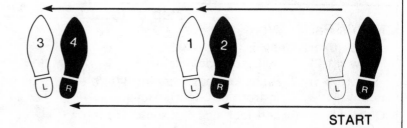

START

Woman's Part:

Time	Beat	Steps
Quick	(1)	1. Right foot side
Quick	(2)	2. Left foot close to right
Quick	(3)	3. Right foot side
Quick	(4)	4. Left foot close to right
Quick	(5)	5. Right foot side
Quick	(6)	6. Left foot close to right

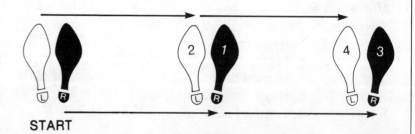

START

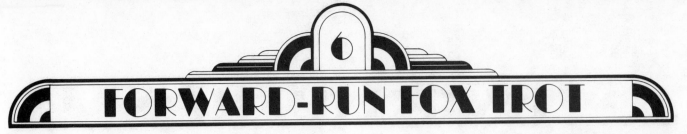

FORWARD-RUN FOX TROT

Although the FORWARD-RUN FOX TROT retains the conventional Fox Trot rhythm (6 beats or 1-1/2 measures of music) and timing (slow/ slow/ quick/ quick), it also contains a few unusual quirks. First of all, the entire pattern is composed of 4 steps: two walk steps, taken on the two slow counts (beats 1-4), followed with two run steps, taken on the two quick counts (beats 5-6). Secondly, unlike most other Fox Trot patterns, the walk steps are *not* followed by brush (close) steps. Thirdly, the man takes all of his steps forward, as the woman takes all of her steps backward. And finally, both the man and the woman will make dual 1/8 left turns (45 degrees counter-clockwise) on each of their four forward or backward steps, as they curve in a circular pattern to their left.

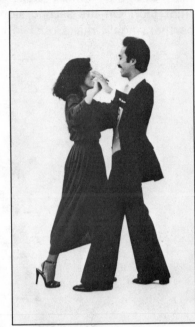

step 1 (beats 1-2)

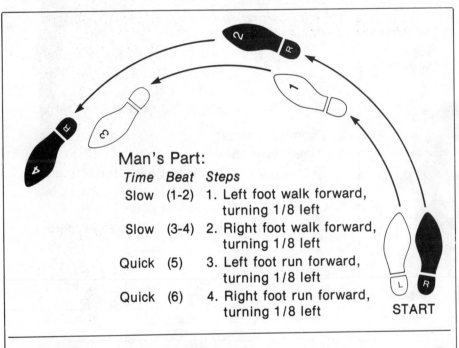

Man's Part:

Time	Beat	Steps
Slow	(1-2)	1. Left foot walk forward, turning 1/8 left
Slow	(3-4)	2. Right foot walk forward, turning 1/8 left
Quick	(5)	3. Left foot run forward, turning 1/8 left
Quick	(6)	4. Right foot run forward, turning 1/8 left

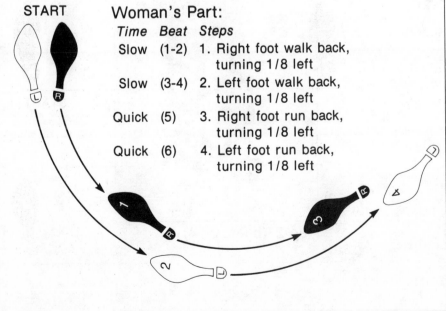

Woman's Part:

Time	Beat	Steps
Slow	(1-2)	1. Right foot walk back, turning 1/8 left
Slow	(3-4)	2. Left foot walk back, turning 1/8 left
Quick	(5)	3. Right foot run back, turning 1/8 left
Quick	(6)	4. Left foot run back, turning 1/8 left

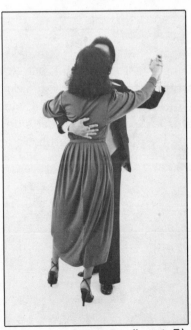

step 3 (beat 5)

FOX TROT

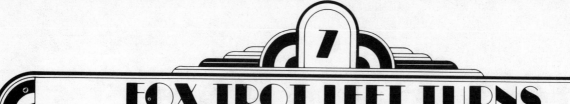

FOX TROT LEFT TURNS

The FOX TROT LEFT TURNS, sometimes called the LEFT HESITATION FOX TROT, add ¼ left turns to each forward or backward step, taken on the slow counts.

On the first slow count, partners make dual left turns, as the man steps forward with his left foot, and the woman steps backward with her right foot. On the second slow count (beats 3-4), partners again make dual left turns, as the man steps backward with his right foot, and the woman steps forward with her left foot. Before initiating these turns, remember to look over your own left shoulder, then let your feet follow the direction in which your nose is pointing. Each of these backward or forward steps must be followed through with a brush (close) step. This pattern concludes on two quick counts with a side step (beat 5), followed with a close step (beat 6).

Man's Part:

Time	Beat	Steps
Slow	(1-2)	1. Left foot forward, turning left
Slow	(3-4)	2. Right foot back, turning left
Quick	(5)	3. Left foot side
Quick	(6)	4. Right foot close to left foot

Woman's Part:

Time	Beat	Steps
Slow	(1-2)	1. Right foot back, turning left
Slow	(3-4)	2. Left foot forward, turning left
Quick	(5)	3. Right foot side
Quick	(6)	4. Left foot close to right foot

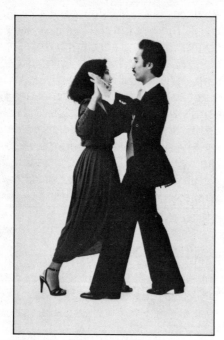

step 1 (beats 1-2)

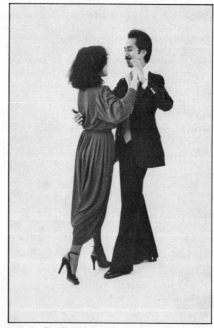

step 2 (beats 3– 4)

CHAPTER 13

TANGO

The TANGO has no clearly defined origins. Different historians have claimed that it may have originated in Argentina, Haiti, Africa, Cuba, Brazil, Spain, or Mexico. According to sociologist Frances Rust, the Tango is an odd mixture of the *tangano* (a dance performed by African slaves brought to Haiti and Cuba in the 18th century) and the habanera (a 19th century Cuban dance). Other authorities insist that the name "Tango," was applied to a version of the *milonga,* a dance originally performed by the Argentinian plainsmen called *gauchos.* Although the Castles standardized the steps in 1914, the Tango did not become the craze in America until the 1920s.

RHYTHM AND PATTERN

The Tango is a highly stylized ballroom dance which combines a staccato progression with pronounced Contrabody Movement. The Tango must be danced with knees slightly flexed, which settles the weight in the lower part of the body and gives one the feeling of closeness to the ground. Footwork must be carefully executed, with the dancer's weight centered over the instep.

All of the basic patterns described in this chapter contain 5 steps, completed in 8 beats (2 measures) of music. "Dance time" for the Tango is counted: slow, slow, quick, quick, slow.

The first two slow counts correspond to walk steps taken forward or backward. Unlike the Fox Trot in which a brush (close) step follows each walk step, the Tango contains a follow through *after* the second beat count. Thus, on the first two slow counts, the dancer walks forward or backward, then holds the position for one beat count, before following through with the opposite foot.

The two quick counts correspond to another walk step forward or backward, followed with a side step. Each step pattern concludes on the final slow count with a "Tango close." Although feet are drawn together in the parallel (close) position, *no* weight is placed on the foot that is brought next to the opposite foot. After drawing feet together, weight remains on the opposite foot, as the dancer pauses or holds the position for one beat of music. On the final slow count, the man balances his weight on his right foot, while the woman balances her weight on her left foot.

The Tango is a progressive dance in which the dancers move around the dance floor in the Line of Direction. On each step, therefore, the dancers turn slightly to their left (counter-clockwise). More important, Contrabody Movement should be emphasized. Thus, whenever the dancer steps forward on his left foot, he pulls his left shoulder back. Conversely, whenever the dancer steps forward on his right foot, he pulls his right shoulder back.

BASIC FORWARD STEP

The BASIC FORWARD STEP IN TANGO consists of 3 walk steps, followed with 1 side step, and concludes with the Tango close. Throughout this entire pattern, partners will be embraced in the Social (Closed) Dance Position. In addition, the Basic Forward Step incorporates the unique rhythm and timing characteristic of most Tango patterns; slow (beats 1-2)/ slow (beats 3-4)/ quick (beat 5)/ quick (beat 6)/ slow (beats 7-8). Each step taken on a slow count is followed with a pause or ''hold'' for one beat of music.

In the Basic Forward Step, the man's part starts with 3 steps forward, followed with 1 step side, and concludes with the Tango close (brush close/hold). The woman's part, which is the natural opposite of the man's part, starts with 3 steps back, followed with 1 step side, and concludes with the Tango close (brush close/hold).

Notice that each of the first two walk steps forward or backward are followed with a pause, in which partners hold the position for one beat of music.

On the Tango close, completed on the last slow count (beats 7-8), do *not* place any weight on the foot that brushes against the opposite foot. Thus, the man lightly touches his left foot next to his right foot, without putting any weight on his left foot, then he holds the position with feet together for one beat of music. The woman on the other hand, lightly touches her right foot next to her left foot, without putting any weight on her right foot, then she holds the position with feet together for one beat of music.

The entire Basic Forward Step should be repeated continuously, as partners progress around the dance floor in the Line of Direction (counter-clockwise). To achieve a smooth and controlled placement of the feet, partners should keep their knees slightly flexed. For true Tango styling, partners should accentuate the Contrabody Movement. 🕺

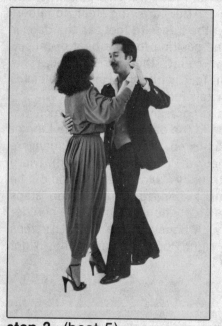

step 3 (beat 5)

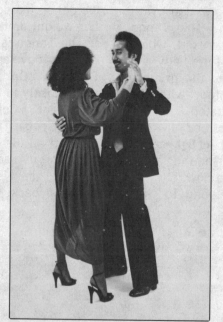

step 4 (beat 6)

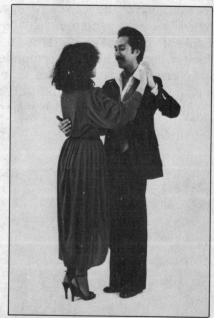

step 5 (beats 7-8)

Man's Part:

Time	Beat	Steps
Slow	(1-2)	1. Left foot forward / Hold
Slow	(3-4)	2. Right foot forward / Hold
Quick	(5)	3. Left foot forward
Quick	(6)	4. Right foot side
Slow	(7-8)	5. Left foot brush next to right foot / Hold

Woman's Part:

Time	Beat	Steps
Slow	(1-2)	1. Right foot back / Hold
Slow	(3-4)	2. Left foot back / Hold
Quick	(5)	3. Right foot back
Quick	(6)	4. Left foot side
Slow	(7-8)	5. Right foot brush next to left foot / Hold

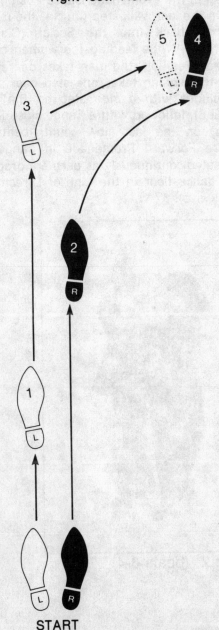

START

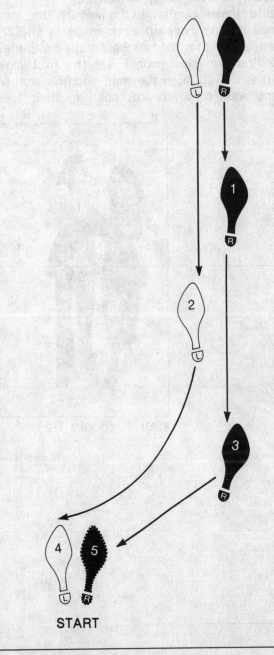

START

TANGO

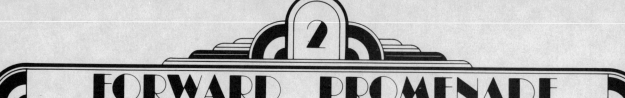

FORWARD PROMENADE

The FORWARD PROMENADE IN TANGO is similar to the Basic Forward Step, in terms of both movement and styling. Both contain step patterns of 5 steps, completed in 8 beats (2 measures) of music. Both maintain the basic Tango rhythm and timing: slow (beats 1-2)/ slow (beats 3-4)/ quick (beat 5)/ quick (beat 6)/ slow (beats 7-8). And finally, throughout both patterns, partners should keep their knees slightly flexed, while they emphasize the Contrabody Movement.

Despite these similarities, however, the step sequence for the Forward Promenade is slightly different, at least for the two walk steps completed on the first two slow counts. On the first slow count (beats 1-2), both the man and the woman take one walk step *forward*, pointing their toes

outward, as they turn slightly away from each other. On this first walk step, partners move into the Promenade Dance Position in which partners are still embraced in the Closed Position, although they both face forward. On the second slow count (beats 3-4), partners continue to walk forward, as they cross one foot in front of the opposite foot (pass forward). A pause or hold for one beat of music follows each of these two forward steps, taken in the Promenade Dance Position.

On the last walk step (quick), the man leads the woman back into the Social (Closed) Dance Position. While leading the woman back into the Closed Position, the man takes one step forward, but the woman takes one step back. The pattern concludes with a side step on the quick count (beat 6), followed with a Tango close (brush close/ hold) on the last slow count (beats 7-8). The entire Forward Promenade in Tango should be repeated continuously as partners progress around the dance floor in the Line of Direction (counter-clockwise).

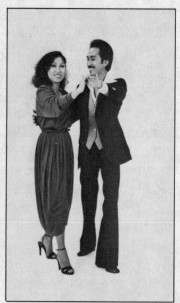

step 1 (beats 1-2)

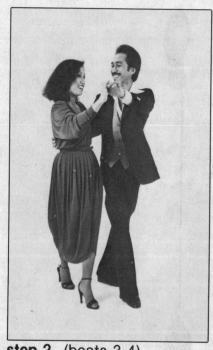

step 2 (beats 3-4)

Man's Part:

Time	Beat	Steps
Slow	(1-2)	1. Left foot forward, turning 1/8 left/ Hold
Slow	(3-4)	2. Right foot pass forward (cross in front of L-foot)/ Hold
Quick	(5)	3. Left foot forward, turning 1/8 right
Quick	(6)	4. Right foot side
Slow	(7-8)	5. Left foot brush next to right foot/ Hold

Woman's Part:

Time	Beat	Steps
Slow	(1-2)	1. Right foot forward, turning 1/8 right/ Hold
Slow	(3-4)	2. Left foot pass forward (cross in front of R-foot)/ Hold
Quick	(5)	3. Right foot back, turning 1/8 left
Quick	(6)	4. Left foot side
Slow	(7-8)	5. Right foot brush next to left foot/ Hold

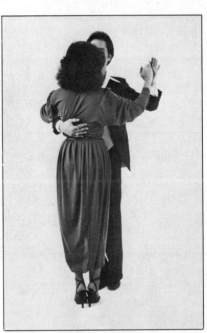

step 5 (beats 7-8)

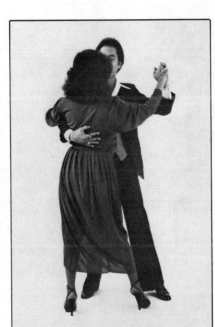

step 4 (beat 6)

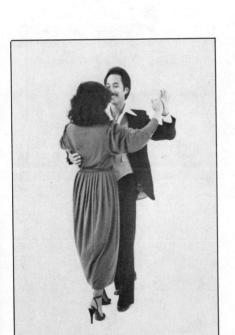

step 3 (beat 5)

TANGO

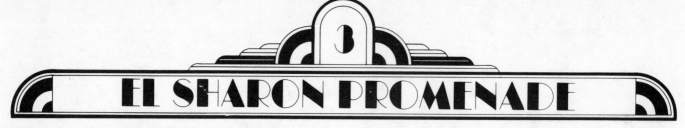

EL SHARON PROMENADE

El SHARON PROMENADE IN TANGO is the basic side step in Tango completed in the Conversation Dance Position. The pattern begins on the first two slow counts with a side step, followed with a pass forward or cross step. On the first slow count (beats 1-2), both the man and the woman take one step side, then hold the position for one beat of music. On the second slow count (beats 3-4), the man releases his left hand from the woman's right hand, as he leads the woman into the Conversation (Open) Dance Position. To move into the Conversation Position, both the man and the woman turn slightly away from each other, as they pass one foot in front of the opposite foot (pass forward), then hold the position for one beat of music.

Although the El Sharon Promenade begins with a side step, followed with a pass or cross step, for the first two slow counts, the pattern concludes like most other Tango patterns. On the last walk step, completed on the quick count (beat 5), the man leads the woman back into the Social (Closed) Dance Position. On the last walk step, the man takes one step forward, leading the woman into the Closed Dance Position, as the woman takes one step backward. The El Sharon Promenade concludes with a side step, completed on the quick count (beat 6), followed with a Tango close on the last slow count (beats 7-8).

On the last walk step, completed on the quick count (beat 5), the man returns the woman to the Social (Closed) Dance Position. As the man takes one step forward, leading the woman back into the Closed Dance Position, the woman takes one step backward. The pattern concludes with a side step (quick), followed by the Tango close (slow).

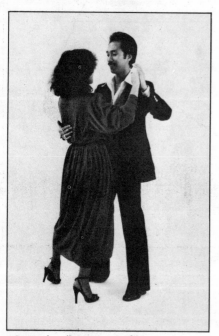

step 1 (beats 1-2)

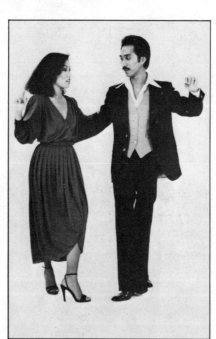

step 2 (beats 3-4)

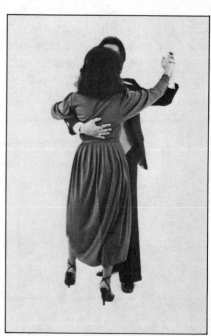

step 3 (beat 5)

Man's Part:

Time	Beat	Steps
Slow	(1-2)	1. Left foot side/ Hold
Slow	(3-4)	2. Right foot pass forward (cross in front of L-foot)/ Hold
Quick	(5)	3. Left foot forward
Quick	(6)	4. Right foot side
Slow	(7-8)	5. Left foot brush next to right foot/ Hold

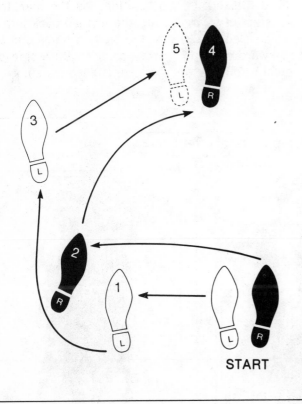

Woman's Part:

Time	Beat	Steps
Slow	(1-2)	1. Right foot side/ Hold
Slow	(3-4)	2. Left foot pass forward (cross in front of R-foot)/ Hold
Quick	(5)	3. Right foot back
Quick	(6)	4. Left foot side
Slow	(7-8)	5. Right foot brush next to left foot/ Hold

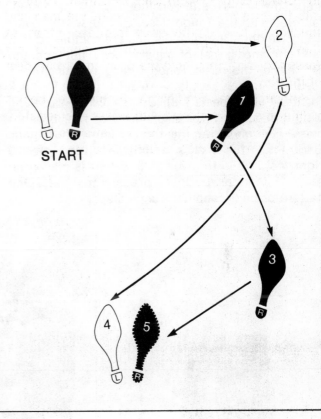

237

TANGO BACK STEP

The TANGO BACK STEP reverses the step direction of the Basic Forward Step, although both rhythm and styling remain the same. Thus, the one and only change evident in this pattern occurs on the first 3 walk steps. As the man takes 3 walk steps backward, starting with his left foot back, the woman takes 3 walk steps forward, starting with her right foot forward. A pause follows each of the first two walk steps, completed on the two slow counts.

Despite the change in direction for the walk steps, the pattern still concludes with a side step, followed with the Tango close. Of course, the basic Tango rhythm, in which 5 steps are completed in 8 beats (2 measures) of music, does not change. Therefore, the basic Tango timing remains: slow (beats 1-2)/ slow (beats 3-4)/ quick (beat 5)/ quick (beat 6)/ slow (beats 7-8). On the Tango close, no weight should be placed on the foot that brushes close. Therefore, at the conclusion of the Tango Back Step, the man's weight is placed on his right foot, while the woman's weight is placed on her left foot, as partners prepare to repeat the pattern or begin another Tango step.

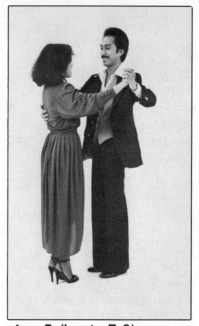

step 5 (beats 7-8)

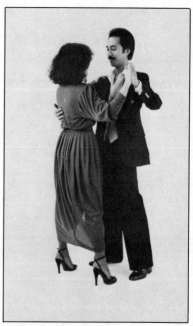

step 4 (beat 6)

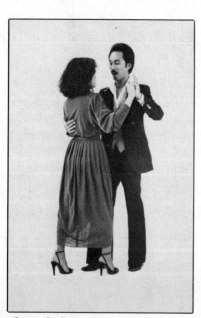

step 1 (beats 1-2)

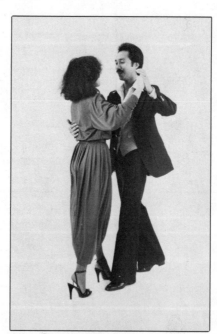

step 2 (beats 3-4)

Man's Part:

Time	Beat	Steps
Slow	(1-2)	1. Left foot back/ Hold
Slow	(3-4)	2. Right foot back/ Hold
Quick	(5)	3. Left foot back
Quick	(6)	4. Right foot side
Slow	(7-8)	5. Left foot brush next to right foot/ Hold

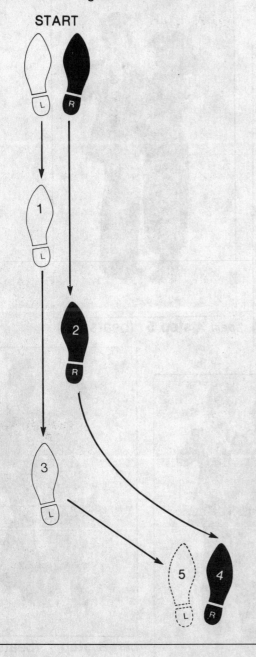

Woman's Part:

Time	Beat	Steps
Slow	(1-2)	1. Right foot forward/ Hold
Slow	(3-4)	2. Left foot forward/ Hold
Quick	(5)	3. Right foot forward/ Hold
Quick	(6)	4. Left foot side
Slow	(7-8)	5. Right foot brush next to left foot/ Hold

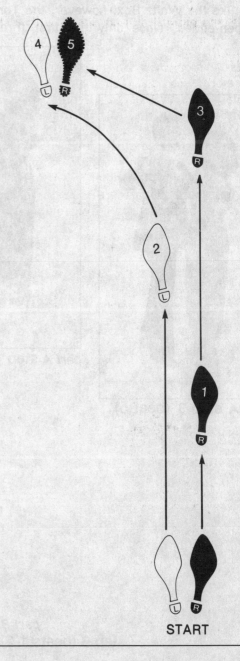

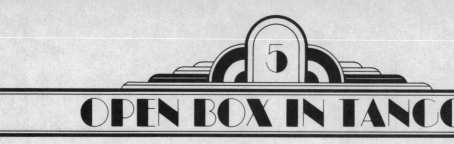

5
OPEN BOX IN TANGO

The OPEN BOX IN TANGO combines the Basic Forward Step with the Tango Back Step to form an elongated, three-sided or open-ended box. Divided into two parts, each part contains a total of five steps, completed in 8 beats (2 measures) of music. Throughout both parts, which combine to form a box configuration, the basic Tango rhythm and timing remain unchanged: slow (beats 1-2)/ slow (beats 3-4)/ quick (beat 5)/ quick (beat 6)/ slow (beats 7-8).

Unlike the Waltz Box, however, the Tango Box is open-ended, since only the first three sides are joined, with the last side left open. The box remains open-ended or three-sided, because the pattern always ends in the same sideways direction, with the man stepping towards his right side, as the woman steps towards her left side. Since the man always starts on his left foot and ends on his right foot, while the woman always starts with her right foot and ends on her left foot, the box can never be closed, for never the twain shall meet. 👫

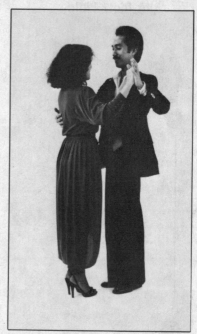

part A **step 5** (beats 7-8)

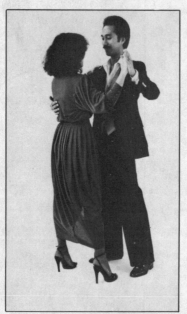

part A **step 4** (beat 6)

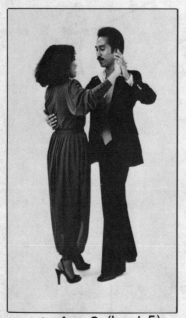

part A **step 3** (beat 5)

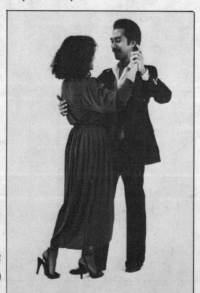

part B
step 6 (beats 1-2)

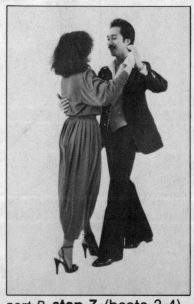

part B **step 7** (beats 3-4)

Man's Part:

Time	Beat	Steps
Slow	(1-2)	1. Left foot forward/ Hold
Slow	(3-4)	2. Right foot forward/ Hold
Quick	(5)	3. Left foot forward
Quick	(6)	4. Right foot side
Slow	(7-8)	5. Left foot brush next to right foot/ Hold

part B

Time	Beat	Steps
Slow	(1-2)	6. Left foot back/ Hold
Slow	(3-4)	7. Right foot back/ Hold
Quick	(5)	8. Left foot back
Quick	(6)	9. Right foot side
Slow	(7-8)	10. Left foot brush next to right foot/ Hold

Woman's Part:

Time	Beat	Steps
Slow	(1-2)	1. Right foot back/ Hold
Slow	(3-4)	2. Left foot back/ Hold
Quick	(5)	3. Right foot back
Quick	(6)	4. Left foot side
Slow	(7-8)	5. Right foot brush next to left foot/ Hold

part B

Time	Beat	Steps
Slow	(1-2)	6. Right foot forward/ Hold
Slow	(3-4)	7. Left foot forward/ Hold
Quick	(5)	8. Right foot forward/ Hold
Quick	(6)	9. Left foot side
Slow	(7-8)	10. Right foot brush next to left foot/ Hold

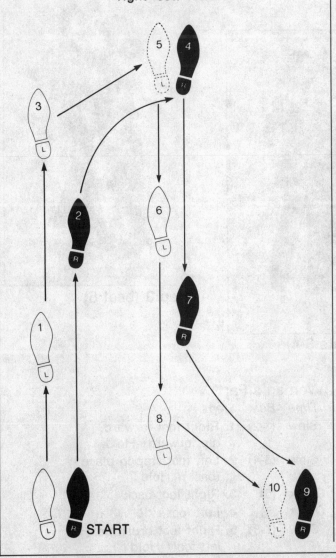

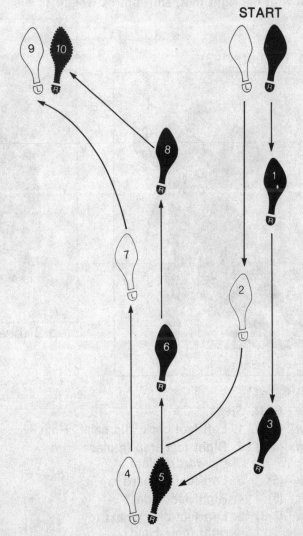

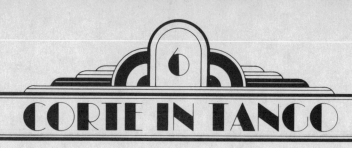

CORTE IN TANGO

The CORTE IN TANGO begins with a dip step. On the first slow count (beats 1-2) the man steps *back*, placing all of his weight on his left foot, while the woman steps *forward*, placing all of her weight on her right foot. To dip, the man bends his left knee, lifts his right foot slightly off the floor, and dips or leans backward. The woman, on the other hand, bends her right knee, lifts her left foot slightly off the floor, and dips or leans slightly forward. To complete the look of the dip step, the shoulders should be angled so that the man's body weight is centered over his left foot, while the woman's body weight is centered over her right foot. Hold the dip position for one beat of music.

On the second slow count (beats 3-4), partners return to an upright position. The man steps in place with his right foot, shifting his weight to his forward foot, and straightening his left knee. Conversely, the woman steps in place with her left foot, shifting her weight to her backward foot, and straightening her right knee. After stepping in place, partners hold the position for one beat of music.

The Corte concludes with the basic pattern, completed in the Social (Closed) Dance Position. On the first quick count (beat 5) the man steps forward with his left foot, while the woman steps backward with her right foot. On the next quick count (beat 6), partners step to the side. On the last slow count (beats 7-8), the pattern concludes with a Tango close (brush close and hold).

step 1 (beats 1-2)

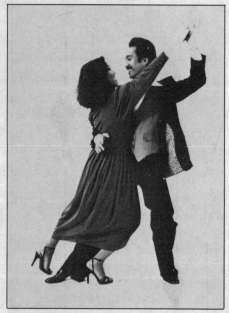

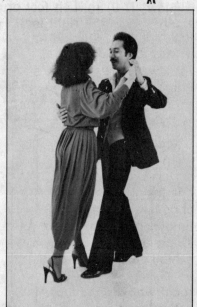

step 2 (beats 3-4)

step 3 (beat 5)

Man's Part:

Time	Beat	Steps
Slow	(1-2)	1. Left foot back, dip back/ Hold
Slow	(3-4)	2. Right foot step in place (forward)/ Hold
Quick	(5)	3. Left foot forward
Quick	(6)	4. Right foot side
Slow	(7-8)	5. Left foot brush next to right foot/ Hold

Woman's Part

Time	Beat	Steps
Slow	(1-2)	1. Right foot forward, dip forward/ Hold
Slow	(3-4)	2. Left foot step in place (back)/ Hold
Quick	(5)	3. Right foot back
Quick	(6)	4. Left foot side
Slow	(7-8)	5. Right foot brush next to left foot/ Hold

CHAPTER 14

AMERICAN SWING

Swing, also known as JITTERBUG or LINDY, originated in America, along with most other jazz forms. Three different Swing variations, lumped under the name Lindy, became particularly popular. Of course, Swing also led to other, more frenetic type dances such as the Charleston, Black Bottom and Shag.

The Jitterbug, a dance performed to swing music, swept the entire country in the mid-30s. The Jitterbug introduced two innovations in Western style dance: the solo or "breakaway" part: and the leap or "air step." In the solo or "breakaway" partners performed individually. On the "air step" the dancers literally jumped off the floor into the air. "The jitterbug was more of a style than a dance," according to Peter Buckman:

A violent, even frenzied athleticism was often employed that made it hazardous for performers and their fellow dancers alike. The name seemed to sum up the movements of its fans, and it became current at the same time as "hepcat," a term used to describe a swing addict. . . Jitterbugging was sexual, exhibitionistic, cathartic, and risky. It could be performed on the spot, or the partners could whirl each other around to take up the entire floor.

BASIC PATTERN AND RHYTHM

Initially, Swing was performed as a modified box step with a distinct shuffling movement. A hint of this shuffle in the form of a brush close step is still evident in Single Rhythm Swing. Swing, however, evolved into three distinct rhythmical patterns — Single Rhythm, Double Rhythm, and Triple Rhythm.

In all three patterns, the timing and beat count remain the same. All contain patterns completed in 6 beats (1-½ measures) of music. All follow the dance timing of slow, slow, quick, quick. And finally, all patterns conclude with a back rock or ball-change steps on the last two beats of music (beats 5-6).

Despite these similarities, there are a few outstanding differences between these Swing patterns. Single Rhythm Swing, which contains four steps, begins with walk steps alternated with brush close steps. Double Rhythm Swing, which contains 6 steps, alternates tap steps with side steps. Triple Rhythm Swing, which contains 8 steps, combines "side-together-side" steps made to alternate sides.

To dance Swing correctly, keep your body relaxed and your knees slightly flexed. The outstanding characteristics of Swing movement are flexible knees, coupled with a slight swaying motion of the upper torso. Because Swing offers such a wide variety of rhythmical patterns, Swing dancers inevitably develop their own unique style. To develop a fantastic style, you might find it helpful to heed the advice of instructor Skippy Blair:

Think of the pattern as being danced in a slot. (This makes for easy maneuvering on a tight floor). The man is the center of the slot. She travels up and down the slot as if she were on roller skates. Her CPB (Center of Balance) is sent back and forth as if on a giant rubber band. The leverage (resistance) consists of changing her direction at given points in the pattern. This interaction between the two bodies produces body flight. 🕺

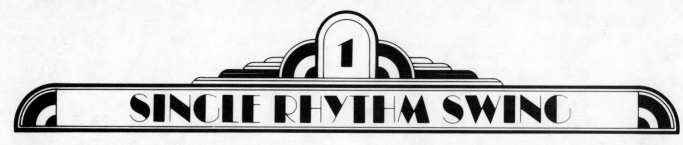

SINGLE RHYTHM SWING

SINGLE RHYTHM SWING contains a basic pattern of 4 steps, completed in 6 beats (1-½ measures) of music. As explained in previous chapters, *Single Rhythm* refers to one step, completed in two beats of music. In Single Rhythm Swing, the basic pattern begins with two side steps, completed in 4 beats of music, although the pattern concludes with a back rock or ball-change steps on the last two beats of music. Moreover, the timing for Single Rhythm Swing is counted: slow (beats 1-2)/ slow (beats 3-4)/ quick (beat 5)/ quick (beat 6). The entire Single Rhythm Swing pattern may be performed in either the Social (Closed) or Holding (Two-Hand) Dance Position.

The basic pattern begins on the two slow counts with two side steps, followed with brush close steps. Each of the two side steps, therefore, is followed with a brush close step in which one foot drifts towards and lightly brushes against the opposite foot, although *no* weight is placed on the foot that brushes. Thus, the side step and the brush close step comprise one inclusive unit, completed in two beats of music.

On the first step (step 1), completed on the first slow count (beats 1-2), the man steps side on his left foot, then lets his right foot drift towards and lightly brush against his left foot, although his weight remains on his left foot. The woman, on the other hand, steps side with her right foot, then lets her left foot drift towards and lightly brush against her right foot, although her weight remains on her right foot.

On the second step (step 2), completed on the

second slow count (beats 3-4), the man and woman switch directions. This time, the man steps side with his right foot, then lets his left foot drift towards and brush lightly against his left foot, although his weight remains on his right foot. Conversely, the woman steps side with her left foot, then lets her right foot drift towards and lightly brush against her left foot, although her weight remains on her left foot.

The basic pattern for Single Rhythm Swing concludes on the two quick counts (beats 5-6) with a back rock or ball-change steps. On beat 5 (step 3), the man steps back on his left foot, as the woman steps back on her right foot. On beat 6 (step 4), the man steps in place on his right foot, as the woman steps in place on her left foot. On the back rock, a slight rocking motion should be emphasized, as weight is shifted from the back foot to the forward foot.

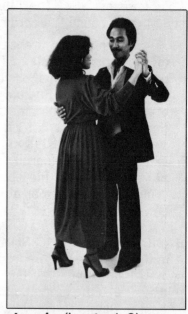

step 1 (beats 1-2)

Man's Part:

Time	Beat	Steps
Slow	(1-2)	1. Left foot side/ (Right foot brush next to left foot)
Slow	(3-4)	2. Right foot side/ (Left foot brush next to right foot)
Quick	(5)	3. Left foot back
Quick	(6)	4. Right foot step in place

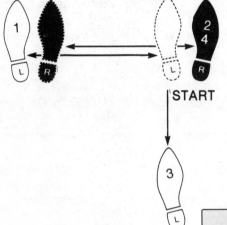

Woman's Part:

Time	Beat	Steps
Slow	(1-2)	1. Right foot side/ (Left foot brush next to right foot)
Slow	(3-4)	2. Left foot side/ (Right foot brush next to left foot)
Quick	(5)	3. Right foot back
Quick	(6)	4. Left foot step in place

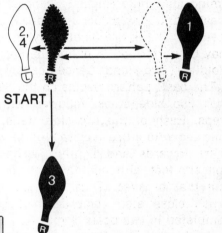

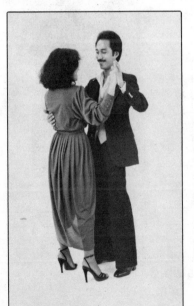

step 2 (beats 3-4)

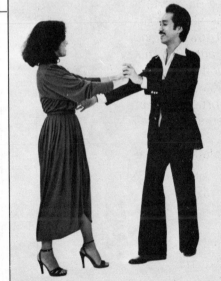

step 3 (beat 5)

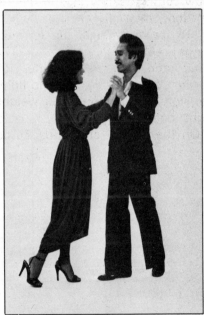

step 4 (beat 6)

AMERICAN SWING

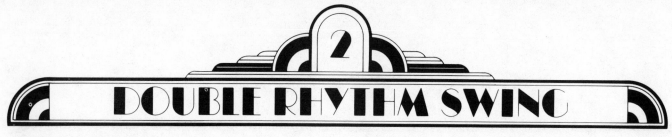
DOUBLE RHYTHM SWING differs from Single Rhythm Swing in two major ways: rhythm and step sequence. As the name suggests, Double Rhythm Swing is an even rhythm unit in which one step is taken on each and every beat of music. Thus, the pattern for Double Rhythm Swing begins with 4 steps, completed in 4 beats of music, although the pattern still concludes with a back rock or ball-change steps. Secondly, in the basic pattern for Double Rhythm Swing, a tap step precedes each walk step, although the pattern still concludes with a back rock or ball-change steps.

Consequently, the basic step pattern for Double Rhythm Swing contains 6 steps, completed in 6 beats (1-½ measures) of music. Nonetheless, the basic timing can still be counted: slow (beats 1-2)/ slow (beats 3-4)/ quick (beat 5)/ quick (beat 6). In addition, Double Rhythm Swing may be performed in either the Social (Closed) Dance Position or in the Holding (Two-Hand) Dance Position.

In Double Rhythm Swing, the basic pattern begins with 4 steps, alternating tap steps with walk steps, although each step is taken on 1 beat of music. On the first two steps (steps 1-2), completed on the first slow count (beats 1-2), the man taps to his left side, then steps to his left side, as the woman taps to her right side, then steps to her right side. On the next two steps (steps 3-4), completed on the second slow count (beats 3-4), the man and woman reverse the direction of their steps. Thus, the man taps to his right side, then steps to his right side, as the woman taps to her left side, then steps to her left side.

The basic step pattern for Double Rhythm Swing concludes with back rock or ball-change steps on the last two quick counts (beats 5-6). On beat 5 (step 5), the man steps back with his left foot, as the woman steps back with her right foot. On beat 6 (step 6), the man steps in place with his right foot, as the woman steps in place with her left foot. A slight rocking motion should be emphasized, whenever weight is shifted from the back foot to the forward foot. ♟

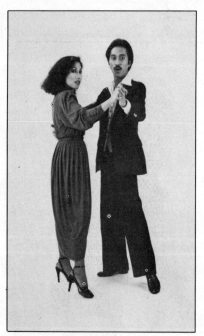

step 1 (beat 1)

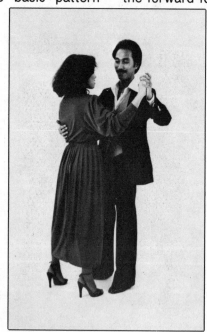

step 2 (beat 2)

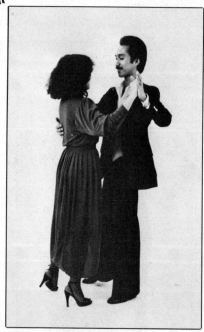

step 3 (beat 3)

Man's Part:

Time	Beat	Steps
Slow	(1)	1. Left foot tap side
	(2)	2. Left foot step side
Slow	(3)	3. Right foot tap side
	(4)	4. Right foot step side
Quick	(5)	5. Left foot step back
Quick	(6)	6. Right foot step in place

Woman's Part:

Time	Beat	Steps
Slow	(1)	1. Right foot tap side
	(2)	2. Right foot step side
Slow	(3)	3. Left foot tap side
	(4)	4. Left foot step side
Quick	(5)	5. Right foot step back
Quick	(6)	6. Left foot step in place

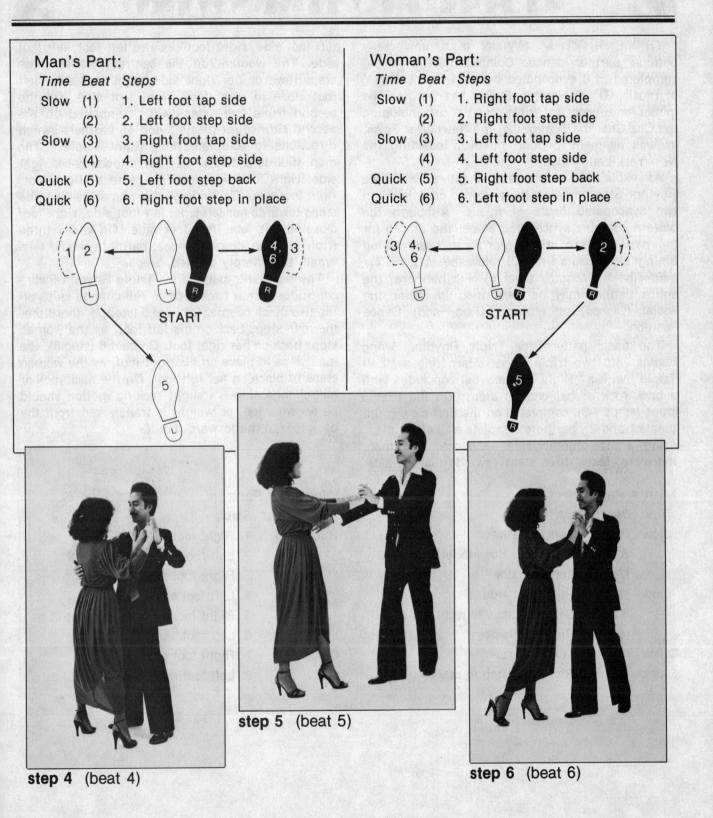

step 4 (beat 4)

step 5 (beat 5)

step 6 (beat 6)

AMERICAN SWING

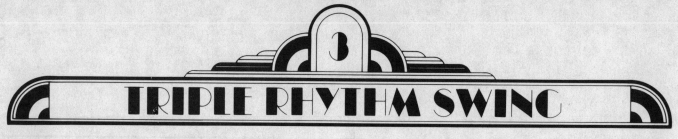

TRIPLE RHYTHM SWING is a universally popular partner dance. Composed of 8 steps, completed in 6 syncopated beats (1-½ measures) of music, Triple Rhythm Swing has become the model for subsequent triple step dances, including the Cha-Cha, the Sugarpush, the Newporter Salsa, as well as many popular hustles, including the New York-Latin Hustle.

As explained in previous chapters, a Triple Rhythm Step contains three steps, completed in two syncopated beats of music. Although the pattern contains syncopated steps, the timing for the basic pattern still conforms to basic Swing timing: slow (beats 1 and 2)/ slow (beats 3 and 4)/ quick (beat 5)/ quick (beat 6). Furthermore, the entire pattern may be performed in either the Social (Closed) or Holding (Two-Hand) Dance Position.

The basic pattern for Triple Rhythm Swing begins with two triple steps, alternating a "Left Triple" with a "Right Triple," but concludes with a back rock or ball-change steps. On the first 3 steps (steps 1-3), completed on the first slow count (beats 1-and-2), partners complete a "Left Triple," using a side-together-side sequence. The man, therefore, takes three steps towards his left side: left foot side, right foot close to left foot, left foot side. The woman, on the contrary, takes three steps towards her right side: right foot side, left foot close to right foot, right foot side. On the second triple step (steps 4-6), completed on the second slow count (beats 3 and 4), partners switch directions to complete the "Right Triple." The man, therefore, takes three steps towards his right side: right foot side, left foot close to right foot, right foot side. Conversely, the woman takes three steps towards her left side: left foot side, right foot close to left foot, left foot side. On these three triple steps to alternate sides, partners should take small, but sharply defined, steps.

The basic step pattern for Triple Rhythm Swing concludes with a back rock or ball-change steps on the two quick counts. On beat 5 (step 7), therefore, the man steps back on his left foot, as the woman steps back on her right foot. On beat 6 (step 8), the man steps in place on his right foot, as the woman steps in place on her left foot. On the back rock or ball-change steps, a slight rocking motion should be accentuated, as weight is transferred from the back foot to the forward foot. ♣

Man's Part:

Time	Beat	Steps
Slow	(1)	1. Left foot side
	(&)	2. Right foot close to left foot
	(2)	3. Left foot side
Slow	(3)	4. Right foot side
	(&)	5. Left foot close to right foot
	(4)	6. Right foot side
Quick	(5)	7. Left foot back
Quick	(6)	8. Right foot step in place

Woman's Part:

Time	Beat	Steps
Slow	(1)	1. Right foot side
	(&)	2. Left foot close to right foot
	(2)	3. Right foot side
Slow	(3)	4. Left foot side
	(&)	5. Right foot close to left foot
	(4)	6. Left foot side
Quick	(5)	7. Right foot back
Quick	(6)	8. Left foot step in place

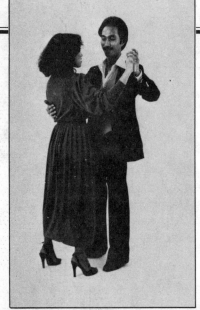

step 3 (beat 2)

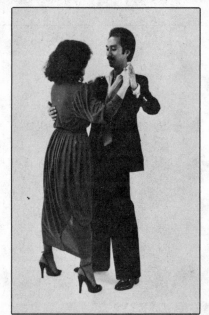

step 4 (beat 3)

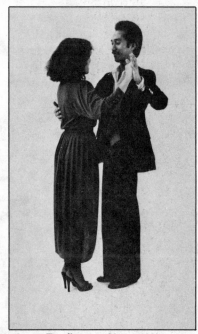

step 5 (beat "and")

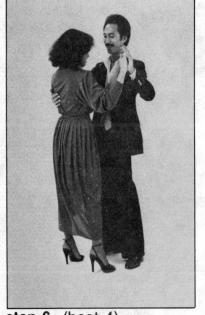

step 6 (beat 4)

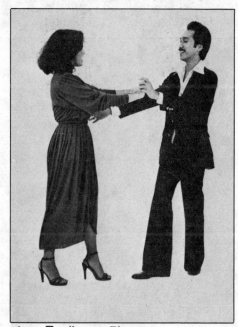

step 7 (beat 5)

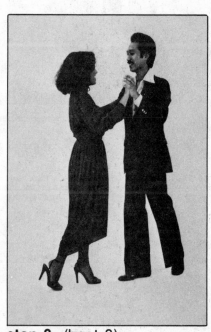

step 8 (beat 6)

AMERICAN SWING

CHAPTER 15

RUMBA

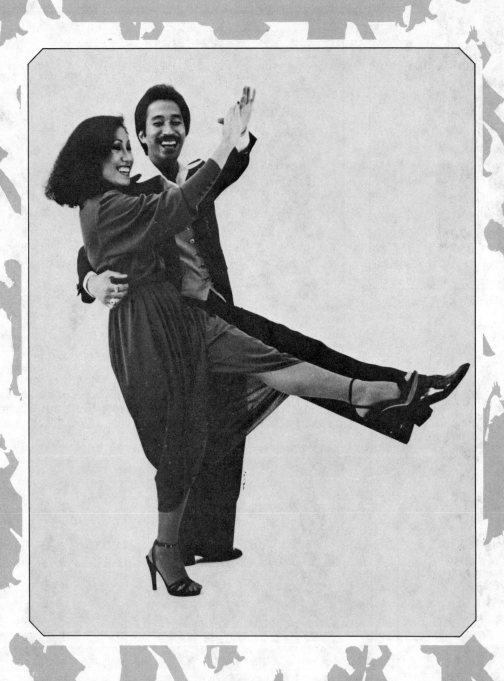

The RUMBA, a dance imported from Cuba to the United States in the late 1920s, combined African and Caribbean rhythms in a frankly erotic dance. "In its most primitive form" according to some critics, "it was an expressive pantomime danced by the natives under the hypnotic spell of elemental music. Even today, in the backcountry of Cuba, this same ritual pantomime is performed."

Because the uninhibited and wild Rumba was considered a bit too risque, a watered down version known as the *son* was the form introduced to European society. After the Castles standardized the steps into a non-progressive box, this dance was jazzed up to produce the Calypso in the 1950s. The Black Waltz, a disco dance popular in some regions of the country, is an up-dated version of the Rumba.

RHYTHM AND PATTERN

In Rumba, the basic step is the Box Step. Unlike the Waltz, however, the Rumba Box begins with a chassé (side step, followed with a close step), but concludes with a forward or backward step. In addition, the Rumba Box contains 6 steps, completed in 8 beats (2 measures) of music.

In "dance time" the Rumba is counted: quick, quick, slow. Each side or close step takes one beat of music. Each forward or backward step, on the other hand, takes two beats of music.

The feeling of the dancer performing the Rumba should be one of effortless floating. This floating sensation is created by the body motion which is concentrated in the hips. To perform this dance correctly, the dancer moves the hips horizontally, while keeping the upper torso relaxed, but motionless. Although the upper torso remains still, the hips sway to the Cuban motion.

As explained in Chapter Two, the Cuban motion involves a pronounced flexing of the knees. As the dancer steps forward on his left foot, he bends his left knee, but balances most of his weight on his right foot, with his right leg straight. While the left knee is bent, the right hip automatically sticks out to the side. Conversely, as the dancer steps forward on his right foot, he bends his right knee, but balances most of his weight on his left foot, with his left leg straight. While the right knee is bent, the left hip automatically sticks out to the side. As weight is placed on the foot, however, the knee straightens, and the body is once again aligned.

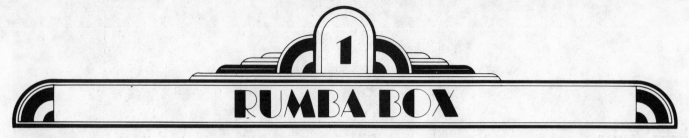

1
RUMBA BOX

The RUMBA BOX, the basic step completed essentially in one small area, contains a series of 6 steps, with a chassé (side step and a close step) preceding each forward or backward step. To add style, partners may turn slightly left (counter-clockwise) on each forward or backward step. This entire pattern, which outlines a square or box on the dance floor, is completed in 8 beats (2 measures) of music, repeating twice the basic Rumba rhythm: quick (beat 1)/ quick (beat 2)/ slow (beats 3-4).

The gentleman begins by stepping to the side with his left foot (quick), closes right foot together with his left foot (quick), and steps forward on his left foot (slow). He then steps to the side with his right foot (quick), closes left foot together with his right foot (quick), and steps backward with his right foot (slow).

The woman's part is a mirror image of the man's part. She steps to the side with her right foot (quick), closes left foot to her right foot (quick), and steps back on her right foot (slow). She then steps to the side with her left foot (quick), closes right foot together with left foot (quick), and steps forward with her left foot (slow).

Without the addition of the Rumba or Cuban motion, the Rumba Box would resemble any other box pattern. Remember, therefore, that the characteristic rhythm and hip motion of this dance is achieved through the knees. When you step with your left foot, your left knee bends forward, straightening as you place your weight on your left foot. When you step with your right foot, bend your right knee forward and straighten it as you place your weight on your right foot.

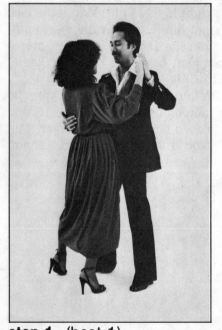

step 1   (beat 1)

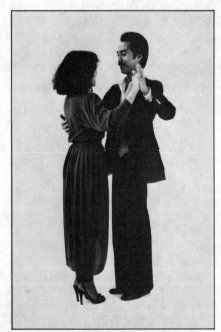

step 2   (beat 2)

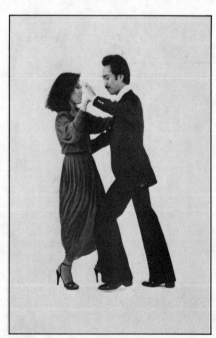

step 3   (beats 3-4)

Man's Part:

Time	Beat	Steps
Quick	(1)	1. Left foot side
Quick	(2)	2. Right foot close to left foot
Slow	(3-4)	3. Left foot forward
Quick	(5)	4. Right foot side
Quick	(6)	5. Left foot close to right foot
Slow	(7-8)	6. Right foot back

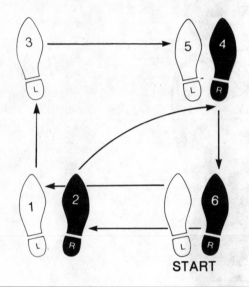

Woman's Part:

Time	Beat	Steps
Quick	(1)	1. Right foot side
Quick	(2)	2. Left foot close to right foot
Slow	(3-4)	3. Right foot back
Quick	(5)	4. Left foot side
Quick	(6)	5. Right foot close to left foot
Slow	(7-8)	6. Left foot forward

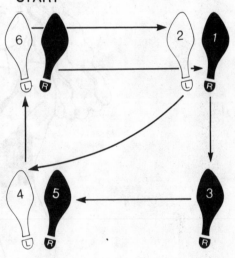

FORWARD PROGRESSIVE STEP

The FORWARD PROGRESSIVE STEP in Rumba combines a succession of walk steps in which the man moves forward, as the woman moves backwards. The man, therefore, steps forward, closes forward (draws feet together), then steps forward again. Conversely, the woman steps back, closes back (draws feet together), then steps back again.

Instead of progressing in a straight line, however, partners may turn slightly to their right or to their left on each forward or back step. Moreover, partners continue to take small, but definite steps, emphasizing the Rumba or Cuban motion. Of course, the entire pattern repeats the basic Rumba rhythm: quick (beat 1)/ quick (beat 2)/ slow (beats 3-4).

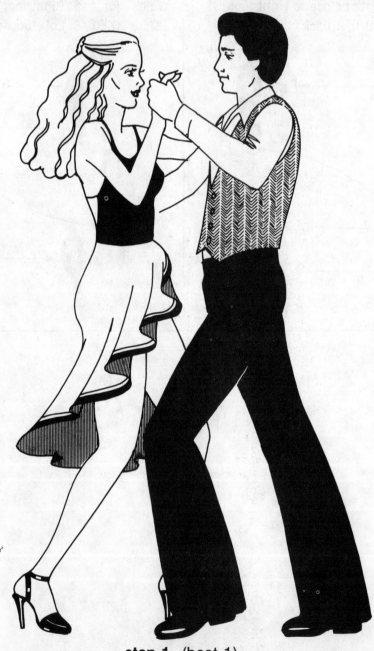

step 1 (beat 1)

Man's Part:

Time	Beat	Steps
Quick	(1)	1. Left foot forward
Quick	(2)	2. Right foot close to left foot
Slow	(3-4)	3. Left foot forward
Quick	(5)	4. Right foot forward
Quick	(6)	5. Left foot close to left foot
Slow	(7-8)	6. Right foot forward

Woman's Part:

Time	Beat	Steps
Quick	(1)	1. Right foot back
Quick	(2)	2. Left foot close to right foot
Slow	(3-4)	3. Right foot back
Quick	(5)	4. Left foot back
Quick	(6)	5. Right foot close to left foot
Slow	(7-8)	6. Left foot back

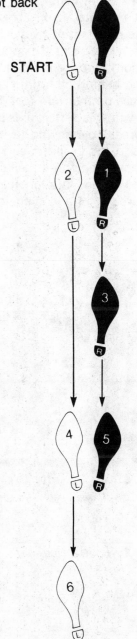

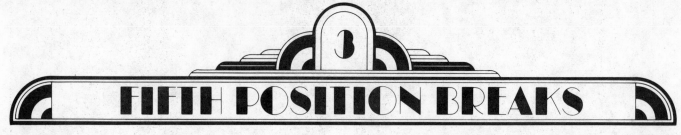

A variation of the Rumba, which creates a side-to-side motion, is called the FIFTH POSITION BREAKS. As explained in previous chapters, a fifth position or pass back step is made by crossing one foot behind the opposite foot. For the Rumba, these fifth position steps are followed with a step in place on the forward foot, but conclude with a step to the side. Despite the slight change in sequence for these Fifth Position Breaks, the basic Rumba timing and rhythm does not change: quick (beat 1)/ quick (beat 2)/ slow (beats 3-4).

The man begins by moving towards his left side, as he takes a small pass back (cross behind or 5th position) step on the ball of his left foot, which is placed behind his right foot (quick). He then steps in place on his right foot (quick), then steps to the side with his left foot (slow). The man continues his breaks by moving towards his right side as he takes a small pass back (cross behind or 5th position) step on the ball of his right foot, which is placed behind his left foot (quick). He concludes his breaks with a step in place on his left foot (quick), then steps side with his right foot (slow).

The woman's part mirrors the man's part. She begins, therefore, by moving towards her right side, as she takes a small back pass back (cross behind or 5th position) step on the ball of her right foot, which is placed behind her left foot (quick). She then steps in place on her left foot (quick), then steps to the side with her right foot (slow). The woman continues her breaks by moving towards her left side, as she takes a small pass back (cross behind or 5th position) step on the ball of her left foot, which is placed behind her right foot (quick). She then concludes her breaks with a step in place on her right foot (quick), then steps side with her left foot (slow).

This pattern can be completed in the Social (Closed) Dance Position, with small steps and slight turns of the body. However, a more stylish version contains larger steps which enable partners to turn into either the Promenade or Conversation Dance Position. For the Promenade Position, partners turn slightly away from each other on the fifth position or pass back steps. Or, to open into the Conversation Dance Position, partners take considerably larger steps, while turning even further away from each other.

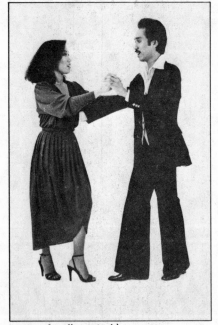

step 1 (beat 1)

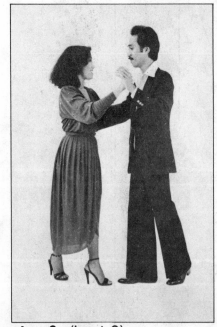

step 2 (beat 2)

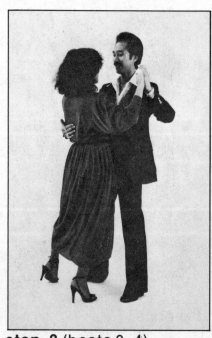

step 3 (beats 3-4)

Man's Part:

Time	Beat	Steps
Quick	(1)	1. Left foot pass back (cross behind right foot)
Quick	(2)	2. Right foot step in place
Slow	(3-4)	3. Left foot side
Quick	(5)	4. Right foot pass back (cross behind left foot)
Quick	(6)	5. Left foot step in place
Slow	(7-8)	6. Right foot side

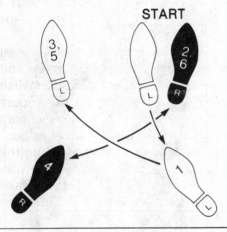

Woman's Part:

Time	Beat	Steps
Quick	(1)	1. Right foot pass back (cross step behind left foot)
Quick	(2)	2. Left foot step in place
Slow	(3-4)	3. Right foot side
Quick	(5)	4. Left foot pass back (cross behind right foot)
Quick	(6)	5. Right foot step in place
Slow	(7-8)	6. Left foot side

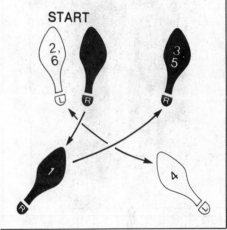

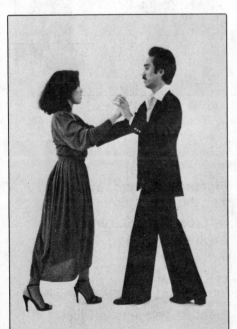

step 4 (beat 5)

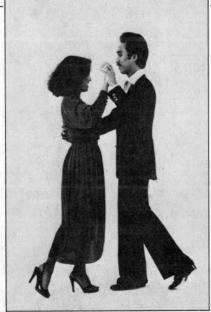

Step 5 (beat 6)

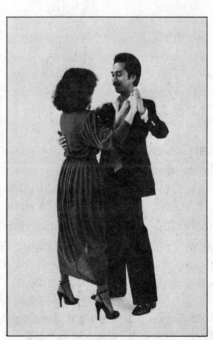

step 6 (beats 7-8)

257

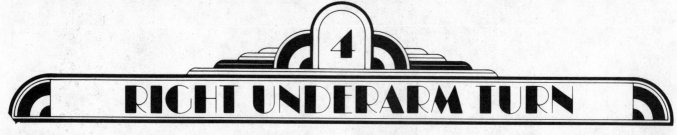
A RIGHT UNDERARM TURN in Rumba adds excitement to the basic Rumba pattern. Similar to other turn variations, the woman begins turning as soon as the man gives her a hand lead for the *right one-hand hold*. The man gives the woman a hand lead by lifting her right hand in his left hand, then he guides her into the turn by exerting slight pressure with his left hand against her back. As the woman makes her Full Right Underarm Turn (360 degrees clockwise) in 3 forward steps, the man continues to do his basic Box Step. After the woman completes her turn, partners resume the Social (Closed) Dance Position and complete their basic Box Step.

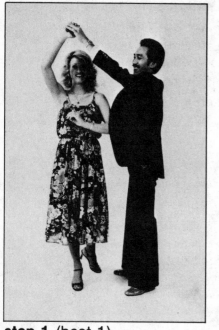

step 1 (beat 1)

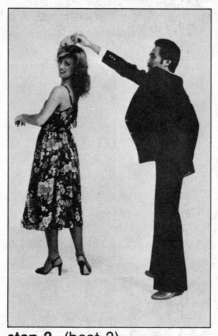

step 2 (beat 2)

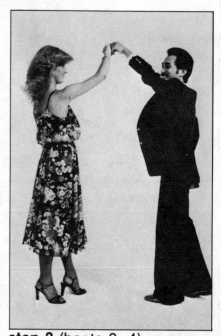

step 3 (beats 3–4)

Man's Part:

Time	Beat	Steps
Quick	(1)	1. Left foot side (lift woman's right hand in man's left hand)
Quick	(2)	2. Right foot close to left foot
Slow	(3-4)	3. Left foot forward (lower woman's right hand in his left hand)
Quick	(5)	4. Right foot side (return to Closed Dance Position)
Quick	(6)	5. Left foot close to right foot
Slow	(7-8)	6. Right foot back

Woman's Part:

Time	Beat	Steps
Quick	(1)	1. Right foot forward, pointing toe, and begin turning right
Quick	(2)	2. Left foot forward, turning right
Slow	(3-4)	3. Right foot forward, completing turn to right
Quick	(5)	4. Left foot side (return to Closed Dance Position)
Quick	(6)	5. Right foot close to left foot
Slow	(7-8)	6. Left foot forward

CHAPTER 16

SAMBA

SAMBA is the Brazilian name for dances originally performed by African slaves. "In Brazil itself," according to historian, Peter Buckman, "there are a number of local sambas or batuques, each with their own variations. These are group dances owing something to the maxixe and the African *lundu.*"

Music for the Samba, first popularized in Rio de Janeiro, combines African and Latin American rhythms. The melody, however, is continually interrupted by the strumming of a guitar or other stringed instrument. Introduced at the 1939 New York World's Fair, the Samba was an instant smash in America. During the 1960s, Brazilian composers and musicians updated the Samba rhythm, which resulted in a dance variation called the "Bossa Nova." In the 1970s, the step sequence was slightly altered and a driving disco beat added to create the Two-Step Hustle. Nevertheless, the key characteristics of the Samba, as performed by Brazilian natives at carnival time, are the bouncy rhythms, springy knee action, and slight pendulum sway.

RHYTHM AND PATTERN

The basic step in Samba is a long narrow box, called the *Caixo.* Similar to the Waltz Box, the *Caixo* begins with a forward or backward step, followed with a chassé (side step, followed with a close step). In Samba, however, the side steps tend to be extremely small, particularly when the music is fast.

Moreover, most music for Samba is written in 2/4 time. The "dance time," therefore, is counted: quick, quick slow. But Samba may also be counted: (1 and 2)/ (3 and 4). Unlike Rumba, the pause in Samba is effected on the close step.

The unique motion characteristic of the Samba is the Pendulum-Bounce. The subtle flexing of the knees up and down produces the bounce effect. The gentle swaying of the body back and forth produces the pendulum effect. In Samba the body motion is down-up-down (up), with a "down" movement on each whole-numbered count, and an "up" movement on each "and" count. The "down" movement is made by bouncing or sinking down on both knees, whereas the "up" movement is made by rising up and straightening the knees.

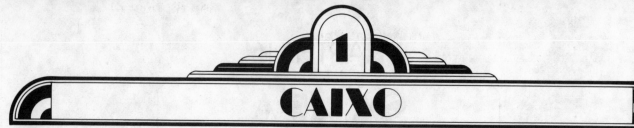

The CAIXO in Samba is a long narrow Box Step. Similar to the Waltz Box, the Caixo is composed of a forward or backward step followed with a side and a close side step. Of course, the woman's part is the natural opposite of the man's part. Thus, the man steps forward, steps side, then closes side, as the woman steps back, steps side and closes side. To complete the Box figure, the man then steps back, steps side, and closes side, as the woman steps forward, steps side, and closes side.

For the Samba Box (Caixo), however, the side and close side steps (the "side together steps") are extremely small steps, particularly when music has a fast tempo! On each step in the pattern partners turn gradually left (counter-clockwise).

Moreover, the timing for the Caixo is still counted: quick/ quick/ slow. Notice, however, that in the Caixo the pause (hold) falls on the closing (feet together) step, rather than on the forward or backward step.

Of course, the basic Samba motion of down-up-down (up) should be used throughout the basic Box Step. Knees should be kept flexed at all times, as you bounce down on every count, but rise up on every "and" between the counts. For the pendulum effect, swing the upper body slightly back on each forward step, but swing the upper body slightly forward on each back step.

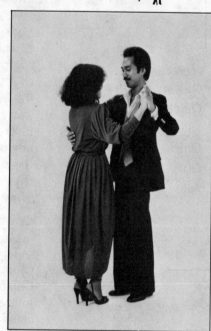

step 3 (beat 2)

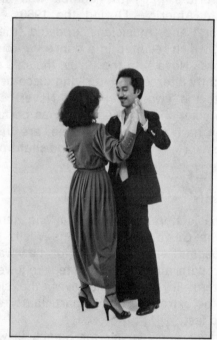

step 2 (beat "and")

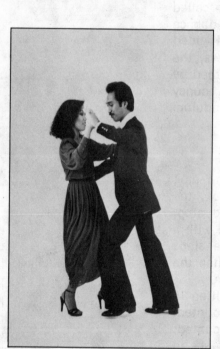

step 1 (beat 1)

step 4 (beat 3)

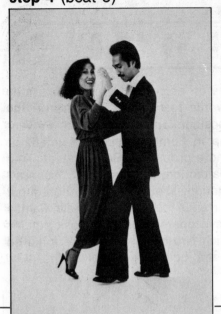

step 5 (beat ''and'')

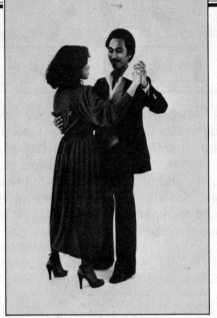

step 6 (beat 4)

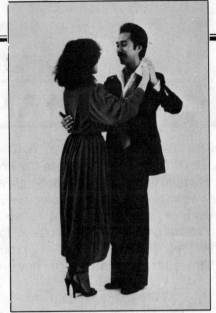

Man's Part:

Time	Beat	Steps
Quick	(1)	1. Left foot forward
Quick	(&)	2. Right foot small step side
Slow	(2)	3. Left foot close to right foot
Quick	(3)	4. Right foot back
Quick	(&)	5. Left foot small step side
Slow	(4)	6. Right foot close to left foot

Woman's Part:

Time	Beat	Steps
Quick	(1)	1. Right foot back
Quick	(&)	2. Left foot small step side
Slow	(2)	3. Right foot close to left foot
Quick	(3)	4. Left foot forward
Quick	(&)	5. Right foot small step side
Slow	(4)	6. Left foot close to right foot

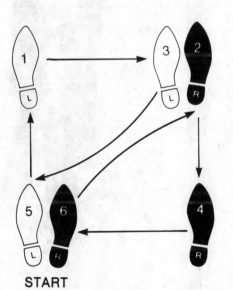

SAMBA

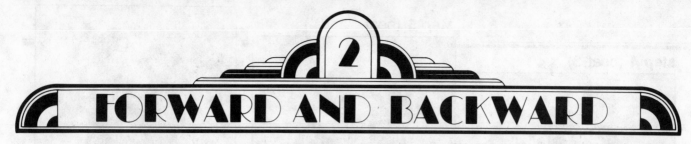

FORWARD AND BACKWARD

The BASIC FORWARD AND BACKWARD STEP IN SAMBA is similar to the Progressive Step in Rumba. As the man steps forward, therefore, the woman steps back. Conversely, as the man steps back, the woman steps forward. In addition, the forward or backward step is followed with a close step in which the feet are brought together.

Unlike the Rumba pattern, however, the Samba pattern concludes on each third step with a step taken in place, while feet remain together in the parallel (close) position. In addition, each forward or backward step in Samba should be small, as opposed to the more prominent Rumba steps. And finally, the Samba motion, with its lilting "bounce" and pendulum motion, should be used throughout this entire pattern. Of course, the basic Samba rhythm with its syncopated beats of music retains the timing in which two quick counts are followed with one slow count: quick/ quick/ slow.

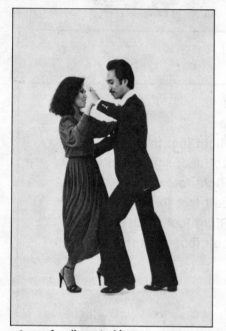

step 1 (beat 1)

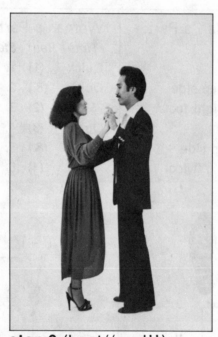

step 2 (beat "and")

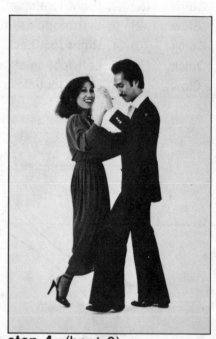

step 4 (beat 3)

Man's Part:

Time	Beat	Steps
Quick	(1)	1. Left foot forward
Quick	(&)	2. Right foot close to left foot
Slow	(2)	3. Left foot step in place
Quick	(3)	4. Right foot back
Quick	(&)	5. Left foot close to right foot
Slow	(4)	6. Right foot step in place

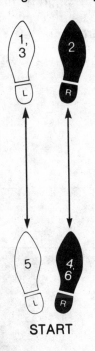

Woman's Part:

Time	Beat	Steps
Quick	(1)	1. Right foot back
Quick	(&)	2. Left foot close to right foot
Slow	(2)	3. Right foot step in place
Quick	(3)	4. Left foot forward
Quick	(&)	5. Right foot close to left foot
Slow	(4)	6. Left foot step in place

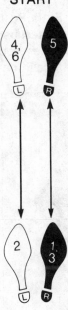

SAMBA

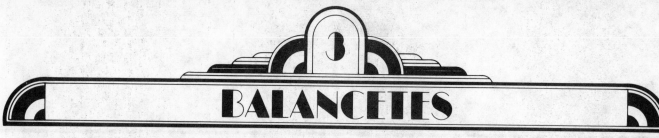

BALANCETES

The BALANCETES or FIFTH POSITION BREAKS in Samba substitute a side-to-side motion for the forward and backward motion of the basic step. Completed in the Closed Dance Position, these Balancetes combine triple steps to alternate sides. A *Balancete Right,* therefore, contains a triple step towards the man's right side (woman's left side). A *Balancete Left,* on the contrary, contains a triple step towards the man's left side (woman's right side). In addition, the second step in each Balancete is a pass back or fifth position step, in which one foot is crossed behind the opposite foot.

Unlike the Rumba Fifth Position Breaks, however, the Samba Balancetes begin with a step to the side (quick). The side step is then followed with a pass back or fifth position step, in which one foot is crossed behind the opposite foot (quick). Each Balancete then concludes with a step in place on the forward foot (slow). Of course, the basic syncopated Samba rhythm is retained throughout the Balancetes: quick/ quick/ slow.

To accentuate the bouncy Samba motion with its pendulum effect, keep your knees flexed as you move your body slightly up and down. Moreover, on the Balancetes, a side-to-side motion should also be emphasized. Thus, as you step to your left side, tilt your body slightly towards your right. Conversely, as you step to your right side, tilt your body slightly towards your left.

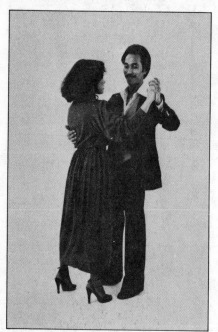

step 1 (beat 1)

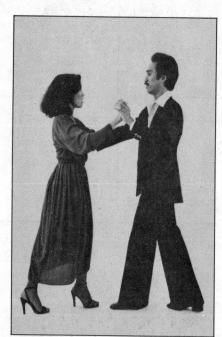

step 2 (beat "and")

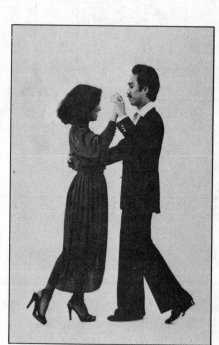

step 3 (beat 2)

step 4 (beat 3)

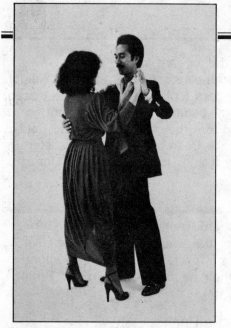

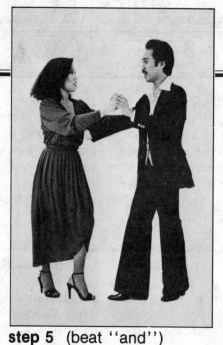

step 5 (beat "and")

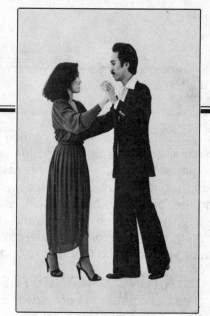

step 6 (beat 4)

Man's Part:

Time	Beat	Steps
Quick	(1)	1. Left foot side
Quick	(&)	2. Right foot pass back (cross behind left foot)
Slow	(2)	3. Left foot step in place
Quick	(3)	4. Right foot side
Quick	(&)	5. Left foot pass back (cross behind right foot)
Slow	(4)	6. Right foot step in place

Woman's Part:

Time	Beat	Steps
Quick	(1)	1. Right foot side
Quick	(&)	2. Left foot pass back (cross behind right foot)
Slow	(2)	3. Right foot step in place
Quick	(3)	4. Left foot side
Quick	(&)	5. Right foot pass back (cross behind left foot)
Slow	(4)	6. Left foot step in place

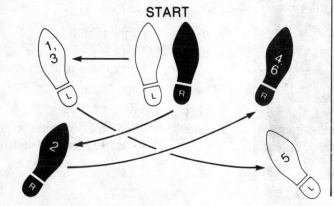

SAMBA

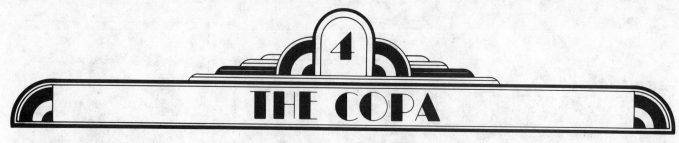

THE COPA

In the COPA, sometimes called the CONVERSA, partners face the same direction and travel forward together. Each Copa is composed of 3 steps: one step forward (quick), followed with a step in place on the foot that is back (quick), and concludes with a step in place on the forward foot (slow). After taking one step forward, therefore, partners shift their weight to the foot that is back, then they shift their weight to the forward foot.

For variety, on the second step, in which weight is shifted to the back foot, one foot may be placed close to, but still behind, the forward foot, with pressure placed on the ball of the foot only. Nevertheless, each Copa concludes with a step in place, in which weight is shifted to the forward foot.

Part A: TWO BALANCETES

The Copa pattern is preceded in Part A with two Balancetes: Balancete Right and Balancete Left. On the second Balancete, the man leads the woman into the Conversation Position. Part A concludes, therefore, with partners standing in the Conversation (Open) Position, with the man's right side parallel to the woman's left side. Some partners prefer, however, to separate only slightly, while keeping their hands clasped in the Promenade Position.

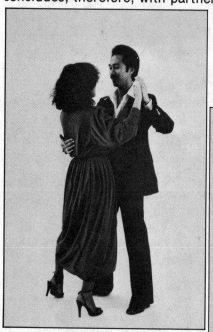

part A **step 1** (beat 1)

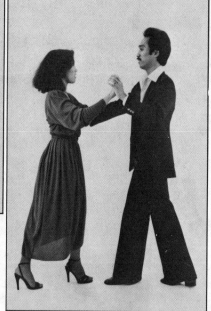

part A **step 2** (beat 2)

Man's Part:

Time	*Beat*	*Steps*
Quick	(1)	1. Left foot side
Quick	(&)	2. Right foot pass back (cross behind left foot)
Slow	(2)	3. Left foot step in place
Quick	(3)	4. Right foot side
Quick	(&)	5. Left foot pass back (cross behind right foot)
Slow	(4)	6. Right foot step in place

Woman's Part:

Time	*Beat*	*Steps*
Quick	(1)	1. Right foot side
Quick	(&)	2. Left foot pass back (cross behind right foot)
Slow	(2)	3. Right foot step in place
Quick	(3)	4. Left foot side
Quick	(&)	5. Right foot pass back (cross behind left foot)
Slow	(4)	6. Left foot step in place

Part B:
TWO COPAS IN CONVERSATION POSITION

In Part B, partners complete two Copas, as both the man and the woman travel forward in either the Conversation or Promenade Dance Position. Although both step forward, then step in place with the back foot, followed with a step in place on the forward foot, the man begins by stepping forward with his left foot, as the woman starts by stepping forward with her right foot. Throughout both Copas, therefore, the man and the woman step on opposite feet, although the forward direction and the movement are the same. 🕺

Man's Part:

Time	Beat	Steps
Quick	(1)	1. Left foot forward
Quick	(&)	2. Right foot step in place
Slow	(2)	3. Left foot step in place
Quick	(3)	4. Right foot forward
Quick	(&)	5. Left foot step in place
Slow	(4)	6. Right foot step in place

Woman's Part:

Time	Beat	Steps
Quick	(1)	1. Right foot forward
Quick	(&)	2. Left foot step in place
Slow	(2)	3. Right foot step in place
Quick	(3)	4. Left foot forward
Quick	(&)	5. Right foot step in place
Slow	(4)	6. Left foot step in place

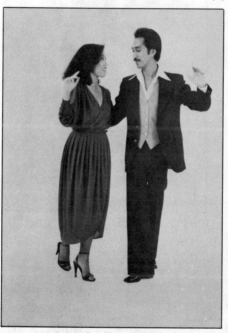 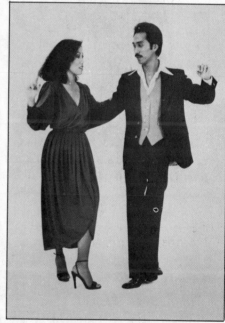

part B **step 4** (beat 3)   *part B* **step 5** (beat ''and'')

SAMBA

Part C:
ONE COPA, RETURNING TO CLOSED DANCE POSITION

In Part C, partners complete one more Copa, then return to the Closed Dance Position with the first half of the Samba Box Step. After completing one more Copa, partners resume the Closed Dance Position, as the man steps forward and the woman steps back. This pattern concludes with a small side step, followed with a close side step in which the feet are drawn together in the parallel (close) position.

Throughout all three parts of the Copa pattern, the Samba rhythm and the Samba motion should be maintained. Although the entire Copa pattern contains a total of 18 steps, the basic Samba timing is still counted: quick/ quick/ slow. To accentuate the Samba motion, keep knees relaxed as you slightly bounce up and down. For the Balancetes in Part A, emphasize the side-to-side motion by tilting your body towards your right as you step to the left side, but tilt your body towards your left, as you step to the right side. On the Copas, partners tilt their torso slightly back on the forward steps, then lean slightly forward on the steps taken in place with the foot that is positioned behind the forward foot. 🕺

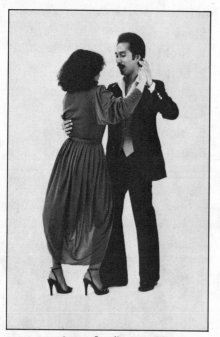

part C **step 4** (beat 3)

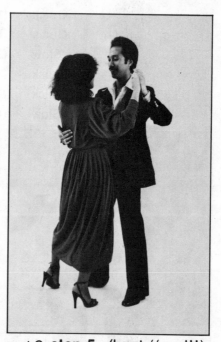

part C **step 5** (beat "and")

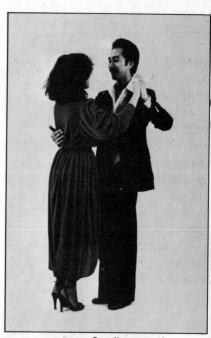

part C **step 6** (beat 4)

Man's Part:

Time	Beat	Steps
Quick	(1)	1. Left foot forward
Quick	(&)	2. Right foot step in place
Slow	(2)	3. Left foot step in place
Quick	(3)	4. Right foot forward
Quick	(&)	5. Left foot side
Slow	(4)	6. Right foot close to left foot

Woman's Part:

Time	Beat	Steps
Quick	(1)	1. Right foot forward
Quick	(&)	2. Left foot step in place
Slow	(2)	3. Right foot step in place
Quick	(3)	4. Left foot back
Quick	(&)	5. Right foot side
Slow	(4)	6. Left foot close to right foot

CHAPTER 17

MERENGUE

The MERENGUE, a Caribbean dance that originated in either Haiti or the Dominican Republic, is still one of the most popular partner dances, performed avidly in contemporary Bahamian discos. According to Abe Peck in *Dancing Madness*, the Merengue "in its early version called for dancers to take a sideward left step then *drag* the right foot toward the left." One popular, perhaps apocryphal legend claims that the dance was created after a military hero from the Dominican Republic, who had one wooden leg, and was forced to limp on every other step. As the crippled officer dragged his lame right leg across the floor, the guests respectfully followed his lead. And thus, from the lame leg of a military man, a unique ballroom dance evolved.

After the Merengue became popular in the United States during the 1950s, the "limp step" was smoothed out, but not eliminated. Moreover, the dance became quite lively, with one step taken on each beat of music. To increase the sensuousness of this dance, plenty of bending knee action, as well as the Cuban (Rumba) hip motion was added.

Although the Merengue was originally danced to Samba music or similar Latin rhythms with a strong beat, the Merengue has once again wiggled its way into some popular disco touch dances. As explained in the chapter on Salsa variations (Chapter 5), there are several disco touch dances— for example, the *Merengue (Single Count) Hustle* or the *Disco Merengue* — that have been taken from Merengue patterns. Therefore, if you would like to spice up your hustle style, try dancing some of these Merengue patterns to your favorite disco song!

BASIC RHYTHM AND MOTION

Most Merengue variations contain step patterns of 8 steps, completed in 8 beats (2 measures) of music. One step is taken, therefore, on every single beat of music. Of course, all Merengue step patterns are made up of 8 quick beats which correspond to the 8 marching steps.

Most important, however, the limp or lame-duck styling is used on the odd-numbered, accented beat counts (beats 1/3/5/7). In addition to the "lame-duck styling," the Cuban or Rumba motion is used throughout all Merengue patterns. Each step is taken, therefore, with knee bent and weight placed on the opposite foot.

Moreover, on all side steps, the shoulder should dip in the direction of the step. On forward steps, however, the body should tilt or lean slightly back. Conversely, on backward steps, the body should tilt or lean slightly forward.

FORWARD PROGRESSIVE STEP

In the BASIC FORWARD PROGRESSIVE STEP the man takes 8 steps forward, starting with his left foot forward, as the woman takes 8 steps backward, starting with her right foot back. On the accented odd beat counts (beats 1/3/5/7) slightly shorter steps will be taken, incorporating the limp or lame duck styling. In addition, as the man steps forward, he will tilt his body slightly back; conversely, as the woman steps back, she will tilt her body slightly forward. Of course, the Cuban or Rumba motion will be used throughout the entire pattern. ♣

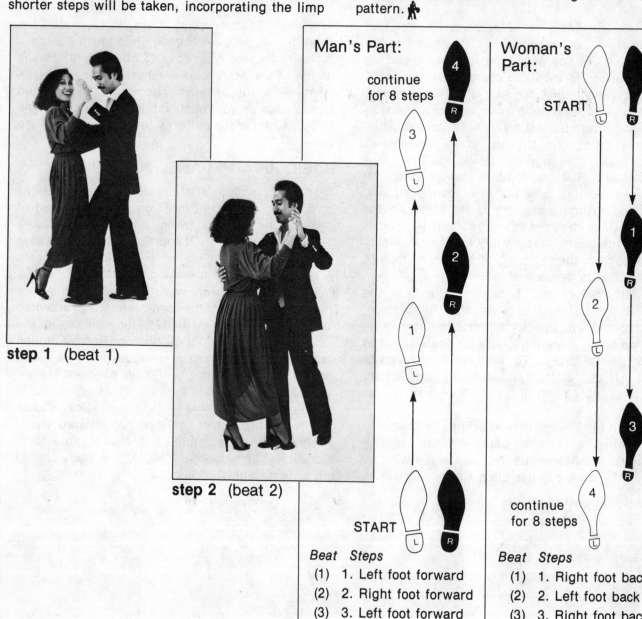

step 1 (beat 1)

step 2 (beat 2)

Man's Part:

continue for 8 steps

START

Woman's Part:

START

continue for 8 steps

Beat	Steps
(1)	1. Left foot forward
(2)	2. Right foot forward
(3)	3. Left foot forward
(4)	4. Right foot forward
(5)	5. Left foot forward
(6)	6. Right foot forward
(7)	7. Left foot forward
(8)	8. Right foot forward

Beat	Steps
(1)	1. Right foot back
(2)	2. Left foot back
(3)	3. Right foot back
(4)	4. Left foot back
(5)	5. Right foot back
(6)	6. Left foot back
(7)	7. Right foot back
(8)	8. Left foot back

BASIC SIDE STEP

The BASIC SIDE STEP contains a series of chassés (side steps, followed by close steps). Although these chasses are similar to those used in other dances, such as the Fox Trot, the Merengue chassés contain one unique feature: namely, the limp or lame duck styling is used on every odd beat (beats 1/3/5/7). In addition, the man steps to his left side, starting with his left foot side, as the woman steps to her right side, starting with her right foot side. Moreover, the Cuban or Rumba motion should be used throughout the entire pattern of 8 steps, completed in 8 beats (2 measures) of music.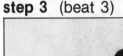

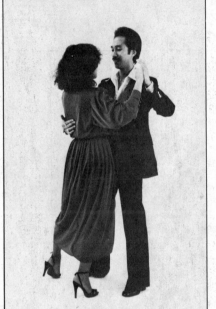

step 1 (beat 1)

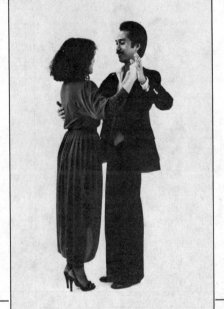

step 2 (beat 2)

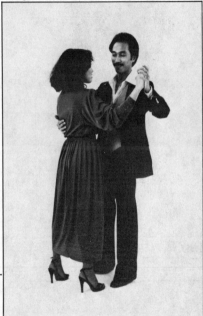

step 3 (beat 3)

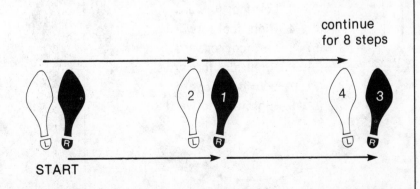

Beat	Steps	Man's Part:
(1)	1.	Left foot side
(2)	2.	Right foot close to left foot
(3)	3.	Left foot side
(4)	4.	Right foot close to left foot
(5)	5.	Left foot side
(6)	6.	Right foot close to left foot
(7)	7.	Left foot side
(8)	8.	Right foot close to left foot

continue for 8 steps

START

Beat	Steps	Woman's Part:
(1)	1.	Right foot side
(2)	2.	Left foot close to right foot
(3)	3.	Right foot side
(4)	4.	Left foot close to right foot
(5)	5.	Right foot side
(6)	6.	Left foot close to right foot
(7)	7.	Right foot side
(8)	8.	Left foot close to right foot

continue for 8 steps

START

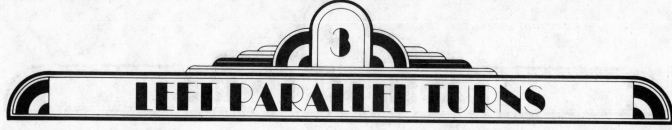
LEFT PARALLEL TURNS add dual left turns to the Basic Forward Step. In this revolving variation both the man and the woman, embraced in the Closed Dance Position, rotate counter-clockwise, although the man takes 8 steps forward, and the woman takes 8 steps back. Of course, the Cuban or Rumba motion should still be used throughout this pattern. 💃

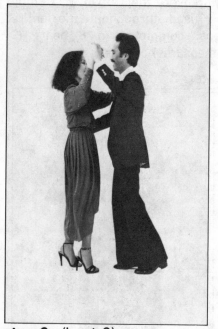

step 2 (beat 2)

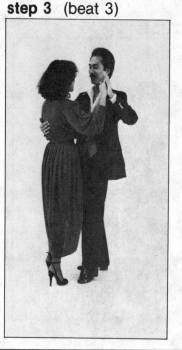

step 3 (beat 3)

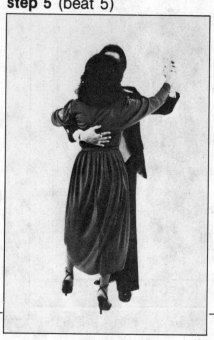

step 5 (beat 5)

Man's Part:

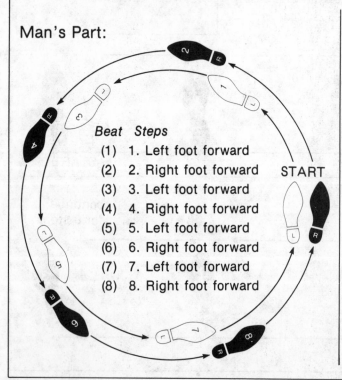

Beat	Steps
(1)	1. Left foot forward
(2)	2. Right foot forward
(3)	3. Left foot forward
(4)	4. Right foot forward
(5)	5. Left foot forward
(6)	6. Right foot forward
(7)	7. Left foot forward
(8)	8. Right foot forward

Woman's Part:

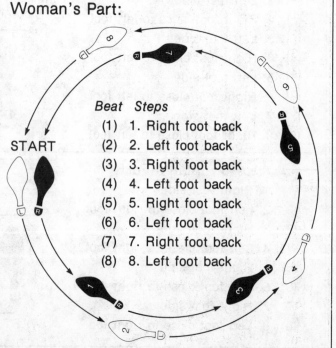

Beat	Steps
(1)	1. Right foot back
(2)	2. Left foot back
(3)	3. Right foot back
(4)	4. Left foot back
(5)	5. Right foot back
(6)	6. Left foot back
(7)	7. Right foot back
(8)	8. Left foot back

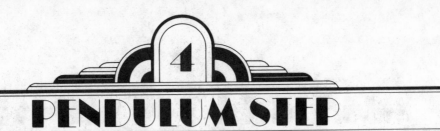

PENDULUM STEP

The PENDULUM STEP in Merengue alternates steps taken diagonally forward with steps taken diagonally backward. In addition, all even beat counts (beats 2/4/6/8) correspond to close steps in which one foot is drawn next to the opposite foot. Nevertheless, the limp or lame duck styling is used only on step 1 and step 5. Moreover, on the forward steps, the body should tilt slightly back; conversely, on the backward steps, the body should tilt slightly forward. Of course, the Cuban or Rumba motion should be used throughout the entire Pendulum Step.

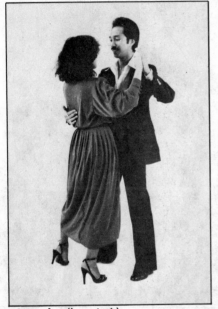

step 1 (beat 1)

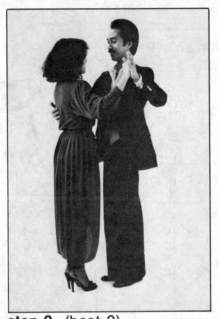

step 2 (beat 2)

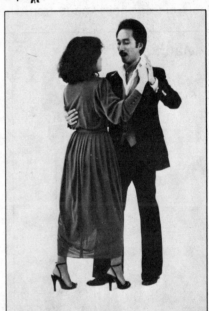

Step 3 (beat 3)

Beat	Steps	Man's Part:
(1)	1. Left foot diagonally forward	
(2)	2. Right foot close to left foot	
(3)	3. Left foot diagonally back	
(4)	4. Right foot close to left foot	
(5)	5. Left foot diagonally forward	
(6)	6. Right foot close to left foot	
(7)	7. Left foot diagonally back	
(8)	8. Right foot close to left foot	

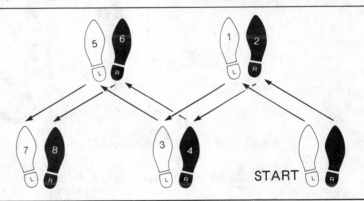

Beat	Steps	Woman's Part:
(1)	1. Right foot diagonally back	
(2)	2. Left foot close to right foot	
(3)	3. Right foot diagonally forward	
(4)	4. Left foot close to right foot	
(5)	5. Right foot diagonally back	
(6)	6. Left foot close to right foot	
(7)	7. Right foot diagonally forward	
(8)	8. Left foot close to right foot	

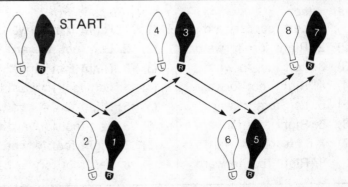

MERENGUE PROMENADE

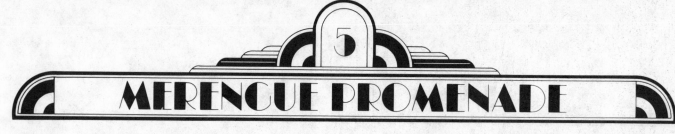

In the MERENGUE PROMENADE, both the man and the woman take 8 steps forward in the Promenade Dance Position. On the first step forward, therefore, partners turn slightly away from each other, until the woman's left hip forms a V-shape with the man's right hip, although they do not release their hands from the Closed Position.

On the next 7 steps, partners continue to move forward. Although the lame-duck styling will not be used for this variation, the Cuban or Rumba hip motion should still be accentuated.

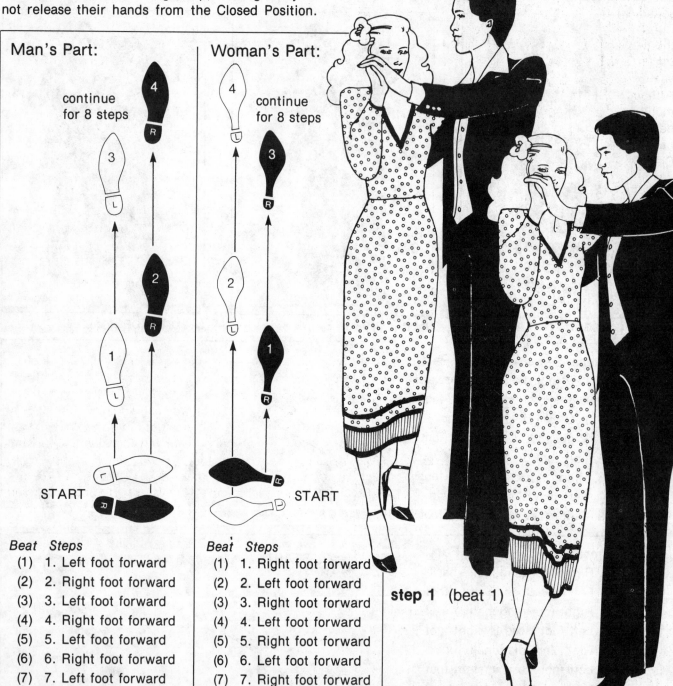

Man's Part:

continue
for 8 steps

4 R
3 L
2 R
1 L
START
L
R

Beat Steps
(1) 1. Left foot forward
(2) 2. Right foot forward
(3) 3. Left foot forward
(4) 4. Right foot forward
(5) 5. Left foot forward
(6) 6. Right foot forward
(7) 7. Left foot forward
(8) 8. Right foot forward

Woman's Part:

continue
for 8 steps

4 L
3 R
2 L
1 R
START
R
L

Beat Steps
(1) 1. Right foot forward
(2) 2. Left foot forward
(3) 3. Right foot forward
(4) 4. Left foot forward
(5) 5. Right foot forward
(6) 6. Left foot forward
(7) 7. Right foot forward
(8) 8. Left foot forward

step 1 (beat 1)

step 2 (beat 2)

CHAPTER 18

CHA-CHA

The CHA-CHA, derived from triple Mambo with just a touch of Swing, is another Cuban import. According to some dance authorities, the name for this Latin American dance came from the "hissing sound made by the heelless slippers worn by Cuban women." During the mid-50s, dancers of the Cha-Cha often broke away from each other to perform a series of sexy body wiggles and hip shakes — a solo style of dance dubbed "shining." Although the Cha-Cha incorporates Cuban hip motion, the steps and movements are more sharply defined. Of course the Cha-Cha Hustle, a disco partner dance, has infused new life into the old Cha-Cha.

BASIC CHA-CHA
RHYTHM AND MOTION

As a modification of the Mambo, the CHA-CHA, with its slower tempo, uses more foot movement and a gentler hip sway. Nevertheless, Cha-Cha is not a smooth flowing dance. Like the Mambo, it emphasizes the off-beat, which gives it a staccato feeling. Thus, a good Cha-Cha should be done with sharp, precise footwork, and plenty of Rumba or Cuban hip motion.

Each half of the basic Cha-Cha pattern consists of five steps, completed in 4 syncopated beats of music. Since pattern variations may begin on either half, it is important to think of each half as a separate unit. In dance lingo, each half of the basic pattern refers to either a "Left Unit" or a "Right Unit," named for the foot on which the man begins the unit.

The five steps which comprise each half of the basic Cha-Cha pattern are completed within the framework of 4 syncopated beats (1 measure) of music. The pattern begins on steps 1-2 (on beats 2-3) with either a forward rock or a back rock. On the forward rock, step forward with one foot, then step in place on the foot that is back. On the back rock, step back with one foot, then step in place on the foot that is forward. Notice that the rock step is *always* made up of two steps in which a weight change is effected, as the weight is placed on one foot, then shifted to the opposite foot.

Each half of the basic pattern concludes with three small steps in succession, steps 3-5, taken in two syncopated beats of music (on beats 4-and-1). These three quick steps or triple rhythm steps compose the "cha-cha-cha." Notice, however, that the first two "cha-cha" steps end on one measure of music (beats 4-and), but the last or third "cha-cha" step begins on the next measure of music (beat 1).

For this reason the Cha-Cha may be counted in either one of two ways. The footwork is often counted as "2-3-4-and-1." Some dancers prefer, however, to count the steps as "1-2-cha-cha-cha." Whichever way you prefer to count the Cha-Cha, remember that each half of the Cha-Cha pattern begins with a rock step (on beats 2-3), but concludes with three quick "cha-cha-cha" steps (on beats 4-&-1).

In addition, on the three small "cha-cha-cha" steps, you should accentuate the hip movement. A simple guideline to remember is that when you step on your left foot, you should relax and slightly bend your left knee, straightening the knee as you place your weight on your left foot. When you step on your right foot, bend your right knee, straightening the knee as you place your weight on your right foot. This is the Rumba or Cuban motion, although in the Cha-Cha, it is sharper and more syncopated, since you should be taking small, quick steps on the "cha-cha-cha" (on beats 4-and-1).

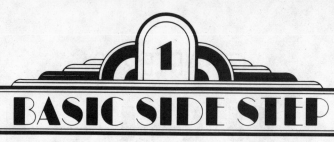

BASIC SIDE STEP

The BASIC SIDE STEP IN CHA-CHA is the step pattern most frequently used for almost all other Cha-Cha variations, including the Crossover Break and/or the Fall Away Breaks. The Basic Side Step in Cha-Cha contains a step sequence of 10 steps that, for all practical purposes, can be divided into two separate parts. Each part contains 5 steps, completed in 4 syncopated beats (1 measure) of music. Part A, the first half of the pattern, contains the 5 steps for the "Left Unit," which is followed in Part B, the second half of the pattern, with the 5 steps for the "Right Unit."

In Part A, the "Left Unit," the man begins on his left foot, although the woman begins on her right foot. In Part B, the "Right Unit," the parts for the man and the woman are reversed, as the man begins on his right foot, and the woman begins on her left foot. Nevertheless, both parts contain similar sequences of steps. For instance, both begin on steps 1-2 (beats 2-3) with rock steps. Furthermore, both conclude on the triple or "cha-cha-cha" steps with side-together-side steps.

Each step taken in either the "Left Unit" or the "Right Unit" should be small, but sharply defined. Moreover, on the rock step a slight rocking motion should be emphasized, as weight is transferred from one foot to the other foot. On the three small "cha-cha-cha" steps, the Rumba or Cuban hip motion should be accentuated. Thus, the left knee should be bent, whenever a step is taken with the left foot. Conversely, the right knee should be bent, whenever a step is taken with the right foot.

Part A:
"LEFT UNIT" OF BASIC SIDE STEP

Man's Part:

Beat		Steps
	(2)	1. Left foot forward
	(3)	2. Right foot step in place
Cha	(4)	3. Left foot side
Cha	(&)	4. Right foot close to left foot
Cha	(1)	5. Left foot side

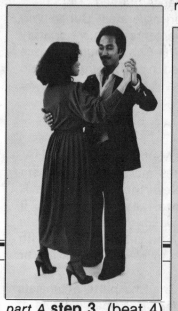

part A **step 3** (beat 4)   **step 4** (beat "and")

Beat		Steps
	(2)	1. Right foot back
	(3)	2. Left foot step in place
Cha	(4)	3. Right foot side
Cha	(&)	4. Left foot close to right foot
Cha	(1)	5. Right foot side

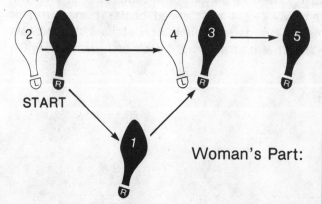

Woman's Part:

Part B:
"RIGHT UNIT"
OF BASIC SIDE STEP

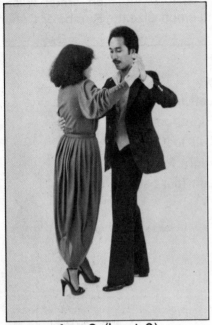

part B **step 2** (beat 3)

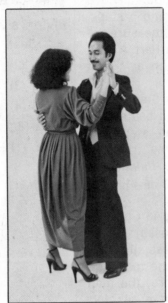

part B **step 3** (beat 4)

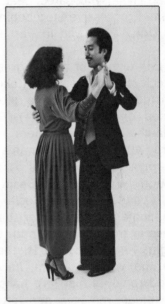

part B
step 4 (beat "and")

Man's Part:

Beat   Steps

(2)	1.	Right foot back
(3)	2.	Left foot step in place
Cha (4)	3.	Right foot side
Cha (&)	4.	Left foot close to right foot
Cha (1)	5.	Right foot side

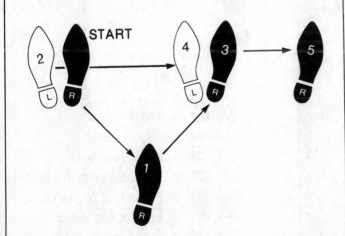

Woman's Part:

Beat   Steps

(2)	1.	Left foot forward
(3)	2.	Right foot step in place
Cha (4)	3.	Left foot side
Cha (&)	4.	Right foot close to left foot
Cha (1)	5.	Left foot side

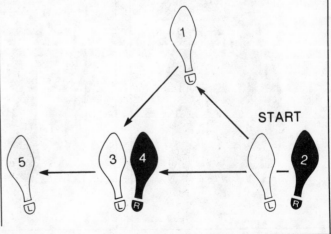

CHA CHA

The PROGRESSIVE BASIC STEP IN CHA-CHA gives partners the chance to move forward and backward, instead of from side to side. Divided into two parts, with each part containing 5 steps, completed in 4 syncopated beats (1 measure) of music, the Progressive Step begins in Part A with a "Left Unit," followed in Part B with a "Right Unit."

Each unit or part of the Progressive Step begins with a rock step on steps 1-2 (taken on beats 2-3), but concludes with a triple step on steps 3-5 (completed on beats 4-and-1). On the triple or "cha-cha-cha" steps, partners move forward or backward, although the woman's part is still the natural opposite of the man's part.

Although the Progressive Basic Step in Cha-Cha is usually danced in the Social (Closed) Dance Position, some partners prefer to release all hands and dance in the *Apart Position*. On the rock step that begins Part A or Part B, therefore, the man releases the woman's right hand from his left hand, and removes his right hand from her back, as the woman removes her left hand from the man's shoulder. In the Apart Dance Position,

partners are free to swing their arms, twist their shoulders, and emphasize the Rumba or Cuban hip motion.

Part A:
"LEFT UNIT" OF THE
PROGRESSIVE BASIC STEP

Man's Part:

Beat		Steps
(2)	1.	Left foot forward
(3)	2.	Right foot step in place
Cha (4)	3.	Left foot back
Cha (&)	4.	Right foot back
Cha (1)	5.	Left foot back

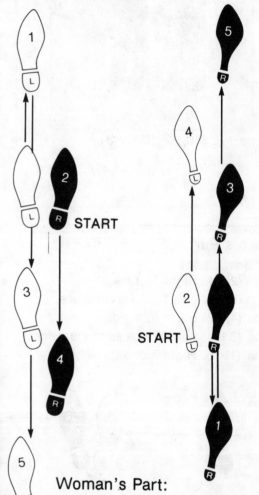

Woman's Part:

Beat		Steps
(2)	1.	Right foot back
(3)	2.	Left foot step in place
Cha (4)	3.	Right foot forward
Cha (&)	4.	Left foot forward
Cha (1)	5.	Right foot forward

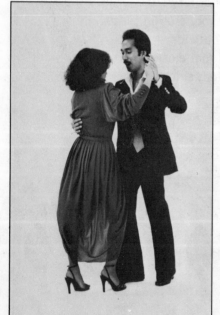

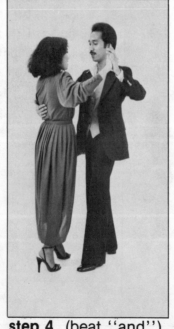

part A **step 3** (beat 4)   **step 4** (beat "and")

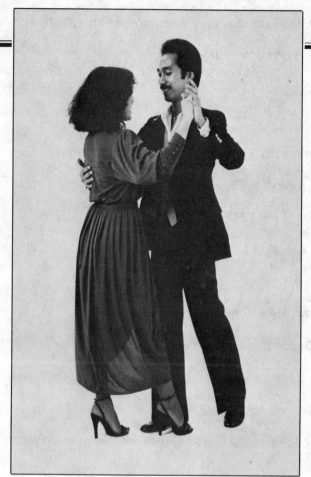

part B **step 3** (beat 4)

PART B:
"RIGHT UNIT" OF THE PROGRESSIVE
BASIC STEP

Man's Part:
Beat   Steps

    (2) 1. Right foot back
    (3) 2. Left foot step in place
Cha (4) 3. Right foot forward
Cha (&) 4. Left foot forward
Cha (1) 5. Right foot forward

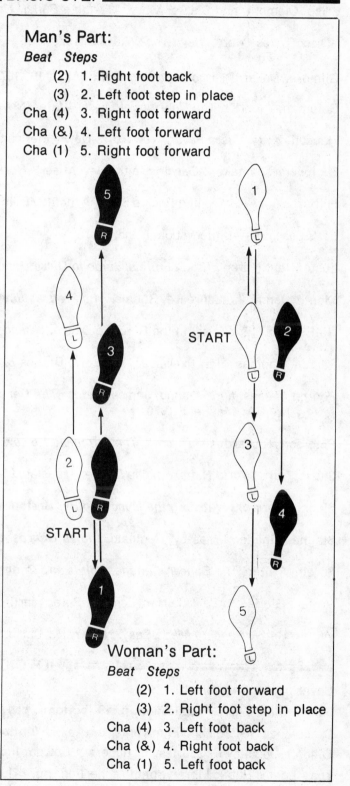

Woman's Part:
Beat   Steps

    (2) 1. Left foot forward
    (3) 2. Right foot step in place
Cha (4) 3. Left foot back
Cha (&) 4. Right foot back
Cha (1) 5. Left foot back

CHA CHA

BIBLIOGRAPHY

Blair, Skippy. *Disco to Tango and Back.* Downey, CA: Blair, 1978.

Buckman, Peter. *Let's Dance: Social, Ballroom, and Folk Dancing.* London: Paddington Press, 1978.

Crisp, Clement, and Clarke, Mary. *Making a Ballet.* New York: Macmillan, 1976.

"Disco Takes Over," *Newsweek* (April 2, 1979).

Gilmore, Mikal. "Disco." *Rolling Stone* (April 19, 1979).

Goldman, Albert. "The Delirium of Disco." *Life* (November 1978).

Hanson, Kitty. *Disco Fever.* New York: New American Library, 1978.

Highwater, Jamake. "Dancing in the Seventies." *Horizon* (May 1977).

Hilburn, Robert. "Telling Rock's Story without Missing a Beat." *L.A. Times* (Feb. 4, 1979).

Let's Disco. K-tel International, Inc., 1978.

Lustgarten, Karen. *The Complete Guide to Disco Dancing*. New York: Warner Books, 1978.

Monte, John, and Laurence, Bobbie. *The Fred Astaire Dance Book.* New York: Simon and Schuster, 1978.

Nettl, Paul. "Exoticism in the Baroque Dance." *Dance* (May 1948).

Parson, Thomas. *How to Dance.* New York: Barnes & Noble Books, 1947.

Penrod, James, and Plastino, Janice Gudde. *The Dancer Prepares: Modern Dance for Beginners.* Palo Alto, CA: Mayfield, 1970.

Peterson, Richard A. "Disco!" *The Chronicle Review* (October 2, 1978).

Sachs, Curt. *World History of the Dance.* Translated by Bessie Schoonberg. New York, 1937.

Siegel, Maria B. *Watching the Dance Go By.* Boston: Houghton Mifflin, 1977.

Singha, Rina, and Massey, Reginald. *Indian Dances.* London: Faber and Faber, 1971.

Sorell, Walter. *The Dancer's Image: Points and Counterpoints.* New York: Columbia University Press, 1971.

Varley, Gloria. *To Be a Dancer.* London: Peter Martin, 1971.

White, Betty. *Dancing Made Easy.* New York: David McKay Co., 1970.

PHOTO CREDITS